Current Progress in Otolaryngology Research

Current Progress in Otolaryngology Research

Edited by Adrien Butler

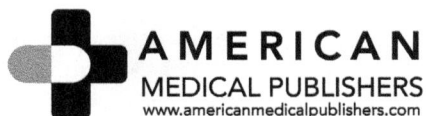

AMERICAN
MEDICAL PUBLISHERS
www.americanmedicalpublishers.com

American Medical Publishers,
41 Flatbush Avenue,
1st Floor, New York,
NY 11217, USA

Visit us on the World Wide Web at:
www.americanmedicalpublishers.com

ISBN: 978-1-63927-407-9

Cataloging-in-Publication Data

Current progress in otolaryngology research / edited by Adrien Butler.
    p. cm.
Includes bibliographical references and index.
ISBN 978-1-63927-407-9
1. Otolaryngology. 2. Otolaryngology--Practice. 3. Otolaryngology--Research. I. Butler, Adrien.
RF46 .C87 2022
617.51--dc23

Table of Contents

Preface

Over the recent decade, advancements and applications have progressed exponentially. This has led to the increased interest in this field and projects are being conducted to enhance knowledge. The main objective of this book is to present some of the critical challenges and provide insights into possible solutions. This book will answer the varied questions that arise in the field and also provide an increased scope for furthering studies.

Otolaryngology is a branch of medicine that uses surgical procedures to deal with the conditions of ear, nose and throat. It also deals with the treatment of head and neck. There are various sub-specialties of otolaryngology such as head and neck oncological surgery, rhinology and sinus surgery, and neurotology. Head and neck oncological surgery include microvascular reconstruction, endocrine surgery, surgical oncology and endoscopic surgery. It also includes the treatment of oral cancer, skin cancer, thyroid cancer, and salivary gland cancer. Rhinology and sinus surgery deals with sinusitis allergy and anterior skull base. While, neurotology focuses on the middle and inner ear, temporal bone, skull base surgery, dizziness and cochlear implant. This book explores all the important aspects of otolaryngology in the present day scenario. It aims to present researches that have transformed this discipline and aided its advancement For someone with an interest and eye for detail, this book covers the most significant topics in the field of otolaryngology.

I hope that this book, with its visionary approach, will be a valuable addition and will promote interest among readers. Each of the authors has provided their extraordinary competence in their specific fields by providing different perspectives as they come from diverse nations and regions. I thank them for their contributions.

Editor

Benign Parapharyngeal Tumours: Surgical Intricacies by Transcervical Approach

Simple Patadia[1]*, Amitkumar Keshri[2]*, Saurin Shah[1] and Arun Shrivastava[3]

[1]MS ENT, SR Neuro-otology, Department of Neurosurgery, SGPGIMS, India
[2]MS ENT, Assistant Professor, Department of Neurosurgery, Neuro-otology, SGPGIMS, India
[3]MCh Neurosurgery, Associate Professor, Department of Neurosurgery, SGPGIMS, India

Abstract

Introduction: Parapharyngeal space (PPS) is one of potential confined fascial planes of head and neck that may be involved by various pathological processes. Being rare, they represent an ominous challenge in its clinical assessment and appropriate surgical intervention.

Material and methods: A study of 14 cases of parapharngeal space tumors (PPST) which presented to our tertiary care Institute from January 2013 to January 2015, were included in this study. All cases were studied by their clinical examination, fine needle aspiration cytology, radiology (computerized tomography and magnetic resonance imaging), extent of excision, postoperative complications and definitive biopsy. All patients underwent surgery by transcervical approach and were followed up for a minimum period of 6 months.

Results: The most common tumour of the parapharyngeal space was pleomorphic adenoma (n=7), followed by schwannomas (n=5), and carotid body tumour (paraganglioma) (n=2). Twelve patients were operated via extracapsular dissection (ECD), and two patients with intracapsular dissection (ICD). Post-operative complications were vocal cord palsy in two cases, marginal mandibular palsy, horner's syndrome, hypoglossal palsy in one case respectively.

Conclusion: The transcervical approach is a versatile approach for complete excision of tumours with excellent surgical exposure and minimum morbidity. It can also be combined with excision of submandibular gland in order to improve exposure. In cases of large schwannomas, ICD is recommended to favor a complete excision.

Keywords: Parapharyngeal space tumours; Imaging; Intracapsular dissection

Introduction

Parapharyngeal space (PPS) is an inverted pyramidal space with its apex towards the hyoid bone. It is bounded medially by buccopharyngeal fascia, posteriorly by the prevertebral fascia and laterally by the medial pterygoid muscle and mandible. The tensor styloid vascular fascia divides the parapharyngeal space into pre-styloid and post-styloid compartment. The prestyloid space contains the retromandibular portion of deep lobe of parotid, minor or ectopic salivary gland, 5th cranial nerve supplying the tensor veli palitini, ascending pharyngeal artery along with venous plexus and fat. The postsyloid space is potential because of its major neurovascular contents like carotid sheath and cranial nerves 9th to 12th. According to its location the differential diagnosis of the pathology of this space are considered as: prestyloid: salivary gland neoplasm, lipoma, neurogenic tumours; poststyloid: schwannoma, paraganglioma, neurofibroma [1-3]. Primary tumours of PPS are rare and account for 0.5% of head and neck neoplasms [1-3]. Because of the location of this space, the clinical examination as well as the appropriate surgical approach is a considerable challenge. Computerized Tomography (CT) and Magnetic Resonance Imaging with MRA- MR Angiography both are important in preoperative diagnosis. Preservation of the fat plane between the mass and the parotid gland strongly suggests an extraparotid origin of tumour. Poststyloid tumours will push the carotid sheath anteromedially; whie posterolateral displacement of carotid sheath is seen in prestyloid

tumours [3,4]. The surgical approaches to access parapharyngeal space tumours (PPST) are traditionally transoral-transcervical, transcervical, transcervical transparotid with and without mandibulotomy [5]. Recent advances have considered the use of endoscopes, microdebriders, neuronavigation, and robotic surgery to facilitate better tumour removal [6]. The experience of PPST in our institiute via transcervical approach is highlighted in this study.

Methods and Materiology

A retrospective study of 14 patients, who were primarily diagnosed as PPST and underwent excision via transcervical approach between January 2013 to January 2015 was done. The data obtained were reviewed on basis of patients clinical details, presenting symptoms, imaging characteristics, fine needle aspiration cytology, surgical approach, postoperative complications, and histological confirmation (Table 1).

Transcervical approach

A curvilinear skin crease incision was given 2.5 cm below the lower border of mandible. In cases of large tumours some modification in the incision was done as shown in (Figures 1 and 2). Subplatysmal skin

*Corresponding authors: Simple Patadia, SR Neuro-otology, Department of Neurosurgery, SGPGIMS, Uttar Pradesh, India; E-mail: simplepatadia@gmail.com

Department of Neurosurgery, Neuro-otology, SGPGIMS, India; E-mail: amitkeshri2000@yahoo.com

Patient	Age	Sex	Presenting complaint	FNAC	Imaging	Displacement of great vessels	Surgery	Postoperative complications	Histopathology
1	42	M	Neck swelling	PA	CT	Posterior	ECD	Marginal mandibular palsy	PA (Fig 7)
2	55	M	Neck swelling	PA	CT	Posterolateral	ECD	Nil	PA
3	47	F	Neck swelling	Inconclusive	CT+MRI	posteriomedial	ECD	Nil	Schwannoma
4	32	F	Neck swelling	Nerve sheath tumour	MRI	Splaying	ICD	Nil	Schwannoma (Fig 8)
5	35	F	Neck swelling	Spindle Cell Tumour	MRI	Splaying	ECD	Hoarseness of voice	Schwannoma (Fig 9)
6	67	M	Neck swelling	Inflammatory cells	MRI	Posterior	ECD	Nil	PA
7	40	F	Intra-oral swelling	Haemorrhagic material	CT+ MRI + MRA	Splaying	ECD	Hoarseness of voice	CBT
8	42	F	Neck swelling	Schwannoma	MRI + MRA	Splaying	ECD	Nil	Schwannoma
9	34	F	Neck swelling	PA	MRI	Posteriolateral	ECD	Nil	PA
10	28	F	Neck swelling	Schwannoma	MRI	Anteriorly	ICD	Hoarseness of voice	Schwannoma
11	49	F	Neck swelling	Inconclusive	MRI	Posterior	ECD	Nil	PA
12	54	M	Neck swelling	Inconclusive	MRI+ MRA	Splaying	ECD	Nil	CBT
13	30	F	Neck swelling	PA	MRI	Posterior	ECD	Nil	PA
14	38	M	Neck swelling	PA	MRI	Posteriolateral	ECD	Nil	PA

FNAC: Fine Needle Aspiration Cytology; PA: Pleomorphic Adenoma; CBT: carotid Body Tumour; ECD: Extracapsullar Dissection; ICD: Intracapsular Dissection

Table 1: Details of patients presenting with parapharyngeal mass.

flaps were elevated. Cervical fascia was incised and sternocleidomastoid muscle was delineated. Great vessels of neck were identified (secured with loops). Posterior belly of digastric was identified and retracted posteriorly. Facial vessels were ligated, if required. Lower cranial nerves were identified (Figure 3). The tumour once identified was dissected extracapsularly and freed from its surrounding attachments (Figure 4). In cases of large or high positioned tumours, the posterior belly of digastric, stylohyoid muscle and stylomandibular ligament were transected for wider exposure. Submandibular gland was also mobilized anteriorly, if required. In three cases, the submandibular gland was removed completely for better visualization. For posterior-medial dissection the tumour was dissected bimanually with one finger intraorally in the parapharyngeal space and the other hand separating the capsule from the operative field. In one case, the sternocleidomastoid muscle was cut below Erb's point for better visualization. Hemostasis was achieved and a drain was inserted. The final view of intraoperative site after tumour removal is shown in (Figure 5) and the removed specimen (schwannoma) is shown in (Figure 6). If the tumour was at the carotid bifurcation and causing splaying of the carotids, careful dissection was done in the carotid sheath and the tumour was followed extracapsularly, with special considerations, not to injure lower cranial nerves. If the capsule was adherent to the carotids, adventitial dissection was carried out. Intracapsular enucleation was done in two cases of suspected cystic schwannomas which were difficult to approach superiorly and medially (Figures 7-9).

Results

Most common presenting complaint was a unilateral neck mass (92.8%). The mean age at presentation was 42.4 years (Range: 28-67 years). The study group had five males (35%) and nine females (65%). FNAC (Fine Needle Aspiration Cytology) was done in all cases. Positive Predictive Value (PPV) of FNAC was 57.14%. Three patients had CT alone, two had both CT and MRI scanning, and the remaining 9 were investigated by MRI imaging. All patients had tumour size greater than 4 cm on imaging studies. Displacement of great vessels is as described (Table 1). All patients underwent tumour excision via transcervical approach. Submandibular gland was removed to improve exposure in four cases and in one case it was retracted anteriorly.

Extracapsular dissection was done in twelve (85.71%) cases, while intracapsular debulking was required in two cases (14.28%).Complete tumour excision was done in all cases. Intraoperative blood transfusion was not required in any case. Post-operative complications included marginal mandibular weakness in one case, vocal cord palsy in two cases (14.28%), horner syndrome in one case and hypoglossal palsy in one case (Table 1). None of the patients developed wound infection or hematoma. Histopathological diagnosis confirmed plemorphic adenoma in seven cases, schwanomma in five cases, paraganglioma in two cases. No cases have tumour recurrences till present.

Discussion

Histologically and anatomically, the most common tumour of the parapharyngeal space is parotid pleomorphic adenoma [7,8]. Our study shows similar finding, with schwannoma being the second most common tumour, followed by paraganglioma. Pleomorphic adenoma occurs in the prestyloid compartment, and arises from either the deep lobe of parotid gland or minor salivary ectopic tissues [9,10]. Schwannomas in PPS arise from lower cranial nerves or from the sympathetic plexus. Paragangliomas, however, are rare; and slow growing tumours of neural crest origin. The other tumors in PPS are neurofibroma, meningioma and lymphoma. The PPV of FNAC was 57.14% in our study which is quite lower than found in literature [11]. One of the reasons of low accuracy of FNAC in our study is the fear of complex anatomy of this region and situation of tumours surrounding the great vessels. Both CT and MRI are highly useful for diagnosis and planning surgical intervention in PPST. The imaging modality of choice according to our study is MRI as it better delineates origin (prestyloid/poststyloid compartment), character (benign/malignant), vascularity, and also shows relation with the deep lobe of parotid and the great vessels. ICA being a component of post styloid space, all tumours in pre-styloid compartment has a tendency to displace it posteriorly. Any tumour inside the carotid sheath may cause splaying of carotids, as seen in our study. High index of suspicion should be kept to rule out schwannoma vs carotid body tumour as FNAC is highly inconclusive. We advise MR with angiography for suspicious tumours in carotid sheath. Vagal schwannomas have a tendency to splay carotids while cervical sympathetic schwannoma will cause anterior displacement of

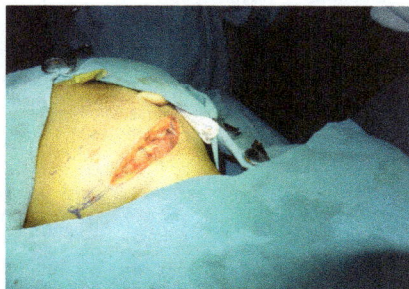

Figure 1: Incision and elevation of subplatysmal flap.

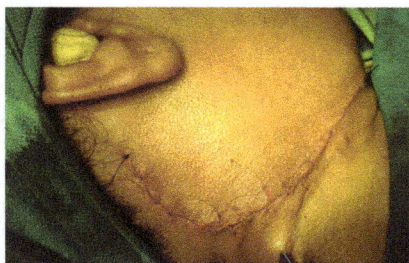

Figure 2: Modification in incision according to the extention of tumour in parapharyngeal space.

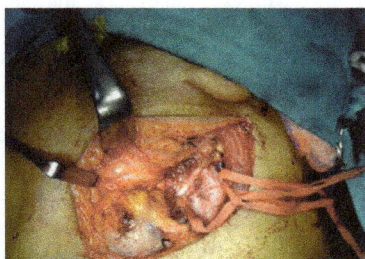

Figure 3: Tumour exposure. Submandibular gland anteriorly, sternocleidomastoid muscle and posterior belly of digastrics posteriorly. Note the glossopharyngeal nerve traversing above the hidden tumour.

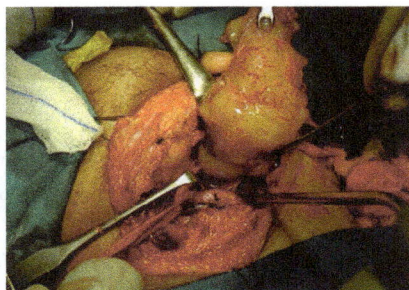

Figure 4: Tumour Removal. Submandibular gland removed for exposure.

carotids. Transcervical approach not only gives excellent exposure both in pre-styloid and post-styloid spaces, but also prevents any undue injury to vessels and nerves. The trans-parotid approach for tumours of deep lobe of parotid are considered having a higher risk of facial

palsy and the transoral approach is not useful for large tumours with extention into neck. However, if required, the trancervical approach can always be combined with parotidectomy and mandibulotomy. Table 2 summarizes the various approaches to PPS and its advantages of transcervical approach over other approaches. The key to prevent

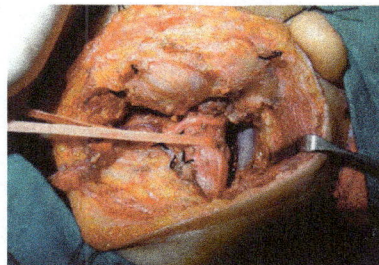

Figure 5: Final view after removal of tumour.

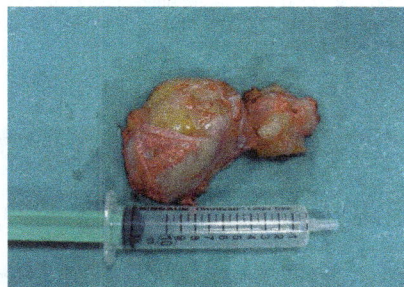

Figure 6: Tumour removed: Histopathological confirmation: Schwannoma.

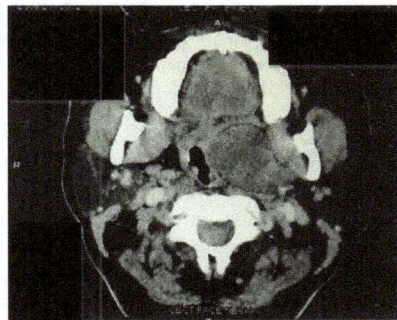

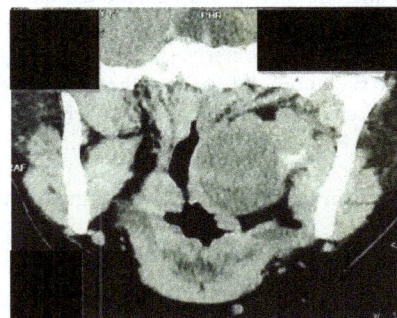

Figure 7 a, b: Coronal CT showing a prestyloid parapharyngeal mass on left side, displacing the pharyngeal mucosa medially. Note the linear displacement of fat surrounding the tumour on axial scan (b).

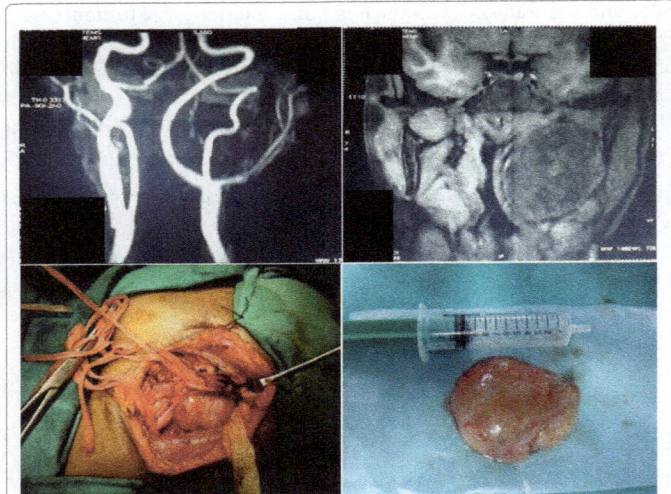

Figure 8 a, b, c, d: Mri Imaging with Angiography showing a parapharyngeal schwannoma between the two forks of carotid causing its splaying in post styloid space. Fig c showing the intaoperative dissection of tumour, taking control of the great vessels. Also note the hypoglossal nerve overlying the tumour. Fig d showing the tumour which was delivered out.

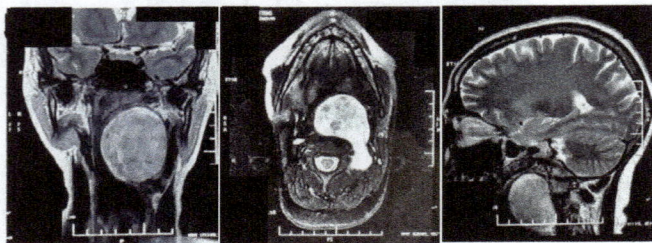

Figure 9: a, b, c: Preoperative Imaging findings in Schwannoma of post styloid space from skull base till carotid bifurcation causing splaying of carotids. Also note a posterolateral extention of the lesion into left c2 foramen. Here the ICA is displaced laterally.

Approaches	Indications	Advantages	Disadvantages
Trans-cervical	Inferior placed tumours	Can be combined with other approaches Intracapsular dissection in case of schwannomas	Blind exposure superior and medially
Trans-parotid	Deep lobe of parotid and minor salivary gland tumours	Better exposure Cuff of parotid can be removed along with tumour for better clearance	Inadequate exposure for medial extention of tumours towards skull base Risk of facial palsy
Trans-cervical with mandibulotomy	Very large, recurrent, superiorly placed tumours	Direct exposure	Mandibular malunion/nonunion Dental trauma Temporo-mandibular joint dislocation Need for tracheostomy

Table 2: Approaches to parapharyngeal space.

vessels. The transcervical approach is a versatile approach for complete excision of tumours with excellent exposure and minimum morbidity. It can also be combined with excision of submandibular gland in order to improve exposure. Intracapsular debulking is recommended in cases of schwannomas, which can provide better neural preservation rate.

any complications during surgery is to perform blunt dissection along the tumour capsule (extracapsular dissection) and avoid its rupture. However in cases with large suspected schwannomas with difficult dissection superiorly and medially, internal enucleation and debulking of tumour is recommended by us to avoid mandibulotomy. Functional preservation of peripheral nerves by intracapsular enucleation has been reported in literature [12,13]. In our study we encountered two vagal, one hypoglossal and one cervical sympathetic schwannoma. We were able to preserve vagal nerve function in one patient. A nerve monitor can also be a useful tool to preserve the nerve of origin. Kim et al. concluded that no significant difference in the recurrence rate between the total tumour removal including nerve fibers and intracapsular enucleation exists [14]. In cases of tumours splaying the carotids, high index of suspicion for carotid body tumour should be kept in mind and careful dissection from the adventitial layer of the carotids should be carried out.

Conclusion

Tumours of parapharyngeal space are challenging and have important surgical considerations due to their close relation to neurovascular structures and deep lobe of parotid gland. Imaging plays a crucial role to delineate origin, vascularity and relation with the great

References

1. Fagan, Johan (2014) Open access atlas of otolaryngology, head & neck operative surgery.

2. Olsen KD (1994) Tumors and surgery of the parapharyngeal space. Laryngoscope 104: 1-28.

3. Tom BM, Rao VM, Guglielmo F (1991) Imaging of the parapharyngeal space: anatomy and pathology. Crit Rev Diagn Imaging 31: 315-356.

4. Chong VF, Fan YF (1998) Radiology of the parapharyngeal space. Australas Radiol 42: 278-283.

5. Bozza F, Vigili MG, Ruscito P, Marzetti A, Marzetti F (2009) Surgical management of parapharyngeal space tumours: results of 10-year follow-up. Acta Otorhinolaryngol Ital 29: 10-15.

6. Paderno A, Piazza C, Nicolai P (2015) Recent advances in surgical management of parapharyngeal space tumors. Current Opinion in Otolaryngology & Head and Neck Surgery 23: 83-90.

7. Bass RM (1982) Approaches to the diagnosis and treatment of tumors of the parapharyngeal space. Head Neck Surg 4: 281-289.

8. Allison RS, Van der Waal I, Snow GB (1989) Parapharyngeal tumours: a review of 23 cases. Clin Otolaryngol Allied Sci 14: 199-203.

9. Kassel EE (1982) Parapharyngeal and deep lobe parotid tumors. J Otolaryngol Suppl 12: 25-35.

10. Carrau RL, Myers EN, Johnson JT (1990) Management of tumors arising in the parapharyngeal space. Laryngoscope 100: 583-589.

11. Mondal P, Basu N, Gupta SS, Bhattacharya N, Mallick MG (2009) Fine needle aspiration cytology of parapharyngeal tumors. J Cytol 26: 102-104.

12. Paderno A, Piazza C, Nicolai P (2015) Recent advances in surgical management of parapharyngeal space tumors. Curr Opin Otolaryngol Head Neck Surg 23: 83-90.

Central Primary Fibrosarcoma Maxilla - A Rare Presentation

Neelam Sood* and **Nisha Sehrawat**

Department of Pathology, Deen Dayal Upadhyay Hospital, New Delhi, India

*****Corresponding author:** Neelam Sood, Department of Pathology, Deen Dayal Upadhyay Hospital, B 337, Ground floor, PaschimVihar, New Delhi- 110063, India;
E-mail: neesu1234@hotmail. com

Abstract

Fibrosarcoma is a malignant neoplasm of fibroblastic origin and rarely affects the maxilla. This case of primary fibrosarcoma maxilla in a 60 year old male describes histopathological pattern and its differential diagnosis with IHC. The patient was treated with partial maxillectomy. The patient presented with recurrence after 8 months of resection. This case is being submitted for its rarity.

Keywords: Maxilla; Herringbone pattern; CT-scan (Computed Tomography-Scan); MRI (Magnetic resonance imaging); IHC (Immunohistochemistry)

Introduction

Fibrosarcoma (FS) is a malignant mesenchymal tumour with fibroblastic proliferation and variable amount of collagen production. In classical cases, herringbone architecture is seen [1]. FS essentially, is a diagnosis of exclusion, thus exact incidence rate cannot be assessed. It mostly accounts for 1-3% of adult sarcomas [1]. It is more frequently seen in soft tissue but primary intraosseous origin has been described in 5% of all cases [2,3]. It rarely affects head and neck region (10%). Mandible is the more common site of involvement in this region [4]. Maxilla is rarely involved and accounts for only 0 to 6.1% cases [5]. Involvement of maxillary antrum is rarely seen [3]. FS of jaw can be periosteal (peripheral) or endosteal (central) [4].

Secondary FS may arise in pre-existing fibrous dysplasia, paget's disease, bone infarct, cyst andosteomyelitis or may present as malignant transformation of pre-existing giant cell tumors of bone or transformation of ameloblastic fibroma [6,7]. It has also been documented to be induced by prior history of irradiation [4].

Case Report

A 60 year old male patient presented with 10 months history of swelling and pain in left cheek region. On intraoral examination an ulceroproliferative growth was seen in the left premolar region with palatal and anterolateral extension as soft tissue swelling in the cheek. The premolar teeth were missing, which according to patient were extracted earlier as were loose. CT scan showed mass lesion in maxilla, with destruction of anterolateral wall and extension into anterior soft tissue as well as into the maxillary antrum (Figure 1a).

Incisional biopsy showed proliferation of spindle shaped cells arranged in proliferating bundles, fascicles and "herringbone pattern", suggestive of Fibrosarcoma. Left partial maxillectomy was performed. Specimen of left partial maxillectomy measuring 10*4*2.5 cm was received. Grossly, an ulceroproliferative, firm, grey white growth measuring 5*3*3 cm on the alveolar ridge extending into maxillary antrum, eroding anterolateral and inferior wall of maxillawith absent overlying premolarteeth was noted. (Figure 1b) It was 4.5 cm away from posterior mucosal and 1. 8 cm from anterior mucosal margins.

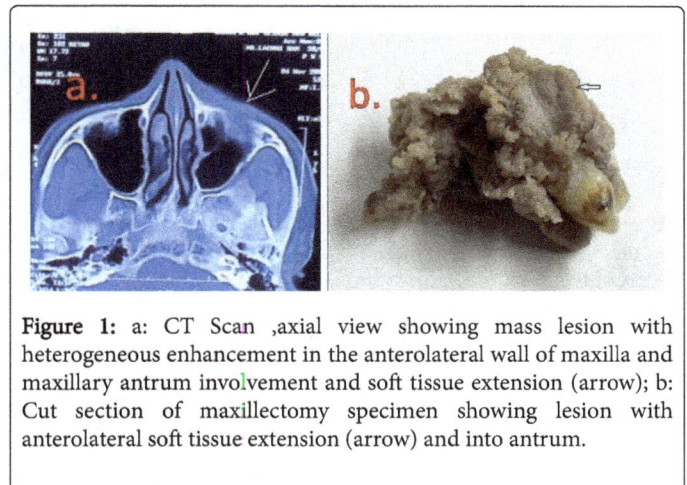

Figure 1: a: CT Scan ,axial view showing mass lesion with heterogeneous enhancement in the anterolateral wall of maxilla and maxillary antrum involvement and soft tissue extension (arrow); b: Cut section of maxillectomy specimen showing lesion with anterolateral soft tissue extension (arrow) and into antrum.

Multiple sections of tumour were taken and stained with Hematoxylin and Eosin (H&E). Sections showed spindle cells arranged in proliferating bundles, fascicles and "herringbone pattern". Tumour cells showed elongated nuclei, coarse chromatin and tapering eosinophilic cytoplasm. Tiny focal loose myxoid areas were also seen. Tumour showed rich vascularity, focal necrosis, moderate degree of pleomorphism and 1-2 mitosis per high power field. Immunohistochemical stains stained were performed. Tumor cells showed positive staining for vimentin ((Biocare, RTU, V9) and ki-67 (Biocare, RTU, Mc-5, Ig G1) proliferation index was estimated at 10%.

The tumor cells were negative for S-100 (Biocare, RTU, 15E2E2), smooth muscle actin (SMA) (Biocare, RTU, 1A4) and Epithelial Membrane Antigen (EMA) (Biocare, RTU, Mc-5, Ig G1), HMB45 (Dako, RTU, HMB45, Ig G1D3), CD34 (Biocare, RTU, QBEnd/10), CD99 (Biocare, RTU, HO36-1. 1, IgG1)and Pan CK (Dako, RTU, AE1/3). Thus a final diagnosis of FS of maxilla (intermediate grade) was given Figure 2.

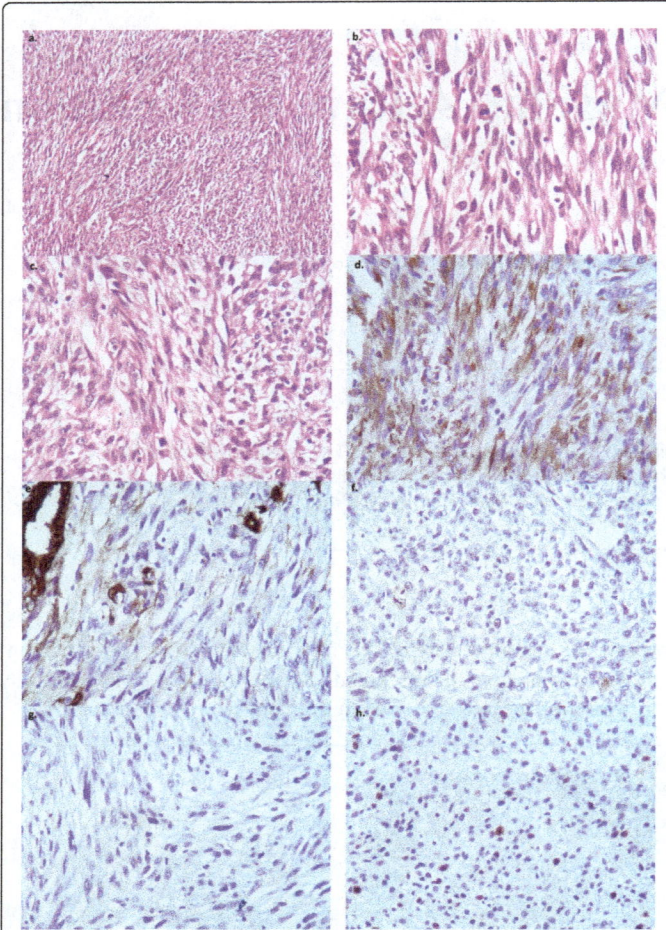

Figure 2: a: Microphotograph showing florid spindle cell proliferation in bundles and fascicles (H & E, 10X); b: Microphotograph depicting frequent mitosis (H & E, 40X); c: Microphotograph showing classical herring bone pattern (H & E, 40X); d: IHC showing strong expression of vimentin (Biocare, RTU, V9, 40X); e: IHC showing tumour cells with negative staining for Smooth muscle actin with positive internal control (Biocare, RTU, 1A4,40X); f: IHC showing tumour cells with negative staining for S 100 (Biocare, RTU, 15E2E2, 40X); g: IHC showing tumour cells with negative staining for Epithelial membrane antigen (Biocare, RTU, Mc-5, Ig G1 40X); h: IHC showing tumour cell with 10% positivity forKi-67 (Biocare, RTU, SP6, Rabbit Ig G, 40X).

Discussion

FS is malignant fibroblastic tumour, which rarely affects maxilla. It is more often seen to involve mandible than maxilla. Only in 0-6.1% cases, it involves maxilla [5]. It is more common in 5-6th decade, with equal sex predilection. However, an occasional case has been reported in pediatric age group too [6]. Patients are mostly asymptomatic. In 30% cases only, it may be symptomatic [2]. Patients mostly present with complain of swelling in jaw with or without pain. Other complaints are loosening of teeth, trismus, fracture and paresthesia [3,5,6].

Radiologically, it presents as osteolytic lesion with ill-defined margins, lacking any internal structures [8]. Thus in absence of any characteristic feature, it is difficult to distinguish it from other central malignant osteolytic lesion including carcinoma and myeloma, when no enlargement of jaw is noted. In some cases it may present as cystic lesion or with well circumscribed margins as documented by a few authors and then the differential of infected dental cyst and central desmoplastic fibroma arise. Ameloblastic fibrosarcoma, Ewing's sarcoma, and radiolucent osteosarcoma can also show similar features [6,9,10]. On Computerized Tomography Scan (CT) it may present as destructive bony lesion, commonly associated with extra osseous soft tissue mass, as seen in this case[11]. Magnetic Resonant Imaging (MRI) shows low to intermediate signal intensity with inhomogeneous enhancement on both T1- and T2-weighted images with an inhomogeneous pattern of contrast enhancement [11].

The histopathological examination plays a very crucial role in identifying this tumour. Although, FS is essentially a diagnosis of exclusion but presence of certain definitive morphological features comprising of spindle shaped cells arranged in interlacing bundles, fascicles and "herringbone pattern" with variable amount of collagen deposition are helpful in reaching the diagnosis. Characteristically cells are spindle with elongated oval to round hyperchromatic nuclei, varying in size. Myxomatous, pseudomyxomatous and cartilaginous areas may also be noted [1-4].

Other malignant tumors which can be considered in its differential are spindle cell carcinoma, monomorphic synovial sarcoma, malignant fibrous histiocytoma, malignant nerve sheath tumors, leiomyosarcoma, and malignantamelanotic melanoma. Malignant peripheral nerve sheath tumour commonly shows spindle cells with serpentine nuclei with high mitotic rate and definitive S-100 positivity [12]. Monomorphic synovial sarcoma is a very close differential diagnosis and especially when it presents with sarcomatous spindle cell component, with co-expression of vimentin, CK and CD 99, absence of which rules its diagnosis [13]. Leiomyosarcoma comprises of fascicles of spindle-shaped cells with blunt ended vesicular nuclei, which are strongly positive for vimentin and smooth muscle actin [14]. Amelanotic melanomas can pose a problem but IHC helps in presence of HMB45, S100 [15]. Spindle cell carcinoma is usually biphasic and shows a strong positivity for EMA and Pancytokeratin [16]. Ameloblastic FS is also biphasic, showing presence odentogenic epithelial elements in some focus atleast. On Immunohistochemistry (IHC), strong vimentin positivity and negative S-100, SMA, desmin, EMA, CD99, CD34, CK, HMB45 help in ruling out other differential diagnosis and reach a conclusive diagnosis [12-16].

Tumour can be graded on the basis of their histological appearances by Broders' method. Grade I (well differentiated) comprises of tumour cells with uniform nuclear appearance with appreciable amount of collagenous intracellular substance. Giant cell and mitotic figures are absent. Grade II (intermediate) comprises of tumour with increased cellularity and decreased amount of intracellular collagenous substance. Tumour cells have closely packed, uniform nuclei. Classical herring bone pattern is prominent with occasional mitotic figures. Grade III (high) comprises of anaplastic tumour cells with increased giant cells and mitotic figures. Our cases falls into intermediate grade with prominent herring bone pattern and uniform closely packed tumour nuclei [1,2]. Depending on the number of mitotic figures, tumor differentiation, and the presence of tumornecrosis, French Fédération Nationale des Centres de Lutte Contre le Cancer

(FNCLCC) grading system is currently, the most widely accepted and according to this it was scored as grade 2 [1].

Management and follow up

Unlike soft tissue FS, osseous FS of bone has a poorer prognosis with 5year survival rate of only 4.231.7% [17]. A Primary vs. secondary site of origin and histological grading, play an important role in the prognosis of FS. Secondary FS usually have an aggressive course [3,8,18]. A difference in clinical course between FS of jaw and its long bone counterpart has been reported by many authors. A favourable prognosis of FS of jaw has been observed during the 5-20 year follow up observation period as compared with long bone fibrosarcoma [17]. FS of oral cavity also have lower rate of metastasis as compared to long bones [4]. The local recurrence has been reported has been reported as 50-60% and metastases in 20-25%, irrespective of the tumour grade. FS of long bones have 5 year survival rate of 4.3% to 31.7% whereas, in case of oral cavity it is 60% for soft tissue and 27% for medullary origin. Degree of differentiation has inverse relation with survival rate, higher grade of differentiation being associated with worse survival [4].

Preferred treatment modality is surgical resection with wide margin. In the FS that is not possible to excise completely, either due to their location or extreme size, postoperative radiotherapy of 60007, 000 cGy and postoperative adjunctive chemotherapy is suggested, to treat potential subclinical or microscopic metastasis especially in grade III FS [17]. However the role of adjuvant radiotherapy and/ or chemotherapy in the treatment is not very clear [4]. This case underwent surgical resection. His recovery was uneventful but subsequently presented with recurrence after 8 months and was referred for further treatment and subsequently lost for follow up.

Conclusion

FS is a malignant tumour of fibroblastic origin, which rarely affect maxillofacial region. Histopathological examination plays an important role. However in absence of classical herring bone pattern, differentiating it from other spindle cell lesions becomes a diagnostic dilemma. In such cases IHC plays a very important role by ruling out other differentials and planning the appropriate treatment.

References

1. Fisher C, Van Den Berg E, Molenaar WM (2002) World Health Organization classification of tumours. Pathology and genetics of tumours of soft tissue and bone. Lyon, France: IARC Press.

2. Huvos AG, Higinbotham NL (1975) Primary fibrosarcoma of bone. A clinicopathologic study of 130 patients. Cancer 35: 837-847.

3. Mansouri H, Rzin M, Marjani M, Sifat H, Hadadi K, et al. (2006) Fibrosarcoma of maxillary sinus. Indian Journal of Otolaryngology and head and neck surgery 58:104-105.

4. Angiero F, Rizzuti T, Crippa R, Stefani M (2007) Fibrosarcoma of the jaws: Two cases of primary tumors with intraosseous growth. Anticancer Res 27: 2573-2581.

5. Khanna S, Singh NN, Singh A, Purwar A (2014) Fibrosarcoma of maxilla with extension into maxillary sinus: A rare case report. Oral MaxillofacPatho J 5: 462-465.

6. Swain N, Kumar SV, Dhariwal R, Routray S (2013) Primary fibrosarcoma of maxilla in an 8 year old child: A rare entity. J Oral Maxillofac Pathol 478.

7. Reichart PA, Zobl H (1978) Transformation of ameloblastic fibroma to fibrosarcoma. Int J Oral Surg 7: 503-507.

8. Rajendran A, Sivapathasundharam B (2012) Shafer's Textbook of Oral Pathology (7thedn) Elsevier.

9. White SC, Pharoah MJ (2000) Oral Radiology: Principles and Interpretation (4thedn) St Louis, MO: Mosby.

10. Khalili M, Shakib PA (2013) Ameloblastic fibrosarcoma of the upper jaw: Report of a rare case with long-term follow-up. Dent Res J (Isfahan) 10: 112-115.

11. Razek AA (2011) Imaging appearance of bone tumors of the maxillofacial region. World J Radiol 3: 125-134.

12. Das SR, Dash S, Pradhan B, Sahu MC, Padhy RN (2015) Malignant peripheral nerve sheath tumour of nose and paranasal sinuses with orbital extension Journal of Taibah University Medical Sciences 10: 238-242.

13. Khalili M, Eshghyar N, Ensani F, Shakib PA (2012) Synovial sarcoma of the mandible. Journal of Research in Medical Sciences? The Official Journal of Isfahan University of Medical Sciences 17: 1082-1085.

14. Chew YK, Noorizan Y, Khir A, Brito MS (2009) Leiomyosarcoma of the maxillary sinus. Med J Malaysia 64: 174-175.

15. Saghravanian N, Pazouki M, Zamanzadeh M (2014) Oral amelanotic melanoma of the maxilla. J Dent (Tehran) 11: 721-725.

16. Rath R, Das BK, Das SN, Baisakh MJ (2014) Spindle cell carcinoma of maxilla: Histomorphological and immunohistochemical analysis of a case Oral Maxillofac Pathol18: 256–261.

17. Marx RE, Stern D (2002) Oral and maxillofacial pathology: A rationale for treatment. Hanover Park, IL: Quintessence Publishing.

18. Slootweg PJ, Müller H (1984) Fibrosarcoma of the jaws. A study of 7 cases. J Maxillofac Surg 12: 157-162.

Clinical Evaluation of Mucin-1 (MUC1) and P16 in Laryngeal Cancer

Irmi Wiest[1#], Christoph Alexiou[2*#], Klaus Friese[1], Doris Mayr[3], Christoph Freier[1,4], Annika Stiasny[1], Peter Betz[5], Marina Pöttler[2], Jutta Tübel[6], Steffen Goletz[7], Tobias Weißenbacher[1], Darius Dian[1], Udo Jeschke[1] and Bernd Kost[1]

[1]Department of Obstetrics and Gynecology – Klinikum Innenstadt, Germany

[2]Department of Otorhinolaryngology, Head and Neck Surgery, Section for Experimental Oncology and Nanomedicine (SEON), Germany

[3]Department of Pathology, LMU, Germany

[4]Division of Clinical Pharmacology, LMU, Germany

[5]Department of Legal Medicine, FAU, Germany

[6]Department of Orthopedics, TUM, Germany

[7]Glycotope, Germany

# Author contributed equally

*Corresponding author: Christoph Alexiou, Department of Otorhinolaryngology, Head and Neck Surgery, Section for Experimental Oncology and Nanomedicine (SEON), Else Kröner-Fresenius-Stiftung-Professorship, University Hospital Erlangen, Glückstr. 10a, Erlangen, Germany; E-mail: christoph.alexiou@uk-erlangen.de

Abstract

Background: Adapted from results in the field of cervical cancer, a direct connection between HPV infection and oropharyngeal carcinoma development could be established. Aim of this study was to evaluate p16 and TA-MUC1 in laryngeal cancer and their correlation to diagnostic, since TA-MUC1 is primarily restricted to malignancies.

Methods: Paraffin-embedded laryngeal cancer specimens (n=129) and normal tissue (n=5) were analyzed for TA-MUC1 expression using hPankoMab-GEXTM antibody and evaluated according the immunoreactive score. Survival was assessed via log-rank test and Kaplan-Meier-survival analysis.

Results: Significant correlation with tumor grading and staging was exhibited by TA-MUC1staining, while being negative in normal tissues. Expression of p16 significantly increased in T4 compared to T1 tumors. Significant differences in overall survival were found in correlation to TNM-classification, grading and relapse. TA-MUC1 showed a positive trend correlating to p16.

Conclusion: Because of this positive trend, we suggest a HPV association in head and neck tumors. Most likely due to an insufficient quantity of HPV-positive patients, no statistical significance could be established. However, targeting TA-MUC1 would improve tumor therapy by linking hPankoMab-GEXTM to the overexpressed galectin. Systematic analysis of HPV-association should be performed generally in laryngeal cancer to gain further information about the interaction of HPV and malignancies.

Keywords: MUC-1; Laryngeal cancer; TA-MUC1; p16; Human papilloma virus (HPV); Head and neck squamous cell carcinoma (HNSCC); hPankoMab-GEXTM

Abbreviations

MUC: Mucin-1; TA-MUC1: Tumor-Associated MUC1; HPV: Human Papilloma Virus; RTK: Receptor Tyrosin Kinase; SLeX: Sialyl Lewis x; SLeA: Sialyl Lewis a; LeY: Lewis Y; TF: Thomsen-Friedenreich Antigen; Gal-1: Galectin-1; DAB: Diaminobenzidine; HNSCC: Head and Neck Squamous Cell Carcinoma, pRb: Retinoblastoma Protein; uVIN: Usual-Type Vulvar Intraepithelial Neoplasia; ADCC: Antibody Dependent Cellular Cytotoxicity

Introduction

Malignant neoplasms of the larynx belong to the most frequent cancer entities in the upper aero digestive tract and squamous cell carcinomas are most common. Treatment decisions depend on stage of disease. Surgery or definitive irradiation with a curative intent is performed often in early stages, whereas more advanced disease stages are usually treated with surgery, radio chemotherapy or radio chemotherapy/radio immunotherapy. Accurate determination of tumor size and localization, as well as detailed knowledge of the presence of lymph node metastases is obligatory for an individualized therapy [1].

HPV in head and neck cancer

Human papillomavirus (HPV) is one of the most investigated pathogenic DNA viruses. Primarily HPV was held responsible only for cervical cancer, but in the last two decades it appeared as a major cause for head and neck cancer as well [2,3]. A total of 28% of all laryngeal carcinomas are associated with HPV [4,5]. More affected by HPV is the oropharyngeal cancer. The publicized numbers of entities range between 25% and 60%, sometimes up to 90% [6]. Patients suffering from head and neck cancer associated with HPV feature a 30% better survivability because of younger patients [7], less relapse [8] and better response to therapies [9]. The cell cycle regulation protein p16 is overexpressed in HPV infected epithelial cells and its verification is still the most common proof of a HPV infection [10,11].

TA-MUC1

Mucin 1 (MUC1) is a high molecular weight transmembrane glycoprotein and expressed on the surface of epithelia all over. In addition its intracellular part is an active receptor tyrosine kinase (RTK) and so it is involved in different signaling pathways [12-14]. In malignant processes MUC1 becomes a carrier protein for oncofetal carbohydrates such as sialyl Lewis x (SLeX), sialyl Lewis a (SLeA), Lewis Y (LeY) and the Thomsen-Friedenreich Antigen (TF) [15]. Expression of the described antigens in benign tissue is mainly restricted to epithelial tissue of human reproduction [16]. Laryngeal cancer shows high expression of SLeA, Gal-1 and TF in contrast to normal tissue of tongue, vocal cord, pharynx, epiglottis and larynx [17]. The latest established epitope of MUC1 is the exclusively tumor related TA-MUC1 [18]. This tumor specific epitope stays adherent to the cell membrane. The appropriate matching monoclonal humanized antibody hPankoMab-GEXTM is unrivalled compared to all current MUC1 antibodies due to strongest specificity and greatest binding capacity [19]. It reacts with a great number of different carcinomas [18,20,21]. On the other hand, hPankoMab-GEXTM already provided good results in clinical trials, phase 1 and 2, for patients suffering from ovarian cancer (unpublished information from Glycotope GmbH, Berlin, Germany).

The screening of laryngeal cancer patients for HPV and TA-MUC1 might not only provide better assessment of prognosis, but also new approaches for therapy. Therefore the aim of our study was the evaluation of p16, its foundation for HPV diagnosis and staining of TA-MUC1. Second aim was the correlation of evaluated staining results to TNM-classification, grading and relapse and their influence on overall survival.

Materials and Methods

Study population

Laryngeal carcinoma specimens of 129 patients were taken after undergoing surgery and histological classification including TNM staging. Thereof 31 were classified as G1, 58 as G2 and 40 as G3. Complete histological and follow up data of all patients were available (grading, staging, date of surgery, relapse, last contact, viability). Normal material, such as tongue, vocal cord, larynx, pharynx and epiglottis, was taken from autopsies at legal medicine (n=5). Omission of any kind of cancer is assured. All samples were processed anonymously; the study was approved by the Ethics Committee of University Hospital Erlangen with a declaration of no objection on 10.07.2012 for using retrospective data analysis and was carried out in compliance with the guidelines of the Helsinki Declaration.

Immunohistochemistry

TA-MUC1: The peroxidase-labeled humanized monoclonal PankoMab-GEXTM was used in a concentration of 2.7 µg/ml (Glycotope GmbH, Berlin, Germany). Immediately after surgery or autopsy tissue specimens were formalin-fixed and subsequently embedded in paraffin. Paraffin sections of 3 µm were prepared and provided for immunohistochemistry by heating them at 55°C overnight. Slides were deparaffinized and rehydrated step wisely in

ethanol. No antigen retrieval was necessary, but endogenous peroxidase activity was blocked by 3% H_2O_2 in methanol for 20 min. unspecific binding sites were of no consequence because of the purity of the antibody. The sections were incubated with the peroxidase-labeled humanized PankoMab-GEXTM (2.7 µg/ml) for 90 min at room temperature. Color development was done by DAB (diaminobenzidine) and counterstaining by hematoxylin [20]. At each approach ovarian and breast cancer specimen were taken as positive controls and omission of the specific antibody as well as incubation with bovine serum as negative controls. According to the immunoreactive score of Remmele and Steger (IRS) slides were analyzed by two different investigators. Intensity of staining and the percentage of positive cells were multiplied for evaluation.

p16: CINtecHistology, Roche, Mannheim, German Specimens were automatically stained using Ventana Benchmark XT. The slides were evaluated by a pathologist. The staining intensity was disposed in 1=low, 2=moderate, 3=strong. Negative and positive control slides were carried along.

HPV diagnosis: Strong p16 expression (intensity 3) was considered as HPV positive. In accordance to histological norm moderate expression (intensity 2) was assessed as HPV positive only in event of outspread, not only focal immunohistochemically staining of p16.

Statistics

Data were analyzed employing the SPSS (v19, IBM, Armonk, New York) statistic software for MS windows and visualized using Microsoft Office 7. Spearman coefficients were employed to correlate data, while the Mann-Whitney U was applied to test for differences between groups. Differences in survival were assessed by applying the log-rank test and survival curves were plotted in accordance with Kaplan-Meier survival analysis. Statistical significance for all tests was set as $p < 0.05$ and data were expressed in terms of mean ± standard error (SEM).

Results

Evaluation of the hPankoMabTM specificity and staining of breast and ovarian cancer tissue as positive controls

All normal tissues of the upper aero-digestive region, such as vocal cord, pharynx (Figure 1A), larynx (1B), tongue and epiglottis remained completely negative. Human epithelia cancer tissue was used as positive control tissue. We identified an intense staining of TA-MUC1 in breast cancer as well as ovarian cancer tissue (1C). Negative control was performed by omission of hPankoMab-GEX^{TM} and incubation with bovine serum.

The expression of TA-MUC1 is increased in laryngeal tumors related to grading and tumor growth

A total of 22 cases of 31 G1 laryngeal tumors (71%) were completely negative for TA-MUC1 with an IRS=0 and the remaining 9 didn't reach an IRS higher than 2. All of the G1 tumors didn't score an IRS relevant scope (Figure 2A). Only few cases showed faint expression of TA-MUC1 (2B). In contrast to the former latter, G2 (2C) and G3 tumors (2D) showed an enhanced TA-MUC1 staining. G2/G3 graded tumor specimens did not differ in the range of the immunoreactive score (IRS). In large part they appeared positive with an IRS up to 9. Focusing on the tumor staging the expression of TA-MUC1 increased with the tumor growth. On average T3 and T4 tumors reached a higher IRS. According the expression of TA-MUC1 to tumor grading reaches statistical significance (p=0.001). G1 tumors showed significantly less staining compared to G2 (p<0.001) and G3 (Figure 2E, p=0.001) carcinomas. In correlation to the tumor stadium the expression of TA-MUC 1 showed an significant increase of staining in tumors in correlation to staging (Figure 2F, p<0.001).

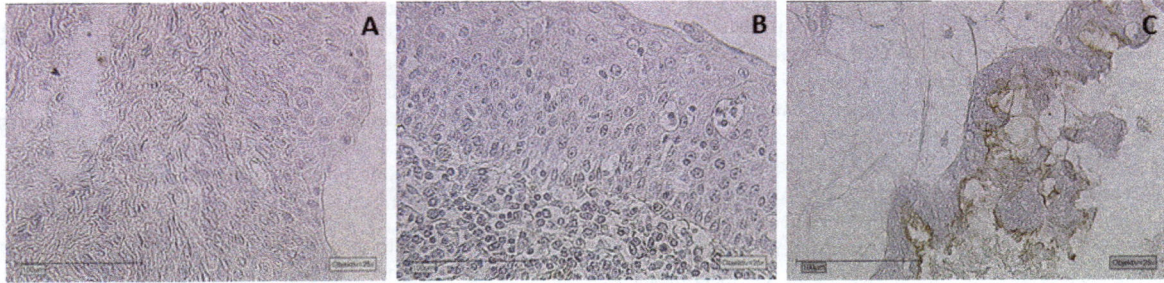

Figure 1: The specificity of the humanized antibody PankoMabTM was tested on non-malignant tissue of pharynx (A) and larynx (B). These tissues showed no positive staining reaction with PankoMabTM. In contrast, ovarian cancer tissue showed intense apical staining of the tumor epithelium (C).

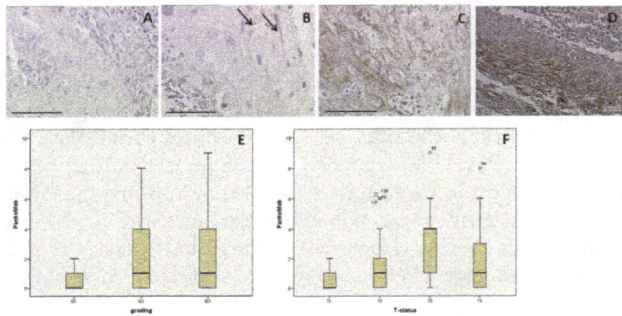

Figure 2: The majority of the laryngeal carcinoma specimens graded G1 showed no staining of TA-MUC1 with PankoMabTM (A). A minor content of G1 carcinomas showed very faint staining of TA-MUC1 (B) marked with to arrows. A significantly greater amount of tumor cells are stained with PankoMabTM in G2 graded carcinomas (C). Again a great amount of tumor cells are stained for TA-MUC1 in G3 graded laryngeal carcinoma specimens (D). A summary of the staining results correlated to grading by Box-Plot graphics is presented in lower section (E). In addition, significant differences of PankoMabTM staining were found regarding T-status of the laryngeal carcinoma specimens. An increase from T1 to T4 tumors is presented as Box Plot (F).

The expression of the HPV-related protein P16 is increased in laryngeal tumors related to tumor growth but not to grading

All G1 laryngeal carcinomas revealed no or only a low expression (intensity 1). G2 and G3 tumors presented mostly a moderate till strong staining level (intensity 2 and 3) in addition of a few cases without an expression (41%). Concerning the tumor staging T1 staged tumor tissue showed faint and non-intense p16 staining (Figure 3A), T2 staged tumors showed more intense but focal p16 expression (3B) an increasing staining intensity can be observed in T3 staged tumor tissue (3C) and a very intense p16 expression was found in T4

carcinomas (3D), which are already spreading and not restricted to the larynx anymore. Summarized 46% of all reviewed paraffin sections remained completely negative. According the expression of p16 to tumor grading doesn`t reach statistical significance. In correlation to the tumor stadium the expression of p16 showed a significant increase of staining in T4 in comparison to T1 tumors (Figure 3F, p=0.034).

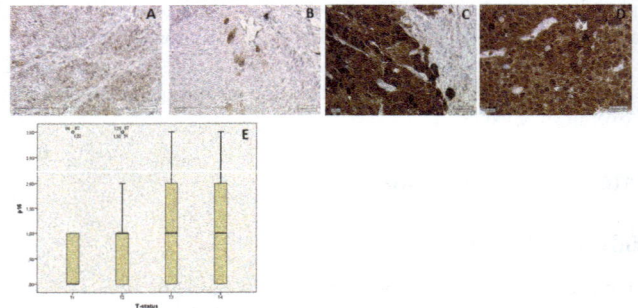

Figure 3: Significant differences in p16 staining and therefore HPV diagnostics in laryngeal carcinoma specimens are found regarding T-status. T1 tumor tissue showed low intense p16 staining with negative HPV status (A). An increase of p16 staining at least in some carcinoma cells was found in T2 staged carcinoma cells (B). T3 staged tumor cells showed very intense p16 staining diagnosed as HPV positive in some cases (C). The same result is found in T4 carcinomas with intense p16 staining and positive HPV diagnoses D). A summary of the staining results correlated to staging by Box-Plot graphics is presented in lower section (E).

Evaluation in laryngeal cancer specimen on the basis of HPV detection

Laryngeal carcinoma tissue slides assessed with staining intensity 3 were rated as HPV positive as well as cases with an outspread moderate stain (intensity 2). Summarized only 23 tumors of a total of 129 (18%) were considered HPV positive.

Correlation analysis of p16, hPankoMabTM and TNM classification

TA-MUC1 showed a strong correlation to the tumor grading (rho=0.247; p=0.002), tumor growth (rho=0.326; p<0.001) and a trend to the p16 staining (rho=0.146, p=0.098). The HPV related protein p16 showed a trend to a positive correlation with grading (rho=0.156; p=0.077) and a significant correlation to tumor growth (rho=199; p=0.023). The T status showed a significant correlation to tumor grading in our group of patients (rho=0.539; p<0.001). A summary is presented in Table 1.

			Correlation analysis					
			p16	HPV	PankoMab	T-Status	Relapse	Grading
Spearman-Rho		Coefficient of correlation	1,000	,627**	,146	,199*	,129	,156
	p16	Sig. (2-tail)	.	,000	,098	,223	,145	,077
		N	129	129	129	129	129	129
		Coefficient of correlation	,627**	1,000	,082	,085	,031	,122
	HPV	Sig. (2-tail)	,000	.	,353	,339	,725	,169
		N	129	129	129	129	129	129
		Coefficient of correlation	,146	,082	1,000	,326**	,051	,274**
	PankoMab	Sig. (2-tail)	,098	,353	.	,000	,565	,002
		N	129	129	129	129	129	129
		Coefficient of correlation	,199*	,085	,326**	1,000	,072	,539**
	T-Status	Sig. (2-tail)	,023	,339	,000	.	,417	,000
		N	129	129	129	129	129	129
		Coefficient of correlation	,129	,031	,051	,072	1,000	,096
	Relapse	Sig. (2-tail)	,145	,725	,565	,417	.	,278
		N	129	129	129	129	129	129
		Coefficient of correlation	,156	,122	,274**	,539**	,096	1,000
	Grading	Sig. (2-tail)	,077	,169	,002	,000	,278	.
		N	129	129	129	129	129	134

Table 1: Spearman Rho analysis revealed positive correlation between p16 staining and T-status (rho=0.199; p=0.023), a trend for a positive correlation was found between p16 and grading (p=0.077) and PankoMabTM staining (p=0.098), PankoMabTM staining is highly significant correlated to both, grading (rho=0.247; p=0.002) and T-status (rho=0.326; p<0.001).

Survival analysis

p=0.034 Kaplan-Meier analysis revealed significant difference in prognosis of laryngeal tumor patients whose tumors showed a higher grading (G2 and 3 compared to G1; p=0.0054). In addition, significant differences in prognosis of laryngeal tumor patients were found in correlation to TNM classification (T<=1 compared to T>1; p=0.007). A third significant parameter in prognosis of laryngeal tumor patients was relapse (no relapse compared to relapse; p<0.001). Kaplan-Meier analysis of TA-MUC1 staining revealed no significant differences (hPankoMab-GEXTM_ IRS<1 compared to hPankoMab-GEXTM IRS >=1; p=0.117). In addition, also p16 staining (p16 IRS <=1 compared to p16 IRS >1; p=0.185) and evaluation of HPV status (HPV negative compared to HPV positive; p=0.292) showed no significant correlation to patient survival. A summary of the survival analysis is presented in Figure 4.

Discussion

Within this study we could show that TA-MUC1 exhibited a strong and significant correlation with tumor grading and staging in head and neck squamous cell carcinomas (HNSCC), but was negative in normal tissues. Expression of p16 as a tool for HPV diagnosis in this type of carcinoma revealed a significant increase of staining in staged T4 tumors in comparison to T1 tumors. TA-MUC1 showed a positive trend in the correlation to p16 staining and therefore HPV involvement. Significant differences in analyses of overall survival were found in correlation to TNM-classification, grading and relapse. The main threat of an ongoing HPV infection is cervical cancer, which is already the third most common type of cancer and also the fourth leading cause of death in women (Symposium "HPV and Cervical Cancer" 2014 DKFZ, Heidelberg, Germany). The number of new cases fell from 9.410 in 1980 to 4.660 in 2010 (Robert-Koch-Institute, Berlin, Germany). The main reason for this decline is undoubtedly the discovery of the interaction of cervical cancer and Human Papilloma Virus (HPV) infection. In addition, the decreasing number of new cases may also be associated with increasing research and better

detection methods [22,23]. Based on newly developed methods, improved screening [24] and preventive vaccination [25] were employed.

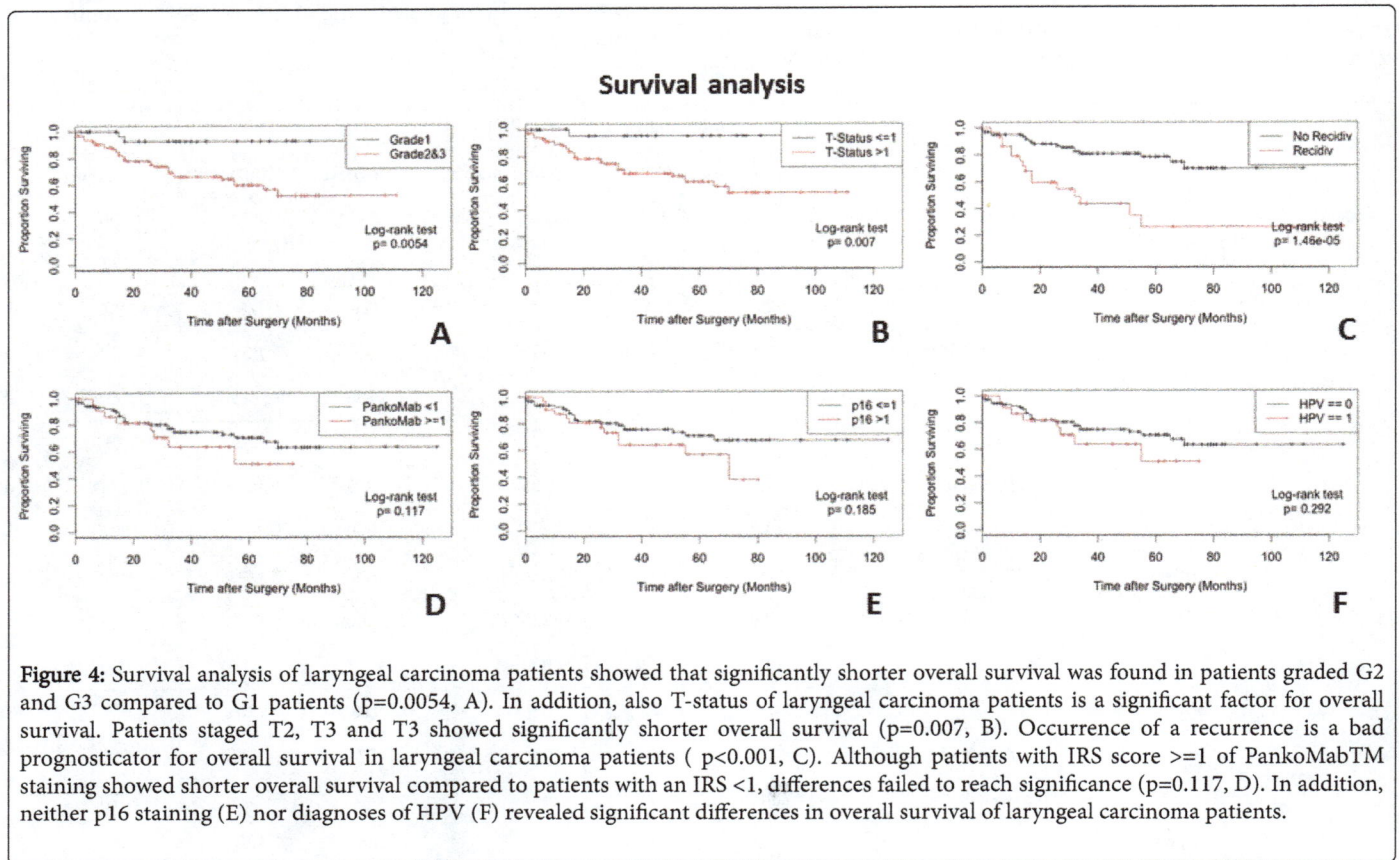

Figure 4: Survival analysis of laryngeal carcinoma patients showed that significantly shorter overall survival was found in patients graded G2 and G3 compared to G1 patients (p=0.0054, A). In addition, also T-status of laryngeal carcinoma patients is a significant factor for overall survival. Patients staged T2, T3 and T3 showed significantly shorter overall survival (p=0.007, B). Occurrence of a recurrence is a bad prognosticator for overall survival in laryngeal carcinoma patients (p<0.001, C). Although patients with IRS score >=1 of PankoMabTM staining showed shorter overall survival compared to patients with an IRS <1, differences failed to reach significance (p=0.117, D). In addition, neither p16 staining (E) nor diagnoses of HPV (F) revealed significant differences in overall survival of laryngeal carcinoma patients.

Adapted from the results in the field of cervical cancer a direct connection between HPV infection and oropharyngeal carcinoma development could be established as well. The virus can be spread through direct skin-to-skin-contact during vaginal, anal and oral sexual intercourse. Therefore, women suffering from cervical cancer carry an increased risk to develop a malignancy also in the upper aerodigestive tract as well as their sexual partner [26,27].

Head and neck squamous cell carcinomas (HNSCC) are the sixth most common cancer worldwide [28]. Formerly tobacco and alcohol abuse used to be the most supposed causes for all tumors of the oral cavity, oropharynx and larynx [29,30]. In 1999, a subset of oropharyngeal cancer was considered HPV associated [31]. Today HPV DNA prevalence for oropharyngeal cancer is found in approximately 50% of all cases. In addition, HPV involvement is estimated in about 25% of the cases of laryngeal and oral cavity cancer [32]. Because there is a strong correlation between HPV positive oropharyngeal cancer and sexual behavior nowadays comprehensive sex education and more information on the benefits of vaccination is indispensable [3,33,34]. Vaccination is most effective, when given before sexual activity starts. Therefore it should be considered for boys as well [35].

Oropharyngeal tumors which are related to HPV infection and p16 overexpression gain better prognosis and overall survival [36,37]. HPV positive patients with an oropharyngeal cancer are on average younger and this cohort shows a distinct reduction in death rate and

progression, furthermore response to radio/chemotherapy is enhanced [38]. HPV associated tumors perpetually express the viral E6 /E7 proteins suggesting that these proteins are required for continued growth of the tumor cells [39,40]. E6 oncoprotein complexes with p53 and as a consequence p53`s growth arrest and DNA repair is disposed. E7 inactivates retinoblastoma tumor suppressor (pRb) pathway. [40,41]. Therefore, DNA damages caused by cytostatic drugs will not be repaired. In addition toxic anticancer treatment of HPV positive cancer cells leads to a strong repression of the oncogenes E6 and E7 [42,43].

The tumor suppressor p16 is able to influence N- and O-glycosylation and galectin (Gal) expression [44,45]. The total number of stromal cells expressing Gal1, Gal3 and Gal9 was significantly higher in human papillomavirus-induced usual-type vulvar intraepithelial neoplasia (uVIN) than in vulvar tissue from healthy women undergoing labial reduction surgery [46]. Among HPV positive cases of laryngeal cancer a higher percentage of specimen showed an increased Gal3 expression than among the HPV negative group [47]. Moreover Gal1 and Gal3 have been proposed as biological markers of aggressiveness in several types of head and neck tumors [17,48,49].

Mucin1 (MUC1) is a receptor for Gal1 and Gal3. MUC1 is a large membrane bound glycoprotein which is expressed on the surface of epithelia [50]. During genesis of malignancies the glycosylation pattern of tumor cells changes [51] while MUC1 acts as a carrier for oncofetal carbohydrates like the Thomsen-Friedenreich antigen and supports invasive growth [52,53]. The recently described MUC1 epitope TA-MUC1 is almost exclusively limited to malign tumors while being overexpressed and remaining adherent to the cell membrane. The newly established antibody hPankoMab-GEXTM recognizes specifically and exclusively the tumor-associated TA-MUC1 [18,19]. Beside its antibody dependent cellular cytotoxicity (ADCC), hPankoMab-GEXTM is able to influence different cell signaling pathways via binding, because the intracellular part of MUC1 is an active receptor tyrosine kinase (RTK) [12,54].

HNSCC have a huge impact upon quality of life and survival. Despite of innovative new treatment implantation such as Laser Surgery, robotic surgery and EGFR antibodies, the overall survival did not improve substantially [55-58].

Within this study, we could demonstrate universal absence of TA-MUC1 in normal tissues of the upper aero digestive tract like larynx, pharynx, vocal-cord, epiglottis and tongue, but overexpression in worse graded laryngeal tumors. The antibody therapy used so far for head and neck carcinoma focuses on inhibition of receptors of the epidermal growth factor family. Side effects like paronychia, abnormalities of hair growth and serious skin irritations are inevitable, because the target is not restricted to malignancies [59]. We were able to show a strong and significant correlation between the TA-MUC1 expression and grading as well as staging. Together with the fact, that TA-MUC1 stays adherent to the cell membrane, this epitope shows great potential being a promising target for an antibody therapy with hPankoMab-GEXTM.

Conclusion

TA-MUC1 and p16 revealed relation by a trend, but we could not show a significant correlation between MUC1 and HPV association. Therefore, we suppose that HPV-associated tumors of head and neck will particularly profit by a TA-MUC1 targeted therapy. This assumption could be due to the fact that after hPankoMab-GEXTM binding the overexpressed Gal1 and GAL3, they cannot act as ligands for MUC1 as a RTK and switch on several signaling pathways. Even though, TA-MUC1 showed a positive trend in correlation to p16 staining a lack of significance is supposedly a problem of an insufficient number of included cases. An analysis of HPV association should be performed generally in laryngeal cancer specimens like in oropharyngeal cancer [60]. Additional data might lead to the conclusion that HPV is also relevant for the onset of laryngeal cancer.

Competing Interests

The authors declare that they have no financial or non-financial competing interests.

Funding

This work was supported by "Forschungsstiftung Medizin am Universitätsklinikum Erlangen", Germany and the "Deutsche Forschungsgemeinschaft" (DFG).

Author's Contribution

IW, CA, KF, DM, CF, AS, PB, MP: Conception and design, performed research, writer, revision and approval of the final version

JT, SG, TW, DD, UJ, BK: Conception and design, revision and approval of the final version.

References

1. Kau RJ, Alexiou C, Stimmer H, Arnold W (2000) Diagnostic procedures for detection of lymph node metastases in cancer of the larynx. ORL J Otorhinolaryngol Relat Spec 62: 199-203.

2. Atula S, Auvinen E, Grenman R, Syrjänen S (1997) Human papilloma virus and Epstein-Barr virus in epithelial carcinomas of the head and neck region. Anticancer Res 17: 4427-4433.

3. Lajer CB, von Buchwald C (2010) The role of human papilloma virus in head and neck cancer. APMIS 118: 510-519.

4. Li XC, Gao Y, Yang F, Zhou M, Li Q, et al. (2014) Systematic review with meta-analysis: The association between human papillomavirus infection and oesophageal cancer. Aliment Pharmacol Ther 39: 270-281.

5. Li X, Gao L, Li H, Gao J, Yang Y, et al. (2013) Human papilloma virus infection and laryngeal cancer risk: A systematic review and meta-analysis. J Infect Dis 207: 479-488.

6. Wittekindt C, Wagner S, Mayer CS, Klußmann JP (2012) [Basics of tumor development and importance of human papilloma virus (HPV) for head and neck cancer]. Laryngorhinootologie 91 Suppl 1: S1-26.

7. Khode SR, Dwivedi RC, Rhys-Evans P, Kazi R (2014) Exploring the link between human papilloma virus and oral and oropharyngeal cancers. J Cancer Res Ther 10: 492-498.

8. Atighechi S, Ahmadpour Baghdadabad MR, Mirvakili SA, Sheikhha MH, Baradaranfar MH, et al. (2014) Human papilloma virus and nasopharyngeal carcinoma: Pathology, prognosis, recurrence and mortality of the disease. Exp Oncol 36: 215-216.

9. Chen AM, Zahra T, Daly ME, Farwell DG, Luu Q, et al. (2013) Definitive radiation therapy without chemotherapy for human papilloma virus-positive head and neck cancer. Head Neck 35: 1652-1656.

10. Mao C, Balasubramanian A, Yu M, Kiviat N, Ridder R, et al. (2007) Evaluation of a new p16(INK4A) ELISA test and a high-risk HPV DNA test for cervical cancer screening: Results from proof-of-concept study. Int J Cancer 120: 2435-2438.

11. Melkane AE, Mirghani H, Auperin A, Saulnier P, Lacroix L, et al. (2014) HPV-related oropharyngeal squamous cell carcinomas: A comparison between three diagnostic approaches. Am J Otolaryngol 35: 25-32.

12. Carraway KL, Ramsauer VP, Haq B, Carothers Carraway CA (2003) Cell signaling through membrane mucins. Bioessays 25: 66-71.

13. Pochampalli MR, el Bejjani RM, Schroeder JA (2007) MUC1 is a novel regulator of ErbB1 receptor trafficking. Oncogene 26: 1693-1701.

14. Singh PK, Hollingsworth MA (2006) Cell surface-associated mucins in signal transduction. Trends Cell Biol 16: 467-476.

15. Croce MV, Rabassa ME, Price MR, Segal-Eiras A (2001) MUC1 mucin and carbohydrate associated antigens as tumor markers in head and neck squamous cell carcinoma. Pathol Oncol Res 7: 284-291.

16. Wiest I, Schulze S, Kuhn C, Seliger, Hausmann R, et al. (2007) Expression of the carbohydrate tumour marker SLeX, SLeA (CA19-9), LeY and Thomsen-Friedenreich (TF) antigen on normal squamous epithelial tissue of the penis and vagina. Anticancer Res 27: 1981-1988.

17. Wiest IC, Alexiou C, Kuhn S, Schulze S, Kunze D, et al. (2012) Expression of different carbohydrate tumour markers and galectins 1 and 3 in normal squamous and malignant epithelia of the upper aaerodigestive tract. Anticancer Res 32: 2023-2029.

18. Fan XN, Karste U, Goletz S, Cao Y (2010) Reactivity of a humanized antibody (hPankoMab) towards a tumor-related MUC1 epitope (TA-MUC1) with various human carcinomas. Pathol Res Pract 206: 585-589.

19. Danielczyk A, Stahn R, Faulstich D, Löffler A, Märten A, et al. (2006) PankoMab: A potent new generation anti-tumour MUC1 antibody. Cancer Immunol Immunother 55: 1337-1347.

20. Dian D, Lenhard M, Mayr D, Heublein S, Karsten U, et al. (2013) Staining of MUC1 in ovarian cancer tissues with PankoMab-GEX detecting the tumour-associated epitope, TA-MUC1, as compared to antibodies HMFG-1 and 115D8. Histol Histopathol 28: 239-244.

21. Dian D, Janni W, Kuhn C, Mayr D, Karsten U, et al. (2009) Evaluation of a novel anti-mucin 1 (MUC1) antibody (PankoMab) as a potential diagnostic tool in human ductal breast cancer; comparison with two established antibodies. Onkologie 32: 238-244.

22. Sano T, Oyama T, Kashiwabara K, Fukuda T, Nakajima T (1998) Expression status of p16 protein is associated with human papilloma virus oncogenic potential in cervical and genital lesions. Am J Pathol 153: 1741-1748.

23. Griffin NR, Bevan IS, Lewis FA, Wells M, Young LS (1990) Demonstration of multiple HPV types in normal cervix and in cervical squamous cell carcinoma using the polymerase chain reaction on paraffin wax embedded material. J Clin Pathol 43: 52-56.

24. Bhatla N, Singla S, Awasthi D (2012) Human papilloma virus deoxyribonucleic acid testing in developed countries. Best Pract Res Clin Obstet Gynaecol 26: 209-220.

25. Sander BB, Rebolj M, Valentiner-Branth P, Lynge E (2012) Introduction of human papilloma virus vaccination in Nordic countries. Vaccine 30: 1425-1433.

26. Hemminki K, Dong C, Frisch M (2000) Tonsillar and other upper aerodigestive tract cancers among cervical cancer patients and their husbands. Eur J Cancer Prev 9: 433-437.

27. Newell GR, Krementz ET, Roberts JD (1975) Excess occurrence of cancer of the oral cavity, lung and bladder following cancer of the cervix. Cancer 36: 2155-2158.

28. Ferlay J, Shin HR, Bray F, Forman D, Mathers C, et al. (2010) Estimates of worldwide burden of cancer in 2008: GLOBOCAN 2008. Int J Cancer 127: 2893-2917.

29. Andréasson L, Björlin G, Hocherman M, Korsgaard R, Trell E (1987) Laryngeal cancer, aryl hydrocarbon hydroxylase inducibility and smoking. A follow-up study. ORL J Otorhinolaryngol Relat Spec 49: 187-192.

30. Maier H, Dietz A, Gewelke U, Seitz HK, Heller WD (1990) [Tobacco- and alcohol-associated cancer risk of the upper respiratory and digestive tract]. Laryngorhinootologie 69: 505-511.

31. zur Hausen H (1999) Papilloma viruses in human cancers. Proc Assoc Am Physicians 111: 581-587.

32. Ndiaye C, Mena M, Alemany L, Arbyn M, Castellsagué X, et al. (2014) HPV DNA, E6/E7 mRNA, and p16INK4a detection in head and neck cancers: A systematic review and meta-analysis. Lancet Oncol 15: 1319-1331.

33. Rettig E, Kiess AP, Fakhry C (2015) The role of sexual behavior in head and neck cancer: Implications for prevention and therapy. Expert Rev Anticancer Ther 15: 35-49.

34. Martín-Hernán F, Sánchez-Hernández JG, Cano J, Campo J, del Romero J (2013) Oral cancer, HPV infection and evidence of sexual transmission. Med Oral Patol Oral Cir Bucal 18: e439-444.

35. Dalianis T (2014) Human papilloma virus (HPV) and oropharyngeal squamous cell carcinoma. Presse Med 43: e429-434.

36. Gronhoj Larsen C, Gyldenlove M, Jensen DH, Therkildsen MH, Kiss K, et al. (2014) Correlation between human papilloma virus and p16 overexpression in oropharyngeal tumours: A systematic review. Br J Cancer 110: 1587-1594.

37. Ang KK, Harris J, Wheeler R, Weber R, Rosenthal DI, et al. (2010) Human papilloma virus and survival of patients with oropharyngeal cancer. N Engl J Med 363: 24-35.

38. Shaughnessy JN, Farghaly H, Wilson L, Redman R, Potts K, et al. (2014) HPV: A factor in organ preservation for locally advanced larynx and hypopharynx cancer? Am J Otolaryngol 35: 19-24.

39. Androphy EJ, Hubbert NL, Schiller JT, Lowy DR (1987) Identification of the HPV-16 E6 protein from transformed mouse cells and human cervical carcinoma cell lines. EMBO J 6: 989-992.

40. Chung CH, Gillison ML (2009) Human papillomavirus in head and neck cancer: Its role in pathogenesis and clinical implications. Clin Cancer Res 15: 6758-6762.

41. Kim MJ, MS Ki, K Kim, HJ Shim, JE Hwang, et al. (2014) Different protein expression associated with chemotherapy response in oropharyngeal cancer according to HPV status. BMC Cancer 14: 824.

42. Butz K, Geisen C, Ullmann A, Spitkovsky D, Hoppe Seyler F (1996) Cellular responses of HPV-positive cancer cells to genotoxic anti-cancer agents: Repression of E6/E7-oncogene expression and induction of apoptosis. Int J Cancer 68: 506-513.

43. Munagala R, Kausar H, Munjal C, Gupta RC (2011) Withaferin A induces p53-dependent apoptosis by repression of HPV oncogenes and upregulation of tumor suppressor proteins in human cervical cancer cells. Carcinogenesis 32: 1697 1705.

44. Amano M, Eriksson H, Manning JC, Detjen KM, Andre S, et al. (2012) Tumour suppressor p16(INK4a)-anoikis-favouring decrease in N/O-glycan/cell surface sialylation by down-regulation of enzymes in sialic acid biosynthesis in tandem in a pancreatic carcinoma model. FEBS J 279: 4062-4080.

45. Sanchez-Ruderisch H, Fischer C, Detjen KM, Welzel M, Wimmel A, et al. (2010) Tumor suppressor p16 INK4a: Downregulation of galectin-3, an endogenous competitor of the pro-anoikis effector galectin-1, in a pancreatic carcinoma model. FEBS J 277: 3552-3563.

46. Van Esch EM, Van Poelgeest MI, Kouwenberg S, Osse EM, Trimbos JB, (2015) Expression of coinhibitory receptors on T cells in the microenvironment of usual vulvar intraepithelial neoplasia is related to proinflammatory effector T cells and an increased recurrence-free survival. Int J Cancer 136: E95-E106.

47. Miranda FA, Hassumi MK, Guimaraes MC, Simoes RT, Silva TG, et al. (2009) Galectin-3 overexpression in invasive laryngeal carcinoma, assessed by computer-assisted analysis. J Histochem Cytochem 57: 665-673.

48. Saussez S, Decaestecker C, Mahillon V, Cludts S, Capouillez A, et al. (2008) Galectin-3 upregulation during tumor progression in head and neck cancer. Laryngoscope 118: 1583-1590.

49. Saussez S, Decaestecker C, Lorfevre F, Chevalier D, Mortuaire G, (2008) Increased expression and altered intracellular distribution of adhesion/growth-regulatory lectins galectins-1 and -7 during tumour progression in hypopharyngeal and laryngeal squamous cell carcinomas. Histopathology 52: 483-493.

50. Mall AS (2008) Analysis of mucins: Role in laboratory diagnosis. J Clin Pathol 61: 1018-1024.

51. Brockhausen I (2006) Mucin-type O-glycans in human colon and breast cancer: Glycodynamics and functions. EMBO Rep 7: 599-604.

52. Mommers EC, Leonhart AM, von Mensdorff-Pouilly S, Schol DJ, Hilgers J, et al. (1999) Aberrant expression of MUC1 mucin in ductal hyperplasia and ductal carcinoma in situ of the breast. Int J Cancer 84: 466-469.

53. Jeschke U, Richter DU, Hammer A, Briese V, Friese K (2002) Expression of the Thomsen-Friedenreich antigen and of its putative carrier protein mucin 1 in the human placenta and in trophoblast cells in vitro. Histochem Cell Biol 117: 219-226.

54. Bitler BG, Menzl I, Huerta CL, Sands B, Knowlton W (2009) Intracellular MUC1 peptides inhibit cancer progression. Clin Cancer Res 15: 100-109.

55. Prince A, Aguirre-Ghizo J, Genden E, Posner M, Sikora A (2010) Head and neck squamous cell carcinoma: New translational therapies. Mt Sinai J Med 77: 684-699.

56. Iro H, Waldfahrer F, Altendorf-Hofmann A, Weidenbecher M, Sauer R, et al. (1998) Transoral laser surgery of supraglottic cancer: Follow-up of 141 patients. Arch Otolaryngol Head Neck Surg 124: 1245-1250.

57. Hans S, Delas B, Gorphe P, Ménard M, Brasnu D (2012) Transoral robotic surgery in head and neck cancer. Eur Ann Otorhinolaryngol Head Neck Dis 129: 32-37.

58. Bonner JA, Harari PM, Giralt J, Azarnia N, Shin DM, et al. (2006) Radiotherapy plus cetuximab for squamous-cell carcinoma of the head and neck. N Engl J Med 354: 567-578.

59. Madke B, Gole P, Kumar P, Khopkar U (2014) Dermatological side effects of epidermal growth factor receptor inhibitors: 'PRIDE' complex. Indian J Dermatol 59: 271-274.

60. Laskaris S, Sengas I, Maragoudakis P, Tsimplaki E, Argyri E, (2014) Prevalence of human papilloma virus infection in Greek patients with squamous cell carcinoma of the larynx. Anticancer Res 34: 5749-5753.

4

Clinical Impact of Chronic Tonsillitis on Weight and Height Parameters in Kosovo children

Beqir Abazi[1], Bajram Shaqiri[1*], Halil Ajvazi[1], Pajtim Lutaj[2] and Pjerin Radovani[2]

[1]Department of ENT – Ophthalmology, Regional Hospital Centre of Gjilan, Kosovo

[2]Department of ENT – Ophthalmology, University Hospital Clinical Centre "Mother Teresa", Tirana, Albania

[*]Corresponding author: Beqir Abazi, Department of Otorhinolaryngology, Regional Hospital Center of Gjilan, Kosovo; E-mail: beqirabazi@yahoo.com

Abstract

Objective: The aim of the study was to determine the association of chronic tonsillitis with physiological parameters, such as the weight and height, before and after the surgical intervention in children.

Methods: This is a cross-sectional study involving 85 children diagnosed with chronic tonsillitis and hospitalized in the Department of Otorhinolaryngology, Regional Hospital Center of Gjilan, Kosovo, from January 2011 to February 2015. All children underwent surgical intervention to correct their condition. Height and weight of participating children was measured before treatment and 6 and 12 months after intervention and their values were compared against each-other and standard reference levels.

Results: The mean age of the participants was 7.15 years (7.11 years for boys and 7.19 years for girls), with no statistically significant difference between boys and girls. Before treatment, the overwhelming majority of children with chronic tonsillitis were under the weight and height standards for their age (95.3% and 98.8%, respectively). For each age-group, there was a positive association between weight and height with time after intervention, even though the statistical significance was achieved only regarding height. One year after the surgical correction of chronic tonsillitis, the proportion of normal weight and normal height children increased from 4.7% to 8.2% (for weight) and from 1.2% to 4.7% (for height).

Conclusions: We propose careful evaluation of young patients with chronic tonsillitis, and monitoring of weight and height for an adequate and timely treatment of it (adenotonsillectomy), as a way to prevent a range of complications including the deteriorating effects on weight and height.

Keywords: Kosovo; Chronic tonsillitis; Growth parameters; Weight; Height

Introduction

Inflammatory changes in the tonsils as a consequence of the local or general disorders in the organism present the clinical entity called Tonsillitis that may be acute or chronic. In addition to local disorders, the inflammatory changes in tonsils, may lead to general disorders in the body. Chronic tonsillitis might be associated with unfavorable changes of weight and weight in patients suffering from this health condition and such clinical changes have been reported in the international literature [1,2]. The tonsils affected by the inflammatory process loose the capability of lymphocytes production causing disorders of T and B-lymphocyte (T-Ly / B-Ly) as well as other effects in the immune-globulins and having direct influence in the cell and hormonal immunity through the hormonal feedback from the hypophysis [3,4]. Some of the local clinical manifestations of chronic tonsillitis include the tonsillogenic, odour (bad smell) from the mouth, difficulty in breathing, continuous coughing, sense of presence of other bodies/entities in the pharynx and irritated angular lymphatic ankle. At the other organs, it is worth mentioning the immunogenic uveitis and general ones like febris rheumatica, systematically skin's disease etc. Chronic tonsillitis, might also have an impact in the patient's weight and height, where the retardation varies about 10% compared to children with normal development [5,6].

In Kosovo there is no information about the influence of chronic tonsillitis on anthropometric parameters of affected children, such as weight and height. Therefore, the aim of this study is to determine the association of chronic tonsillitis with physiological parameters, such as the weight and height, before and after the surgical intervention in a sample of children suffering from this disease in Kosovo.

Methods

Study population and sampling

This is a cross-sectional study involving 85 young patients (37 boys and 48 girls), diagnosed with chronic tonsillitis and presented for specialized treatment at the Department of Otorhinolaryngology (ENT) of the Gjilan Regional Hospital in Kosovo, from January 2011 to February 2015. All participating children were diagnosed with some form of chronic tonsillitis that has not been possible to be addressed through conventional treatment and therefore required a more radical type of treatment. We included all children that showed up at Gjilan Regional Hospital during the aforementioned period of time.

Data collection

We measured the anthropometric parameters of each participating child, such as weight and height, following standard protocols. For the measurement of weight, the children were advised to remove any heavy clothing and shoes whereas for the measurement of height they were instructed to stand in the right position. The measurement of height and weight was performed at the moment the patient showed up at our hospital (that is, before the surgical treatment) and then 6 months and 12 months after the surgical treatment of chronic tonsillitis. The same calibrated weight and height scales were used to measure the weight and height of children in each of the three measurement points of time. Also, we used the standard reference levels of weight and height by age, in order to compare our data against such thresholds.

Data analysis

For categorical variables absolute numbers and the respective percentages were reported. For continuous variables the mean value and the standard deviation of the parameter was reported. To compare the mean values of weight and height in different points in time the student's t-test, through the one-way ANOVA procedure, was used. For categorical variables, the chi-square test was used. The associations were considered as statistically significant if the P-value ≤ 0.05.

All the statistical analysis were carried out using the Statistical Package for Social Science (SPSS) software, version 16.

Results

There were 85 children that participated in the study, of whom 37 were boys (43.5%) and 48 girls (56.5%). The mean age of participants was 7.15 years $\pm$ 1.89 years, without significant difference between boys and girls (P=0.849) (Table 1). The age of the participants ranged from 4 years (8 subjects) to 11 years old (1 subject). Around two-thirds of participating children were pupils (65.9%) whereas the remaining 34.1% were still in kindergarten (Table 1). Also, more than half of participating children resided in urban parts of the country, without statistically significant difference between boys and girls (Table 1).

Variable	Total	Gender		P- value
		Boys (n=37)	Girls (n=48)	
Age (continuous)	7.15 ± 1.89 *	7.11 ± 2.01	7.19 ± 1.82	0.849
Age				
4 years	8 (9.4) †	4 (10.8)	4 (8.3)	
5 years	11 (12.9)	5 (13.5)	6 (12.5)	
6 years	15 (17.6)	7 (18.9)	8 (16.7)	0.913
7 years	13 (15.3)	5 (13.5)	8 (16.7)	
8 years	14 (16.5)	6 (16.2)	8 (16.7)	
9 years	13 (15.3)	4 (10.8)	9 (18.8)	
10 years	10 (11.8)	5 (13.5)	5 (10.4)	
11 years	1 (1.2)	1 (2.7)	0 (0.00)	
Status				
Children	29 (34.1)	14 (37.8)	15 (31.3)	0.525
Pupil	56 (65.9)	23 (62.2)	33 (68.8)	
Residence				
Urban	47 (56.0)	21 (58.3)	26 (54.2)	0.703
Rural	37 (44.0)	15 (41.7)	22 (45.8)	
*Mean value ± standard deviation.				
†Absolute number and column percentage (in paranthesis).				
‡P - value according to student's t-test (for continuous variables) or chi-square test (for categorical variables).				

Table 1: General characteristics for the patients included in the study.

Table 2 displays the mean values of weight and height before the surgical intervention and 6 months and 12 months after it, for boys and girls. It can be noted that there is a positive association of weight and height with the time after surgical treatment of chronic tonsillitis, even though the statistical significance was not achieved. However, in both boys and girls the mean value of weight and height increased 6 and 12 months after operation compared to the period before the intervention.

Variable	Total		Boys (n=37)		Girls (n=48)	
	Mean value ± SD	P- value	Mean value ± SD	P- value	Mean value ± SD	P- value
Weight (in kg)				0.367		0.538
Before the operation	23.86 ± 7.33 24.96 ± 7.39	0.212*	24.27 ± 7.03		23.54 ± 7.61	
6 months after operation	25.87 ± 7.51		25.53 ± 6.99		24.52 ± 7.73	
12 months after operation			26.61 ± 7.20		25.29 ± 7.77	
Height (in cm)		0.012		0.112		0.105
Before the operation	119.9 ± 11.2		120.3 ± 10.6		119.8 ± 11.8	
6 months after operation	122.6 ± 11.5		123.0 ± 11.0		122.4 ± 12.1	
12 months after operation	125.3 ± 11.8		125.8 ± 11.9		125.0 ± 11.9	
*P - value according to one-way ANOVA test.						

Table 2: Mean weight and height accordig to time of the measurement, by gender.

Tables 3 and 4 display the mean values of weight and height by age and gender and time of measurement. In general it can be noted that the mean weight and height of participants is lower than the standard reference levels of weight and height for any given age. On the other hand, the time trends observed are clear: for any given age, there is an increase of mean weight and mean height of participants 6 months and 12 months after the surgical intervention compared to the respective values before the treatment and such trends are observed in boys and girls (Tables 3 and 4). However, in general these time-differences in mean values did not reach statistical significance for weight for both boys and girls (Table 3) but they were mostly significant as regards mean values of height in both boys and girls, when mean values of height 12 months after operation are compared against respective values before operation (Table 4).

Boys						
Variable	Standard mean weight	Mean weight before the operation	Mean weight 6 months after the operation	Mean weight 12 months after the operation	P-value for three periods	P- value before the op. 12 month after op.
Age	20.28	14.13	15.25	16.25	0.076 *	0.033 *
4 years	22.03	17.00	18.40	19.30	0.370	0.198
5 years	23.51	21.86	22.92	23.43	0.408	0.214
6 years	30.90	24.40	26.10	27.20	0.494	0.261
7 years	35.28	27.42	28.50	29.75	0.708	0.421
8 years	40.36	31.00	32.13	33.38	0.686	0.417
9 years	46.16	31.20	32.20	33.80	0.746	0.464
10 years	52.56	37.00	40.00	42.00	-	-
11 years						
Total	31.46	24.27	25.53	26.61	0.367	0.156
Girls						
Age	20.39	14.00	14.50	15.13	0.687 *	0.408 *
4 years	23.75	15.83	16.75	17.67	0.418	0.208
5 years	27.39	16.81	17.63	18.50	0.521	0.267
6 years	31.47	21.31	22.63	23.38	0.329	0.152
7 years	33.55	30.81	31.69	32.25	0.329	0.151
8 years	41.82	28.88	29.87	30.44	0.617	0.341
9 years	48.18	33.50	34.80	36.10	0.831	0.559
10 years						

Total	32.93	23.54	24.52	25.29	0.538	0.267
*P - value according to one-way ANOVA test.						

Table 3: Mean weight of the subject in the study according to age and gender and time of measurement.

Boys						
Variable	Standard mean height	Mean height before the operation	Mean height 6 months after the operation	Mean height 12 months after the operation	P-value for three periods	P- value before the op. 12 month after op.
Age	109.5	102.0	103.9	106.4	0.164 *	0.106 *
4 years	116.8	110.6	112.9	114.7	0.020	0.018
5 years	123.9	116.7	118.2	119.6	0.074	0.031
6 years	131.0	119.2	123.0	125.4	0.017	0.013
7 years	137.8	124.2	128.2	132.5	0.005	0.002
8 years	144.1	130.8	132.8	135.0	0.515	0.287
9 years	149.9	134.6	137.6	141.2	0.176	0.087
10 years	155.5	135.0	140.0	149.0	-	-
11 years						
Total	131.2	120.3	123.0	125.8	0.112	0.032
Girls						
Age	108.4	100.5	102.5	106.8	0.013 *	0.020 *
4 years	116.1	106.8	109.5	112.2	0.017	0.010
5 years	123.9	115.5	116.8	119.4	0.037	0.017
6 years	131.3	116.1	118.6	121.0	0.103	0.044
7 years	137.7	126.4	128.9	130.1	0.086	0.051
8 years	143.8	125.7	129.7	132.6	0.009	0.006
9 years	149.6	142.0	145.0	148.2	0.360	0.145
10 years						
Total	131.6	119.8	122.4	125.0	0.105	0.034
*P - value according to one-way ANOVA test						

Table 4: Mean height of the subject in the study according to age and gender and time of measurement.

Tables 5 and 6 show that the overwhelming majority of study participants are under the standards for weight (95.3%) and under the standards for height (98.8%) for their respective age, thus supporting the findings in Tables 3 and 4. The situation is similar in boys and girls regarding these two parameters, with no statistical significant differences ($P>0.05$).

Variable	Total	Gender		P-value†
		Boys (n=37)	Girls (n=48)	
Weight before operation Under the standard In norm	81 (95.3) * 4 (4.7)	34 (91.9) 3 (8.1)	47 (97.9) 1 (2.1)	0.193
Weight 6 months after operation Under the standard	78 (91.8) 7 (8.2)	32 (86.5) 5 (13.5)	46 (95.8) 2 (4.2)	0.120

In norm				
Weight 12 months after operation Under the standard In norm	78 (91.8) 7 (8.2)	32 (86.5) 5 (13.5)	46 (95.8) 2 (4.2)	0.120
*The absolute number and percentage according to columns (in parenthesis).				
†P - value according to hi square test				

Table 5: The patients' weight in the study compared to standard reference levels.

Variable	Total	Gender		P-value†
		Boys (n=37)	Girls (n=48)	

Height before operation Under the standard In norm	84 (98.8) * 1 (1.2)	37 (100.0) 0 (0.0)	47 (97.9) 1 (2.1)	0.377
Height 6 months after operation Under the standard In norm	84 (98.8) 1 (1.2)	37 (100.0) 0 (0.0)	47 (97.9) 1 (2.1)	0.377
Height 12 months after operation Under the standard In norm	81 (95.3) 4 (4.7)	36 (97.3) 1 (2.7)	45 (93.8) 3 (6.3)	0.444

*The absolute number and percentage according to columns (in parenthesis).

†P - value according to hi square test

Table 6: The patients' height in the study compared to standard reference levels.

Discussion

This is the first study addressing the association of chronic tonsillitis and anthropometric parameters such as weight and height among young children in Kosovo. We noticed that the mean weight and mean height of chronic tonsillitis children was lower than mean standard reference levels, for each age group and in both boys and girls. Also, we evidenced that the surgical treatment of chronic tonsillitis resulted in an improvement of mean weight and mean height of study participants and the improvement was greater about one year after the intervention, whereas for height these differences were significant in most cases. In addition, despite the lack of statistical significance regarding changes of weight, we spotted a clinical significance: the findings indicate that there is a positive association between time after surgical correction of chronic tonsillitis and weight and height of patients, suggesting the improvement of the latter.

The beneficial effects of adenotonsillectomy on weight and height of young children is documented in the international literature. For example, a review of literature and meta-analysis, including children with sleep disordered breathing due to adenotonsillar hypertrophy, reported that adenotonsillectomy was associated with a significantly increased standardized weight and height [1]. Another study involving 96 children reported a similar improvement of weight and height of children following adenoidectomy [7] and yet similar findings were reported by other surveys [8,9].

Adenotonsillar hypertrophy is often associated with growth retardation, maybe due to reduced appetite and caloric intake, nocturnal hypoxemia and respiratory acidosis, with probably the involvement of impaired growth hormone secretion and action, even though the exact mechanisms of how adenotonsillar hypertrophy leads to growth retardation remain still little understood [8]. This finding is in accordance with the findings from our study which reported that all the children observed had mean weight and height lower than standard reference levels, suggesting a possible negative effect of chronic tonsillitis on growth parameters under study. Moreover, even one year after the intervention, this group of patients could not reach the weight and height of normal children whereas another study reported that after the intervention the height of the patient reached those of their peers [8]. The fact that we did not notice this in our

study could suggest a more deep effect of chronic tonsillitis on growth parameters, which cannot be overcome in a one-year period of time. However, such hypothesis has to be confirmed by future studies in Kosovo.

We think that the growth retardation in this group of patients could not be entirely attributed to chronic tonsillitis. The study by Ersoy and colleagues reported that "at the preoperative period, weight of their patients were approximately equivalent to those of their healthy peers", whereas we found that even before the operation the mean weight and height of our patients was much lower compared to standard reference growth levels. This could indicate malnutrition problems in Kosovo children, as suggested by a recent scientific research work [10].

In conclusion, we demonstrated that there is a beneficial effect of adenotonsillectomy on growth parameters of children such as weight and height in Kosovo. Regardless of the cross- sectional nature of the study and the impossibility to establish temporal relationships between events, we think that chronic tonsillitis might play a role in the "slowing down" of these patients regarding to their weight and height. Therefore, the surgical intervention to properly address this disease is very important to improve these parameters. However, the wider picture would require a comprehensive intervention to improve the general conditions and nutrition status of children in order for various interventions to be effective towards normalization of growth parameters of Kosovo children.

References

1. Bonuck KA, Freeman K, Henderson J (2009) Growth and growth biomarker changes after adenotonsillectomy: systematic review and meta-analysis. Arch D s Child 94: 83-91.

2. Costa DJ, Mitchell R (2009) Adenotonsillectomy for obstructive sleep apnea in obese children: a meta-analysis. Otolaryngol Head Neck Surg 140: 455-460.

3. Kang JM, Auo HJ, Yoo YH, Cho JH, Kim BG (2008) Changes in serum levels of IGF-1 and in growth following adenotonsillectomy in children. Int J Pediatr Otorhinolaryngol 72: 1065-1069.

4. Mitchell RB, Boss EF (2009) Pediatric obstructive sleep apnea in obese and normal-weight children: impact of adenotonsillectomy on quality-of-life and behavior. Dev Neuropsychol 34: 650-661.

5. Hakim F, Kheirandish-Gozal L, Gozal D (2015) Obesity and Altered Sleep: A Pathway to Metabolic Derangements in Children. Semin Pediatr Neurol 22: 77-85.

6. Gozal D, Kheirandish-Gozal L (2010) the obesity epidemic and disordered sleep during childhood and adolescence. Adolesc Med State Art Rev 21: 480-490

7. Kiris M, Muderris T, Celebi S, Cankaya H, Bercin S (2010) Changes in serum IGF-1 and IGFBP-3 levels and growth in children following adenoidectomy, tonsillectomy or adenotonsillectomy. Int J Pediatr Otorhinolaryngol 74: 528-531.

8. Ersoy B, Yücetürk AV, Taneli F, Urk V, Uyanik BS (2005) Changes in growth pattern, body composition and biochemical markers of growth after adenotonsillectomy in prepubertal children. Int J Pediatr Otorhinolaryngol 69: 1175-1181.

9. Aydogan M, Toprak D, Hatun S, Yüksel A, Gokalp AS (2007) The effect of recurrent tonsillitis and adenotonsillectomy on growth in childhood. Int J Pediatr Otorhinolaryngol 71: 1737-42.

10. Rysha A (2015) Nutrition in kindergartens in Kosovo. A Doctor thesis. University of Kassel. Faculty 11 Organic Agricultural Sciences. Department of Organic Food Quality and Food Culture.

5

Comparative Study between Partial Surgical Inferior Turbinectomy and Sub-mucosal Diathermy of Inferior Turbinate for Treatment of Inferior Turbinate Hypertrophy

Mohammed A. Gomaa*, Osama G. Abdel Nabi, Abdel Rahim A. Abdel Kerim, and Ahmed Aly

Faculty of Medicine, Minia University, Minia, Egypt

Abstract

Introduction: One of the major causes of chronic nasal obstruction is diseases of inferior turbinate commonly inferior turbinate hypertrophy, which sometimes do not respond to medical treatment and need surgery. Different surgical methods have been achieved for inferior turbinate hypertrophy e.g.: linear cautery, laser cautery, silver nitrate cautery, submucosal diathermy and inferior turbinate trimming. The principle of surgery is diminishing of the inferior turbinate size to decrease the patient's complaint while preserving the function and anatomy of the nasal air passages.

Aim of the work: The current study aims to compare the results in respect of safety and efficacy of sub-mucosal diathermy (SMD) versus partial surgical inferior turbinectomy (PSIT) in terms of postoperative improvement of nasal obstruction, nasal pain, degree of intra-nasal crustations and degree of tissue healing.

Patients and Methods: fifty patients of different age groups and both sexes were involved in the study. Patients were divided in two groups (A and B), each group includes 25 patients. Group A had turbinate reduction through PSIT and group B had turbinate reduction through SMD. In both groups follow up was carried out after two weeks, one month and three months.

Results and conclusion: The current study revealed that SMD is better than PSIT regarding the postoperative nasal pain and degree of intra-nasal crustations after 2 weeks and after 1 month of follow-up, but there was no statistically significant difference between both groups regarding the degree of nasal obstruction and tissue healing throughout the 3 months post-operative follow up period.

Keywords: Inferior turbinate; Sub-mucous diathermy; Surgical turbinectomy

Introduction

Chronic nasal obstruction resulting from inferior turbinate hypertrophy is a common subjective complaint encountered in the practice of rhinology. Allergic rhinitis, vasomotor rhinitis, idiopathic rhinitis and compensatory hypertrophy in septal deviation are the most common causes for the inferior turbinate hypertrophy [1]. Enlargement of the inferior turbinate is mainly due to swelling of the sub-mucosa and rarely due to enlargement of the bone itself. Hypertrophy of inferior turbinate caused by dilation of sub-mucosal venous sinusoids is the cause in intrinsic rhinitis, and responds to decongestant. Sometimes the inferior turbinate enlargement due to sub-mucosal fibrosis does not respond to decongestant [2]. The etiology of turbinate dysfunction is multi factorial. Because the turbinates have a very rich blood supply and are governed by the sympathetic and parasympathetic nervous systems, anything that affects either of these 2 systems affects the turbinates and, hence, the nose [3]. Hammad et al., revealed that turbinoplasty for hypertrophied inferior turbinate not only improve nasal obstruction but also may improve the chronic non-sinogenic headache [4]. The aim of the study was to compare the efficacy of sub-mucosal diathermy and partial surgical inferior turbinectomy in cases of chronic hypertrophic rhinitis regarding the improvement of nasal obstruction, degree of nasal pain, degree of intra-nasal crustations and the degree of tissue Healing and adhesions formation.

Patients and Methods

Our study was approved from Research Ethics Committee of Minia faculty of medicine, Minia University and an informed consent was taken from all patients. The current study is a prospective comparative study that done at the department of Otorhinolaryngology, Minia University hospital from July, 2013 to February, 2014 to evaluate the effects of Sub-mucosal diathermy) SMD (of inferior turbinate versus partial surgical inferior turbinectomy) PSIT (in patients with chronic hypertrophic rhinitis causing nasal obstruction. A total of fifty patients of different age groups and both sexes were involved in the study. Patients were divided in two groups (A and B), each group includes 25 patients. Patients were randomly divided into the two groups. Group (A) had turbinate reduction through PSIT of bone and soft tissue of inferior turbinate and group (B) had turbinate reduction through SMD of inferior turbinate.

Inclusion criteria

We included in our study patients with bilateral nasal obstruction or stuffiness not responding to medical treatment, and all patients didn't have previous nasal surgery with normal nasopharyngeal examination. All the included patients completed their follow-up visits up to 3 months postoperatively.

***Corresponding author:** Mohammed A. Gomaa, Professor of Otorhinolaryngology, Faculty of Medicine, Minia University, ENT Department, Minia, Egypt; E-mail: magomaa67@gmail.com

Exclusion criteria

We excluded from the study any patient with the following exclusion criteria:

1-Patients with other causes of nasal obstruction like: marked deviated nasal septum, concha bullosa or nasal polyps.

2-Patients with hemoglobin less than 10 gm/dl.

3-Patients who lost their follow-up visits.

All patients were subjected to a detailed history of ear, nose and throat with special emphasis on nasal symptoms (nasal obstruction, nasal discharge, sneezing and snoring). Nasal endoscopy (2.7 mm and 4 mm diameter, 0°nasal endoscope, Karl Storz, Germany) was used the endoscope without the use of local decongestants to assess the actual turbinate size pre and postoperatively according to the grading system described. Computed Tomography (CT) was performed for each patient in coronal, axial and sagittal views with the use of local decongestants 10 minutes before the CT examination. Group A had turbinate reduction through partial resection of bone and soft tissue of inferior turbinate and group B had turbinate reduction through sub-mucosal diathermic coagulation of the inferior turbinate.

Partial surgical inferior turbinectomy (PSIT)

The inferior turbinate was infiltrated with ephedrine (1:1000) up to the posterior end. The inferior turbinates were mediatized using a blunt freer type of turbinate elevator then mucosa was crushed at its attachment to lateral nasal wall using an intestinal clamp forceps. Using the turbinectomy scissors, the bulk of the anterior and mid-portion of the inferior turbinate was removed medial to the crush portion. Posterior end of the inferior turbinate was removed with a special scissor which crushes and then cuts the tissue [5].

Sub-mucosa diathermic coagulation of hypertrophied inferior turbinate

Diathermic cautery was performed using an insulated needle electrode. The needle tip is pressed against the anterior end of the inferior turbinate and activated for a short period giving a devascularized zone to reduce bleeding. The needle is then introduced into the sub-mucosa through this zone to the posterior end of the turbinate with special care to stay close to the bone. The mono-polar power diathermy is then turned on whilst the needle is slowly withdrawn over a period of 5 seconds. Three to five such passes were performed for each inferior turbinate at a coagulation current of 70W. If the diathermy current is sufficient, the mucosa of the turbinate blanches and shrinks [6]. After both techniques of turbinate reduction, ribbon gauzes soaked in ephedrine (1:1000) were used to secure hemostasis during the procedure. Intra-nasal septal silastic splints were applied in both sides to prevent occurrence of adhesions between inferior turbinates and nasal septum. Final hemostasis was maintained by using a Merocel nasal pack (Medtronic, California, USA) which usually was removed after 48 hours. The septal splints were removed on the 10th postoperative day. All patients were received antibiotics in the form of cephalosporin (500 mg twice daily) and analgesics in the form of paracetamol (500 mg three times per day) for 7-10 days postoperatively, also patients were instructed to use local nasal decongestants and nasal douche with sodium bicarbonate for 2 weeks postoperatively.

E-Postoperative Follow up

In each visit we compared the two groups regarding the following parameters:

1. Improvement of nasal obstruction.

2. Degree of nasal pain.

3. Extend of intranasal crustations.

4. Degree of tissue Healing and adhesions formation.

Nasal obstruction was analyzed according to VAS (Visual Analogue Score) system by asking the patients to score relief of nasal obstruction post-operatively from 1-10 and was categorized as follow [7]:

• No improvement: VAS (1-3).

• Partial improvement: VAS (4-7).

• Complete improvement: VAS (8-10).

Intranasal pain was also analyzed according to VAS by asking the patients to score the post-operative pain from 1-10 and was categorized as follow [8].

• Mild pain: 1-3

• Moderate pain: 4-7

• Severe pain: 8-10

Extend of intra-nasal crustations was analyzed according to endoscopic scoring of Lund and Kennedy [8], as follow:

• Grade 0: Absence of crustations.

• Grade 1: Mild crustations: partially filling the nasal cavity.

• Grade 2: Severe crustations: fully filling the nasal cavity.

Tissue healing was assessed also according to endoscopic scoring of Lund and kennedy, as follow:

Good healing: Rapid mucosal re-epithelization, minimal crustations, no nasal synechiae, patient feel relief of nasal symptoms.

Moderate healing: Mucosal re-epithelization, mild to moderate crustations, with nasal synechiae, patient feel relief of nasal symptoms.

Poor healing: Delayed mucosal re-epithelization, severe crustations and nasal synechiae, persistent inflammations and infection and patient doesn't feel relief of his/her nasal symptoms.

In both groups Follow up was carried-out on Two weeks, One month and Three Months postoperatively to assess the previous parameters.

Statistical analysis

The Statistical Program SPSS for Windows version 19 was used for data entry and analysis. Graphics were done by Excel Microsoft office 2013. Quantitative data were presented by mean and standard deviation, while qualitative data were presented by frequency distribution. Chi Square test was used to compare between two or more proportions. Student t-test was used to compare two means.

Results

The study was done on fifty patients, 34 (68%) were females and 16 (32%) were males. Patients were in the age range of 16-43 years (mean age 26.1 ± 6.6) with no significant difference between the 2 groups regarding their age and sex distribution (Table 1).

Two weeks of postoperative follow-up: (Table 2)

Nasal pain: Table 2 compares between the 2 groups regarding the

	Partial inferior turbinectomy N=25	Submucosal diathermy N=25	
	Mean ± SD	Mean ± SD	P value
Age (year)	26.1 ± 6.6	26.1 ± 6.8	1.00
	N (%)	N (%)	P value
Sex :			1.00
· Female	17 (68%)	17 (68%)	
· Male	8 (32%)	8 (32%)	

Table 1: Socio-demographic characters of the study patients.

degree of post-operative nasal pain. There was a statistically significant difference (P=0.02) between the two groups regarding the sensation of mild pain, with a lower incidence in patients with PSIT, with no statistically significant difference regarding the sensation of moderate pain. However there was a statistically significant difference (P=0.01) between the two groups regarding the reporting of severe pain with lower incidence in patients with SMD.

Extend of intra-nasal crustations: Table 2 compares between the 2 groups regarding the extend of intra-nasal crustations. There was a statistically significant difference (P=0.02) between the two groups regarding the mild and moderate crustations (P=0.02 and P=0.07 respectively), with a lower incidence in patients with SMD.

Improvement of nasal obstruction: Table 2 compares between the 2 groups regarding the improvement of nasal obstruction with no statistically significant difference between the two groups.

One month post-operatively: (Table 3)

Nasal pain: There was a complete absence of nasal pain in both groups after 1 month.

Extend of intra-nasal crustations: Table 3 compares between the 2 groups regarding the extend of intra-nasal crustations. There was a statistically significant difference (P=0.01) between the 2 groups regarding the presence of mild intra-nasal crustations after 1 month.

Improvement of nasal obstruction: Table 3 compares between the 2 groups regarding the improvement of nasal obstruction with no statistically significant difference between the 2 groups regarding the post-operative improvement of nasal obstruction after 1 month.

Post-operative tissue healing: Table 3 compares between the 2 groups regarding the degree of post-operative tissue healing. There was no statistically significant difference between the 2 groups regarding post-operative tissue healing after 1 month.

Three months postoperatively: (Table 4)

Nasal pain: There was a complete absence of nasal pain in both groups after 3 months post-operatively.

Extend of intra-nasal crustations: Table 4 compares between the 2 groups regarding the extend of intra-nasal crustations. There was no statistically significant difference between the 2 groups regarding the post-operative intra-nasal crustations after 3 months.

Improvement of nasal obstruction: Table 4 compares between the 2 groups regarding the improvement of nasal obstruction. There was no statistically significant difference between two groups regarding the post-operative improvement of nasal obstruction after 3 months.

Post-operative tissue healing: Table 4 compares between the 2 groups regarding the degree of post-operative tissue healing. There was

no statistically significant difference between the 2 groups regarding post-operative tissue healing after 3 month.

Discussions

Nasal obstruction is one of the commonest chronic symptoms encountered in otolaryngology. In most patients the cause is either septal deviation or inferior turbinate hypertrophy due to vasomotor

	Partial inferior turbinectomy N=25	Submucosal diathermy N=25	
	N (%)	N (%)	P value
Nasal obstruction			
· No improvement	0 (0%)	0 (0%)	1.00
· Partial improvement	2 (8%)	5 (20%)	0.4
· Complete improvement	23 (92%)	20 (80%)	0.4
Pain			
· Mild	5 (20%)	14 (56%)	0.02
· Moderate	12 (48%)	11 (44%)	1.00
· Severe	8 (32%)	0 (0%)	0.01
Crustation			
· Absence of crustations	0 (0%)	2 (8%)	0.5
· Mild crustations	20 (80%)	11 (44%)	0.02
· Severe crustations	5 (20%)	12 (48%)	0.07

Table 2: Comparison between both groups at 2 weeks of postoperatively.

	Partial inferior turbinectomy	Submucosal diathermy	P value
Crustation			(0.01)
· Absence of crustations	0 (0%)	5 (20%)	0.06
· Mild crustations			
· Severe crustations	22 (88%)	13 (52%)	0.01
	3 (12%)	7 (28%)	0.3
Obstruction			
· No improvement	0 (0%)	0 (0%)	-0.5
· Partial improvement	3 (12%)	6 (24%)	0.5
· Complete improvement	22 (88%)	19 (76%)	0.5
Healing			
· Good	12 (48%)	18 (72%)	(0.1)
· Moderate	13 (52%)	7 (28%)	0.1
· Poor	0 (0%)	0 (0%)	0.1

Table 3: Comparison between both groups at 1 month postoperatively.

	Partial inferior turbinectomy N=25	Submucosal diathermy N=25	P value
	N (%)	N (%)	
Nasal obstruction			
· No improvement	0 (0%)	0 (0%)	1
· Partial improvement	3 (12%)	3 (12%)	1
· Complete improvement	22 (88%)	22 (88%)	1
Crustation			
· Absence of crustations	21 (84%)	19 (76%)	0.7
· Mild crustations	4 (16%)	6 (24%)	0.7
· Severe crustations	0 (0%)	0 (0%)	1
Healing			
· Good	15 (60%)	21 (84%)	0.1
· Moderate	10 (40%)	4 (16%)	0.1
· Poor	0 (0%)	0 (0%)	1

Table 4: Comparison between both groups at 3 months postoperatively.

rhinitis or allergic rhinitis. The hypertrophy of the inferior turbinate is either due to increased thickness of the medial mucosal layer which could be attributed to the hypertrophy of the lamina propria that houses sub-epithelial inflammatory cells; venous sinusoids and sub-mucosal glands or it could be due to an increase in the size of the bony structure of the inferior turbinate. Surgical treatment is controversial, and variety of surgical procedures is performed for managing inferior turbinate hypertrophy, but there is no completely effective therapy [9]. Surgical reduction of the turbinate can be performed by several different techniques [10]. Partial inferior turbinectomy is a procedure directed at relieving nasal, There are various studies which had shown that partial inferior turbinectomy is as effective procedure in relieving nasal obstruction as total inferior turbinectomy with success rate ranging from 70 to 80% [11]. However partial inferior turbinectomy should be performed cautiously in order to protect anatomical structures and physiological functions of nose Monopolar diathermy is an old technique for the reduction of sub-mucosal tissue of the inferior turbinate, but still widely practiced [9]. The effect of Sub-mucous diathermy is achieved through coagulation of the venous sinusoids within the turbinate, leading to sub- mucosal fibrosis [9]. Although turbinate tissue volume reduction by various techniques leads to shrinkage of the turbinate size, however the epithelial changes of chronic hypertrophic turbinate remains more or less unaltered [9]. Our study results showed that subjective feeling of nasal obstruction was persisted for 2 weeks with no significant difference between the 2 groups. This non-significant difference was persisted for 3 months postoperatively. Our results were different from the results of that the subjective results of nasal obstruction is better in patients with PSIT than patients with SMD, however they also documented that the proper benefit of nasal airflow in SMD is achieved after 2 months, while the dramatic response is obtained within only 2 weeks postoperatively in patients who had inferior turbinectomy. Tables 5 and 6 compare our results with the published data regarding the degree of nasal obstruction. Salzano et al. reported in their study that 20% of SMD group had moderate pain and 80% had mild pain at the end of 2 weeks post-operatively [3]. In our study, 44% of our patients who had SMD had moderate pain while 56% of these patients had mild pain at 2 weeks post-operatively and moderate crustations were noticed in only 48% of SMD patients on the second week postoperatively [7]. Our study results also agree with Imad and Salzano [7,3] studies with 44% of their patients who had SMD complained of moderate degree of intra-nasal crustations. In Imad et al. [7], good nasal tissue healing was reported in 92% of SMD patients compared to 52% of PSIT patients at the end of first postoperative month. In our study, 72% of SMD patients had good healing compared to 48% of PIT patients who had good nasal tissue healing, this difference may be attributed to the fact that when the inferior turbinate transected, this usually expose the edge of the inferior turbinate bone resulting in continuing crusting until the bone is re-covered with a mucosal surface [6]. Our study showed that SMD is better than PSIT regarding nasal pain and intra-nasal crustations after two weeks, but both techniques are equal regarding the improvement of nasal obstruction and degree of tissue healing. Although our study

Study	Year	Method	Nationality	Results
Barbosa Ade et al	2005	(by Acoustic Rhinometry).	Brazil	98%
Fradis et al	2000		USA	96%
Rakover & Rosen	1996		USA	77%
Serrano	1996		France	81.70%
Elwany & Harrison	1990		Egypt	77%
Pollock & Rohrich	1984		USA	90%
Our study	2014	By VAS	Egypt	88%

Table 6: Improvement of nasal airflow in patients with partial inferior turbinectomy in different studies compared to our present study.

represents a relatively small sample of patients, with the use of only subjective assessment parameters, however this study may open a new era for multi-institutional study with more objective assessment parameters of nasal air flow and longer duration of follow up.

References

1. Farmer SE, Eccles R (2006) Chronic inferior turbinate enlargement and the implications for surgical intervention. Rhinology 44: 234-238.

2. Marieb EN (2003) Essential of Human Anatomy and Physiology. (7th edition). Benjamin Cummings, San Francisco.

3. Salzano FA, Mora R, Dellepiane M, Zannis I, Salzano G, et al. (2009) Radiofrequency, high-frequency, and electrocautery treatments vs partial inferior turbinotomy: microscopic and macroscopic effects on nasal mucosa. Arch Otolaryngol Head Neck Surg 135: 752-758.

4. Hammad MS, Gomaa MA (2012) Role of some anatomical nasal abnormalities in rhinogenic headache. Egyptian Journal of Ear, Nose, Throat and Allied Sciences 13: 31-35.

5. Anil H, Mahjabeen B (2014) Comparative Study Between Partial Inferior Turbinectomy and Submucosal Diathermy in the Management of Inferior Turbinate Hypertrophy. G M 3: 2277-8179.

6. Fradis M, Malatskey S, Magamsa I, Golz A (2002) Effect of submucosal diathermy in chronic nasal obstruction due to turbinate enlargement. Am J Otolaryngol 23: 332-336.

7. Imad H, Javed, Sanaullah (2012) Comparison of Submucosal Diathermy with Partial Inferior Turbinectomy: A Fifty Case Study. J Postgrad Med Inst 26: 91-95.

8. Lund VJ, Kennedy DW (1995) Quantification for staging sinusitis. The Staging and Therapy Group. Ann Otol Rhinol Laryngol Suppl 167: 17-21.

9. Gindros G, Kantas I, Balatsouras DG, Kandiloros D, Manthos AK, et al. (2009) Mucosal changes in chronic hypertrophic rhinitis after surgical turbinate reduction. Eur Arch Otorhinolaryngol 266: 1409-1416.

10. Azeem QA, Khalil H, Barlas NB (2002) Is total inferior turbinectomy a reliable answer for nasal obstruction caused by hypertrophied inferior turbinates. Pak Postgrad Med J 13: 120.

11. Ross DA, Nguyen DB (2004) "Inferior turbinectomy in conjunction with septodermoplasty for patients with hereditary hemorrhagic telangiectasia" Laryngoscope 114: 779-781.

Study	Year	Method	Nationality	Results
Luczaj	2007	(by Acoustic Rhinometry).	Poland	98%
Fradis et al	2000		USA	76%
Warwick – Brown	1987		UK	60%
Our study	2014	by VAS	Egypt	88%

Table 5: Improvement of nasal airflow in patients with sub-mucous diathermy in different studies compared to our present study.

6

Dentigerous Cyst or Ameloblastoma in Paediatric Patient: A Diagnostic Dilemma?

Singh G[1], Banda NR[1*], Patel A[2] and Kandya A[1]

[1]Department of Pedodontics and preventive dentistry, Modern dental college and research centre, Indore, India

[2]Department of Oral and maxillofacial surgery, Modern dental college and research centre, Indore, India

*Corresponding author: Banda Naveen Reddy, Department of Pedodontics and preventive Dentistry, Modern dental college and research centre, Gandhinagar, Airport road, Indore, Madhya Pradesh, India, 453112; E-mail: drreddybanda@gmail.com

Abstract

Most of the times paediatric patients report to the clinics with a chief complaint of decayed teeth, associated with pain and sometimes swellings, which regress after proper treatment. But dentist should be aware of unusual and rare pathologic conditions in children. These conditions sometimes are associated with hidden aggressive nature. These unusual and rare kinds of clinical conditions should also be included in differential diagnosis. Present case shows inadvertent finding of Unicystic Ameloblastoma (UA) in paediatric patient, which was asymptomatic and aggressive in nature. This case report shows diagnosis and surgical management of such type of lesions in paediatric patients.

Keywords: Paediatric patient; Unicystic ameloblastoma; Dentigerous cyst

Introduction

Too often, dental practitioners see their responsibility to the patient begin and end with the care and maintenance of the teeth and periodontium. It is also easy to focus strictly on the dental needs of the patient regarding chief complaint and remain oblivious to other things. Subtle or even not so subtle lumps, bumps, swellings or changes in texture or colour of oral mucosa may signify the presence of a reactive or a hamartomatous overgrowth of tissue or a benign or malignant disease. Common intra-oral swellings of jaws which generally are diagnosed in paediatric patients are odontomes, cysts like dentigerous cyst, radicular cyst, eruption cyst odontogenic keratocyst, juvenile ossifying fibroma, ameloblastoma and cysts or swellings of non-odontogenic origin. Some of these swellings have potential to turn up in some severe kind of pathology but these kind of changes are rare. Ameloblastomas are benign tumours which grow slowly but have the potential to enlarge to enormous size even causing deformity of bone [1]. Although, it is one of the most common benign odontogenic tumour, it is considered to be rarity in pediatric age group [2,3].

Here, we report a distinctive case of intra-oral swelling with undefined extra-oral swelling, and which was initially diagnosed as dentigerous cyst.

Case Report

A 10 yr old male patient reported to dept. of pedodontics and preventive dentistry with the chief complain of pain in lower right back tooth region. Past medical history and past dental history was unremarkable. Family history was not significant. Intra-oral examination revealed multiple carious teeth including 53, 54, 55, 63, 64, 65, 73, 74, 75, 83, 84 and 85 and over retained maxillary primary left lateral incisor 62. On extra-oral examination, a slight ill-defined swelling was present on left side below the left eye (Figure 1a). Bird's eye view (Figure 1b) revealed a remarkable swelling on left side. Intra-oral examination revealed an ill-defined swelling on buccal vestibule in maxillary left posterior region (Figure 1c) which was felt hard on palpation, extending from distal to maxillary left primary canine (63) to mesial of maxillary left permanent first molar (26). The swelling was ill defined, firm on palpation, non-tender, extending into left maxillary vestibule. The overlying mucosa was apparently normal with no signs of inflammation or pus discharge. It was not compressible and no pulsation were felt.

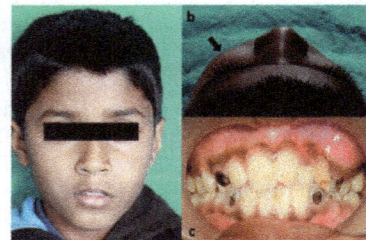

Figure 1: Pre-operative clinical pictures: a: Illdefined extraoral swelling on left cheek; b: Bird's view showing swelling (arrow) on left side of face; c: Intra oral swelling on left posterior vestibular area with multiple carious teeth.

Orthopantamogram (Figure 2a) of the patient revealed radiolucency in relation to the maxillary left primary first and second molar. Computed tomography (Figure 2b) of the patient showed a well-defined radiolucency involving 64, 65 and permanent tooth bud of 24, 25. Occlusal view in 3D CBCT (Figure 2c) showed expansion of buccal and palatal cortical plates of involved area. Based on clinical and radiological findings, a provisional diagnosis of dentigerous cyst was made.

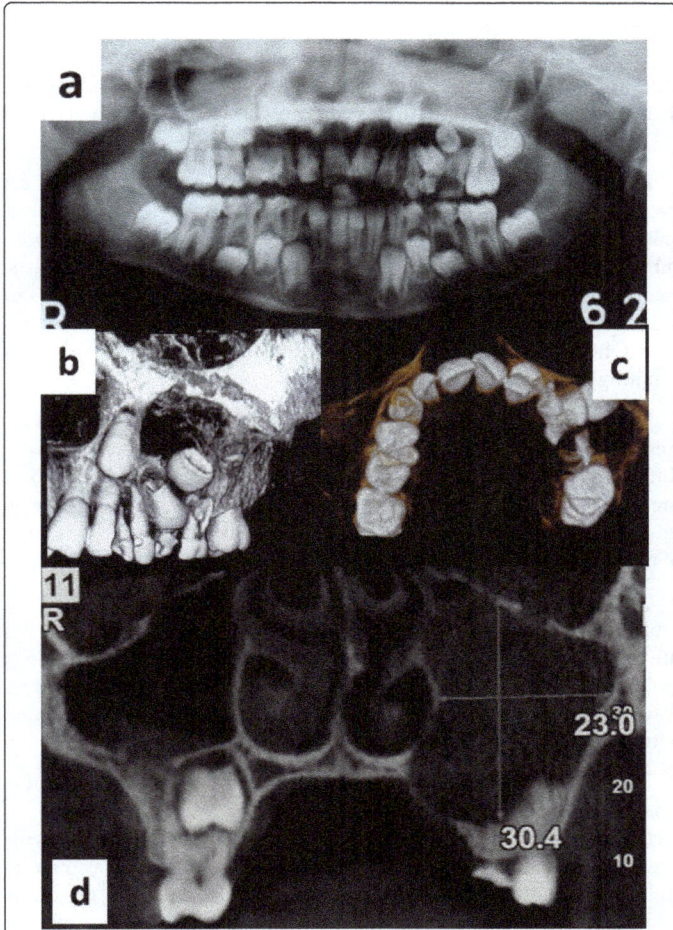

Figure 2: Pre-operative radiographic pictures; a: OPG showing haziness of left maxillary sinus, and rotation of permanent premolars tooth bud; b & c: Images showing expansion of buccal and palatal cortical plates; d: Image showing hyperdensity in left maxillary sinus suggestive of obliteration of sinus.

Under general anesthesia, the surgical area was exposed buccally. Crevicular incision was given from maxillary left permanent central incisor 21 to maxillary left permanent first molar 26 with releasing incision and flap was reflected (Figure 3a). Reflection of flap revealed thinning of buccal cortical plate (Figure 3b) which was removed. After which pathological mass (Figure 3c) was clearly visible with permanent tooth bud. Curettage of cystic lining was done and complete cyst was removed in toto (Figure 3d) along with tooth bud of maxillary left permanent first and second premolar i.e., 24, 25. Extractions of 62, 63, 64, and 65 were also done (Figure 3e). Flap was approximated and sutures were given. Betadiene impregnated gauge was placed inside the hollow cavity. Patient was recalled after 6 days for removal of gauge and cavity was left for secondary healing. Tissue specimen was sent for histopathological examination. Patient was recalled for follow up after every 7 days upto a month. 6 months postoperative follow-up PNS view and OPG showed no evidence of recurrence, clinical picture showed healing of involved area (Figure 4a-4c).

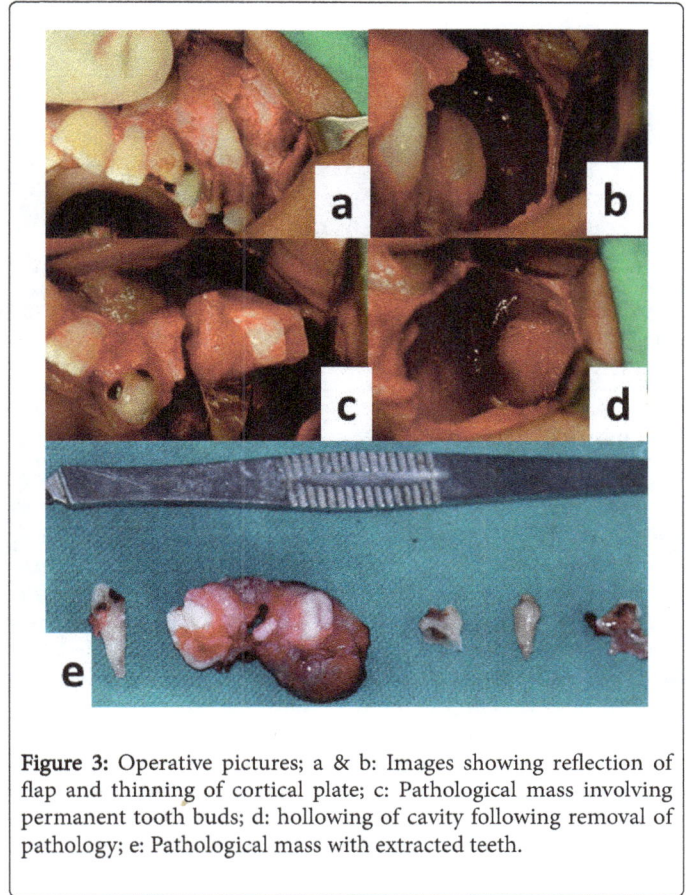

Figure 3: Operative pictures; a & b: Images showing reflection of flap and thinning of cortical plate; c: Pathological mass involving permanent tooth buds; d: hollowing of cavity following removal of pathology; e: Pathological mass with extracted teeth.

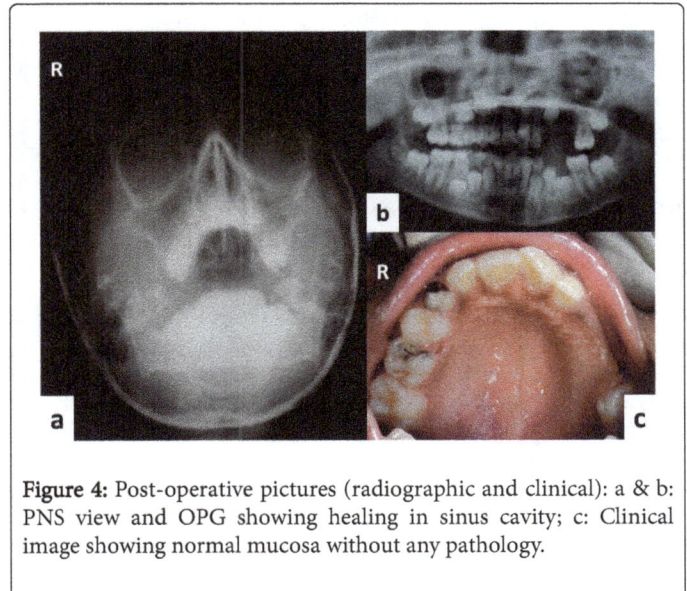

Figure 4: Post-operative pictures (radiographic and clinical): a & b: PNS view and OPG showing healing in sinus cavity; c: Clinical image showing normal mucosa without any pathology.

Histopatholigial report confirmed the diagnosis of intraluminal unicystic ameloblastoma. Multiple histological sections were prepared from the soft tissue specimen. Unicystic ameloblastoma showing typical luminal lining of ameloblast like cells and Intral luminal proliferation of ameloblastic cells were evident in histopathological slides (Figure 5a and 5b).

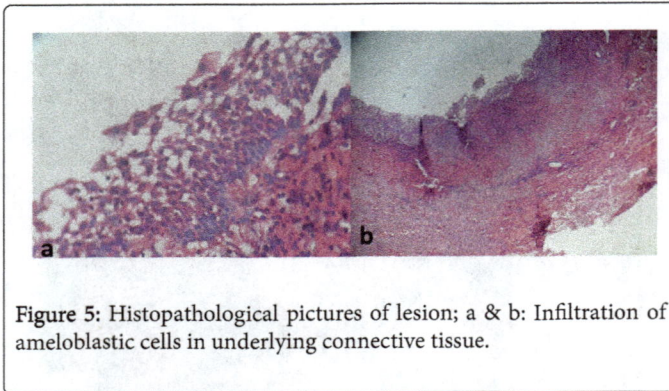

Figure 5: Histopathological pictures of lesion; a & b: Infiltration of ameloblastic cells in underlying connective tissue.

Discussion

Ameloblastoma, with rare exceptions, is a benign and slow growing but relentlessly infiltrative tumour composed of odontogenic epithelium with mature, fibrous stroma without odontogenic ectomesenchyme [4]. The tumour is considered a rarity in paediatric patients, accounting for approximately 10–15% of all reported cases of ameloblastoma [5,6]. It represents 13–54% of all jaw tumours affecting all age groups, with a peak incidence in the third and fourth decade of life [7]. Bansal et al. [3] stated that the occurrence of ameloblastoma was 15.2% (39/256) in patients aged under 18 yrs, similar to Olaitan and Adekeye (14.6%) [8]. The mandible was the most common site of occurrence in all races; 225 (96.6%) tumors were encountered in the mandible and 8 (3.4%) in the maxilla, with an overall mandible:maxilla ratio of 28.1:1 [2].

World Health Organization (WHO), classified ameloblastomas into four groups: (1) solid/multicystic, (2) extraosseous/peripheral, (3) desmoplastic, and (4) unicystic. Robinson & Martinez (1977) first described Unicystic ameloblastoma (UA), usually presenting as unilocular lesion radiographically and appearing cystic in nature microscopically [9]. This special type of ameloblastoma is common in younger age group and respond to conservative treatment [10]. The term unicystic refers to macro and microscopic features of a well-defined monocystic lesion showing cavity with linning that consist of complete or focal areas of odontogenic epithelium [11].

In the present case, the pathology was provisionally diagnosed as dentigerous cyst because multiple deep carious teeth were present on the affected site, which might result in inflammation at the apex of deciduous tooth leading to the development of inflammatory follicular cyst in which premolars are commonly involved. Characteristically, Dentigerous cyst is attached to the neck of unerupted teeth, enveloping its crown. It is important that the definition of dentigerous cyst is applied strictly and that the diagnosis of dentigerous cyst is not made uncritically on radiographic evidence alone [12]. So, the differential diagnosis of OKC was made. OKC sometime remains undiagnosed because it tends to expand in medullary cavity. Occurrence of large OKCs involving maxillary sinus, that led to displacement and distruction of floor of orbit and proptosis of eye have also been mentioned in literature [12]. Radiographically OKC is well demarcated with distinct sclerotic margin and it might be expecting slow growing margins. Clinically it may occur in vital standing tooth giving appearance of radicular cyst. That may imapde the eruption of related teeth, resulting in a dentigerous appearance radiologically and may give rise to misconception [12].

The belief that UA arises either from pre-existing odontogenic cyst like dentigerous cyst or airsing de novo has been debatable. While Robinson and Martinez stated that the possibility of neoplastic transformation of non-neoplastic ameloblastoma though less frequent. The reason being the epithelium of odnotgenic cyst and ameloblastoma are showing common origin [11]. The fact that among all cysts, dentigerous cyst is common in pediatric patients. The occurrence of UA can be supported by this theory.

Prepathogenic mechanisms were proposed by Leider et al for evolution of UA. 1) ameloblastic transformation of reduced enamel epithelium in association with developing tooth, along with subsequent cystic development. 2) Development from neoplastic transition of non-neoplastic ameloblastic epithelium of dentigerous or other odontogenic cysts. 3) Cystic degeneration of ameloblastic islands in a solid ameloblastoma followed by fusion of multiple microcysts resulting in a unicystic lesion [13].

The treatment of ameloblastoma is controversial. In children, the treatment is complicated by three factors: 1) continuing facial growth, different bone physiology (greater percentage of cancellous bone, increased bone turnover and reactive periostium) and presence of unerupted teeth; 2) difficulty in initial diagnosis; and 3) predominance of the unicystic type of ameloblastoma [2].

Unicystic ameloblastoma is radiologically characterized by a unilocular aspect and it is less aggressive than the solid type, but has the potential for recurrence [2] But in the present case, the pathology had involved the left maxillary sinus which is evident in radiograph. And there is greater rotation of permanent tooth bud than that found with a dentigerous cyst.

The treatment of ameloblastoma varies according to type of lesion, from a conservative approach to radical resection. The rate of recurrence following radical treatment is lower than that following conservative treatment. Radical resection of an ameloblastoma in children should be avoided. Such treatment could result in deformity and dysfunction of the face, which is bound to influence both the physical and psychological development of the child later in life [14]. So all the points should be kept in mind while choosing the treatment option, and should end up with functional and aesthetic rehabilitation.

Conclusion

This case report showed how an unsuspected carious lesion led to a cystic lesion which further transformed into a rare, benign tumour i.e., an intraluminal unicystic ameloblastoma. The lesion attained a considerable size without the patient's/ Guardian's awareness. Such cases test the clinicians knowledge and treatment protocol options once the diagnosis is confirmed. The need of the hour for the clinician is to take into consideration, the age of the patient and also the rehabilitative or corrective procedures to establish proper functional and aesthetic restoration of occlusion. Thus, an early diagnosis and appropriate treatment strategy can prevent/decrease the morbidity associated with the same.

References

1. Reddy SK, Rao GS (2011) Unicystic ameloblastoma in 6 year old child and its significance. Worl J Dent 2: 363-366.

2. Zhang J, Gu Z, Jiang L, Zhao J, Tian M, et al. (2010) Ameloblastoma in children and adolescents. Br J Oral Maxillofac Surg 48: 549-554.

3. Bansal S, Desai RS, Shirsat P, Prasad P, Karjodkar F, et al. (2015) The occurrence and pattern of ameloblastoma in children and adolescents: an

Indian institutional study of 41 years and review of the literature. Int J Oral Maxillofac Surg 44: 725-731.

4. Barnes L, Eveson JW, Reichart P, Sidransky D (2005) Pathology and genetics of head and neck tumors. Lyon: IARC Press pp: 1-435.

5. Keszler A, Dominguez FV (1986) Ameloblastoma in childhood. J Oral Maxillofac Surg 44: 609-613.

6. Ueno S, Nakamura S, Mushimoto K, Shirasu R (1986) A clinicopathologic study of ameloblastoma. J Oral Maxillofac Surg 44: 361-365.

7. Reichart PA, Philipsen HP, Sonner S (1995) Ameloblastoma: biological profile of 3677 cases. Eur J Cancer B Oral Oncol 31B: 86-99.

8. Olaitan AA, Adekeye EO (1996) Clinical features and management of ameloblastoma of the mandible in children and adolescents. Br J Oral Maxillofac Surg 34: 248-251.

9. Robinson L, Martinez MG (1977) Unicystic ameloblastoma: a prognostically distinct entity. Cancer 40: 2278-2285.

10. Lau SL, Samman N (2006) Recurrence related to treatment modalities of unicystic ameloblastoma: a systematic review. Int J Oral Maxillofac Surg 35: 681-690.

11. Gabhane M, Kulkarni M, Mahajan A (2011) Unicystic ameloblastoma of mandible: a case report. Indian J Stomatal 2: 273-276.

12. Shear M, Speight PM (2008) In Dentigerous cyst: Cysts of the oral & maxillofacial regions (4th edn.). Blackwell munksgaard.

13. Leider AS, Eversole LR, Barkin ME (1985) Cystic ameloblastoma. A clinicopathologic analysis. Oral Surg Oral Med Oral Pathol 60: 624-630.

14. Scariot R, da Silva RV, da Silva FW Jr, da Costa DJ, Rebellato NL (2012) Conservative treatment of ameloblastoma in child: a case report. Stomatologija 14: 33-36.

7

Differences in Acetic Acid Ototoxicity in Guinea Pigs are Dependent on Maturity

Takafumi Yamano[1,2*], Hitomi Higuchi[2], Tetsuko Ueno[2], Takashi Nakagawa[2] and Tetsuo Morizono[3]

[1]Section of Otorhinolaryngology, Department of Medicine, Fukuoka Dental College, Japan
[2]Department of Otorhinolaryngology, Fukuoka University School of Medicine, Japan
[3]Department of Otorhinolaryngology, Fukuoka University School of Medicine Nishi Fukuoka Hospital, Japan

Abstract

Objectives: The objective was to study if the difference exist in drug ototoxicity between less mature and mature guinea pigs.

Methods: The matured animal group had a body weight of 400 g and the less mature animal group had a body weight of 200 g. After compound action potential of the eight cranial nerves was measured, the middle ear cavity was filled with acetic acid.

Results: The less mature animal group was more sensitive to the acetic acid treatment than the more mature animal group.

Conclusion: We suggest that a difference in ototoxicity of certain otic drop treatments may exist between pediatric and adult patients.

Keywords: Ototoxicity; Acetic acid, maturity; Guinea pig

Introduction

Otic drops have been used worldwide for the treatment of acute and chronic otitis media. However, the possibility of ototoxicity when utilizing ear drops is always a concern of clinical otologists. In the past, we have examined the ototoxicity of commercially available ear drops [1] and disinfectants used within the middle ear cavity for treatment [2-4].

Ear drops containing acetic acid have been shown to have ototoxic effects, as reported in our previous studies [5,6].

Although the maturity of an animal may influence the ototoxicity of ear drops, previous studies have evaluated only the ototoxic effects on adult guinea pigs. Therefore, the goal of this study was to examine the effect of the maturity of an animal on ototoxicity.

Materials and Methods

Animals

The animals used in this study were albino Hartley guinea pigs with a normal Preyer's reflex. The mature animal group (n=5) had a mean body weight of 400 g and the less mature animal group (n=4) had a mean body weight of 200 g. According to a growth curve of guinea pigs' weight and age, 400 g body weight was equivalent to 7 weeks old and 200 g body weight to 2.5 weeks old.

Drug

The drug utilized in this study was acetic acid at a pH of 5.0. Acetic acid can be found at various concentrations in Burow's solution (pH 3.5), Vo-Sol (pH 4.08), and other types of ear drop. A previous study in our laboratory indicated that acetic acid at a pH of 4.0 or less had strong ototoxicity when applied to the middle ear cavity of adult guinea pigs [5,6].

Anesthesia

The animals were secured in a custom-made head holder and anesthetized with sodium pentobarbital (30 mg/kg). The surgical area was treated with Xylocaine (0.5%) prior to making the skin incision necessary for access to the middle ear cavity.

Surgery

The bulla was exposed using a retroauricular incision. A small hole, about 2 mm in diameter, was made into the bulla using a dental drill. The round window membrane was visualized with a surgical microscope at a magnification of 40X.

Sound system

The guinea pigs were stimulated with asynchronous tone bursts of 4 kHz and 8 kHz (1-ms rise and fall time, followed by a 10-ms plateau time) as well as click sounds. Stimuli were given at a pulse rate of 20 per sec, from 80 dB (re 20 µPa) to thresholds at 10 dB decrements. The speaker used was a Telephonics TDH-39P and the sound source was placed 10 cm from the auricle. The free field sound pressure was monitored and calibrated using a Bruel and Kjær 0.5 in condenser microphone.

Recording system and measurement of the compound action potentials (CAP) of the eight cranial nerves

A 0.08 mm diameter, Teflon Insulated silver wire with an exposed ball tip was carefully mounted on a micromanipulator utilizing the peripheral round window membrane. An Ag-AgCl reference electrode

*Corresponding author: Takafumi Yamano, Section of Otorhinolaryngology, Department of Medicine, Fukuoka Dental College, Japan; E-mail: yamano@college.fdcnet.ac.jp

was placed within the neck muscles. The Traveler Express ER-22 (Biologic Systems Corp., Santa Rosa, CA, USA) was utilized to average (200 times) CAP responses.

Drug application

After the initial CAP was measured, the middle ear cavity was filled with acetic acid at a pH of 5.0. The amount of fluid necessary to fill the middle ear cavity was about 0.2 mL. After 30 min, the middle ear cavity was thoroughly dried using a tissue paper wick and a second CAP measurement was made. Second and initial CAP measurements were compared. Figure 1 is a block diagram of the experimental approach utilized in this study.

Histopathology

After measurements were completed, the temporal bones were harvested for histopathologic study. Celloidin-embedded specimens were cut into 20 μm thick slices and histopathologic changes were evaluated.

Analysis of data

A threshold response was defined as an N1-P1 signal with an amplitude of 10 μV. Change in the sound pressure level of dB measurements before and after drug application was defined as a change in hearing. The threshold changes before and after drug application were compared and a paired t-test was used to assess statistical significance. This protocol was approved by the Fukuoka University Animal Ethics Committee.

Results

In the less mature animal group, a statistically significant elevation of the CAP threshold was noted for click sounds ($P < 0.05$) and for tone bursts of 4 kHz ($P < 0.05$) (Figure 2A and 2B). For tone bursts of 8 kHz, an elevation of the CAP threshold was noted in the less mature group, but was not statistically significant (Figure 2C). The CAP amplitude for click sounds and tone bursts of 4 kHz and 8 kHz at 60 dB, there

was a statistically significant reduction in the less mature group (Figure 3A-3C). In the less mature animal group, both CAP thresholds and CAP amplitudes had greater sensitivity to the acetic acid treatment. To measure the amplitude, we utilized a sound pressure of 60 dB SPL. We specifically utilized this sound pressure because a sound pressure within this range yields a clear waveform, which improves the analysis of the amplitude. Figure 4 is a histopathology image taken from a less mature animal (body weight 200 g). After 30 min, no histopathologic finding was observed at the organ of Corti, stria vascularis, or where the spiral ganglion cells reside (Figure 4). The Figure 4 is the cross section of the cochlea at the basal turn. (Magnification×200).

Discussion

With the exception of a previous study from our laboratory performed by Ichibangase et al. [2], no study has reported differences in the ototoxicty of ototopical drugs in experimental animals of varying levels of maturity. Age-dependent changes in susceptibility to ototoxic drugs were addressed by Prieve and Yanz [7]. This group injected kanamycin and bumetanide intravenously into 18 and 38-year-old mice. Their results indicated that younger of the two animal groups had a reduction in the CAP; however, this change was not observed in the older group. The authors postulated that the damage was due to the hair cells. Ichibangase et al. [2] studied the ototoxic effect of povidone-iodine, a topical drug, in guinea pigs ranging in age from an infant group (body weight: 100 ± 10 g), a young group (body weight 200 ± 20 g), to an adult group (body weight 400 ± 30 g). The authors reported that the age of the animals influenced the ototoxicity of this treatment.

The present study supports previous studies in that we found that less mature animals were more vulnerable to ototopically applied drugs than mature animals. We used a human testing system for CAP measurements. For the guinea pig, we used a relatively low frequency range (4–8 kHz). Furthermore, the click stimulus that we used stimulated the entire cochlea, meaning that comparisons of the CAP response for the click before and after drug application represent changes in total cochlear function. Certainly, higher-frequency testing

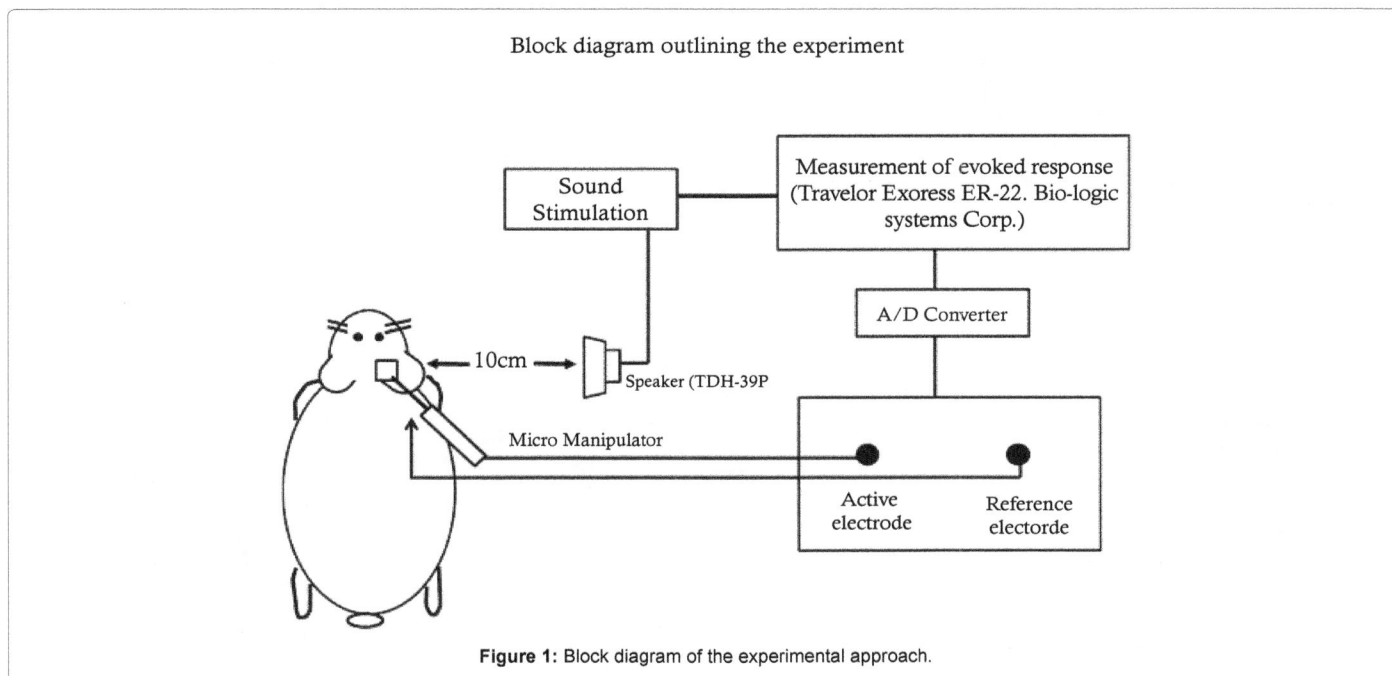

Block diagram outlining the experiment

Figure 1: Block diagram of the experimental approach.

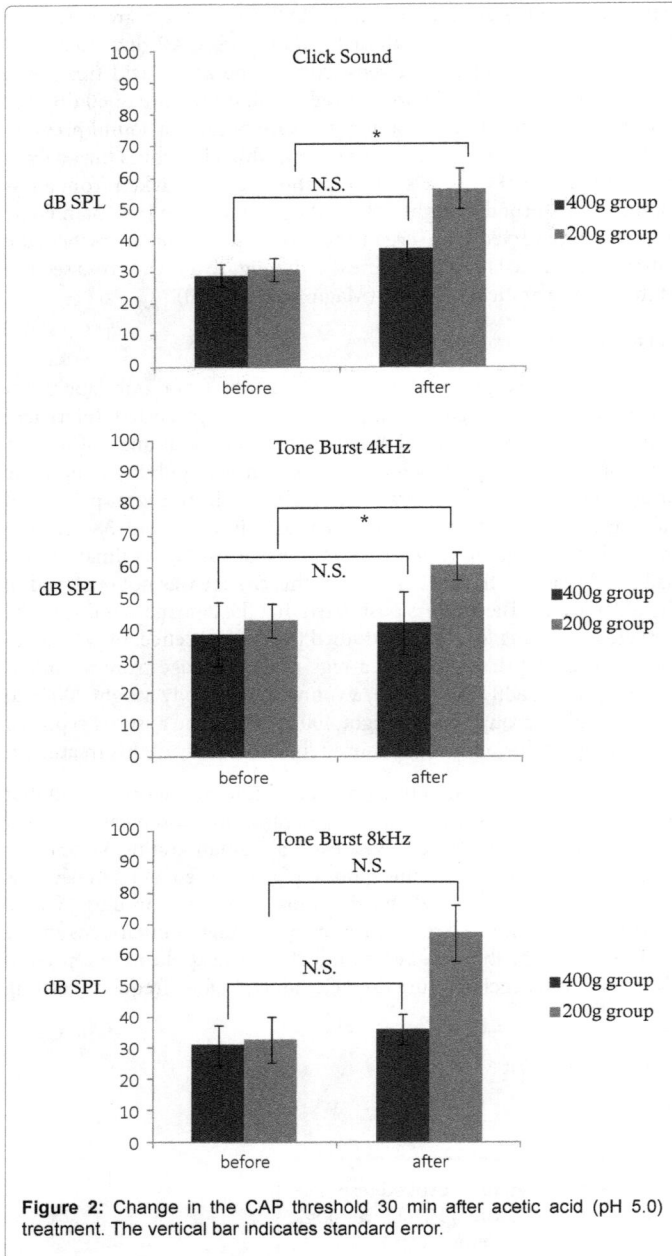

Figure 2: Change in the CAP threshold 30 min after acetic acid (pH 5.0) treatment. The vertical bar indicates standard error.

in humans to the passive diffusion of a drug from the middle ear to the inner ear. However, these results could also suggest that rodent models are a more sensitive sentinel model for ototoxicity, or perhaps, better represent pediatric rather than adult patients. Ear drops were given to infected ears in which the middle ear cavity was often filled with mucopurulent exudates. The round window membrane may be covered with fluids and the membrane itself may thicken due to mucosal edema. Thus, the membrane may offer an additional mechanical barrier. Experimental data in a chinchilla with otitis media showed decreased permeability of the RWM to horseradish peroxidase [12] and reduced ototoxic effects to cortisporin [13]. Sahni et al. [14] documented the increased thickness of the RWM in humans with various types of otitis media. Although our data are sound, it is of importance to proceed with caution when making human assumptions from animal data.

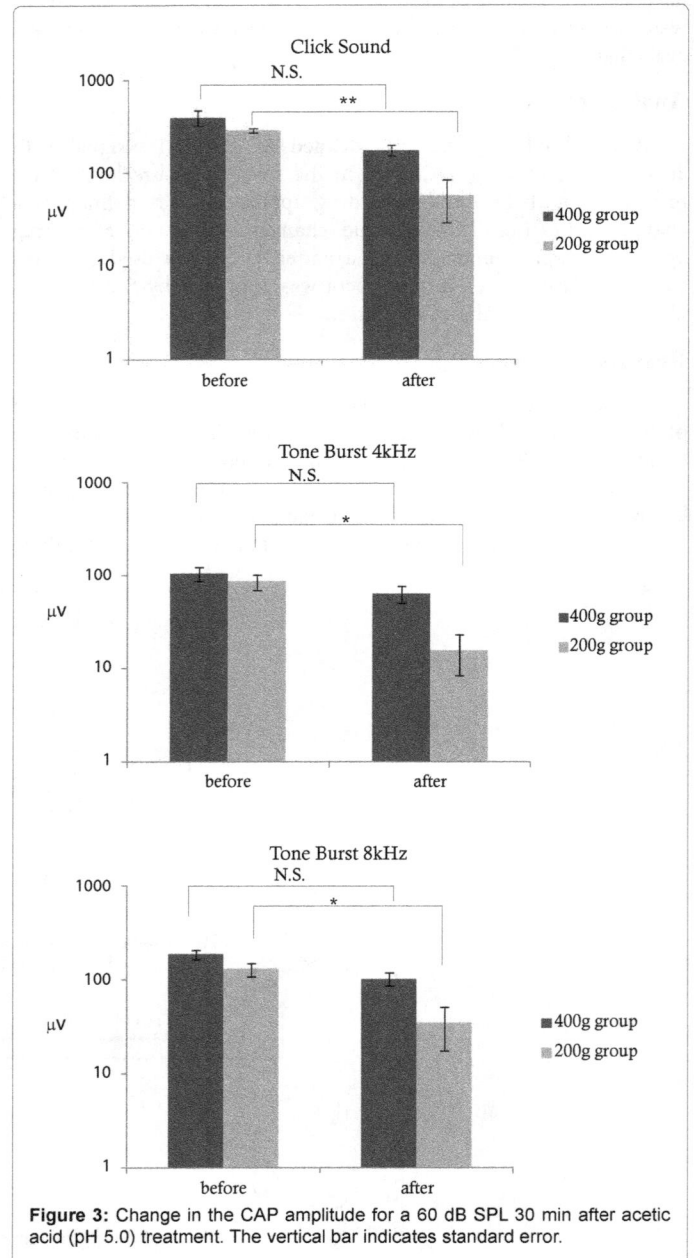

Figure 3: Change in the CAP amplitude for a 60 dB SPL 30 min after acetic acid (pH 5.0) treatment. The vertical bar indicates standard error.

may be more desirable. However, in our previous experiments, these tone ranges resulted in massive reductions in the CAP even as early as 10 min of the following: cortisporin, colimycin, Vo-Sol ear drops, or Povidone Scrub application on the round window [8-10]. Thus, indicating to us, that this is a reasonable range of frequencies to use in comparative evaluations. The two most common laboratory animals used for ototoxicity studies are the guinea pig and chinchilla. Both species have a round window that is vulnerably exposed in the middle ear cavity. This is unlike the human round window, which is deeply recessed in a narrow niche. Perhaps, more important is the difference in the thickness of the RWM between humans and rodents. The human membrane is approximately sixfold thicker and has a greater collagen density than the rodent membrane. Nomura et al. reported that a pseudo-membrane often drapes the human round window [11]. The above-mentioned anatomical differences could afford a greater barrier

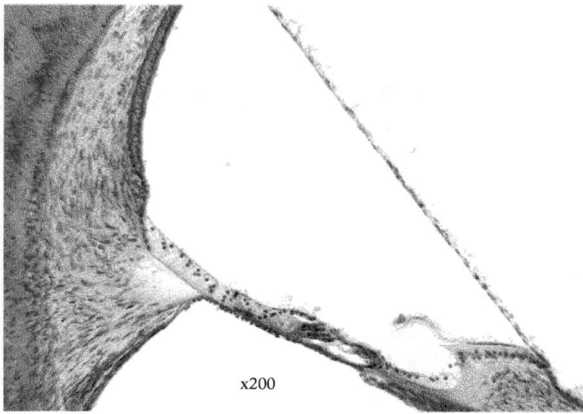

Figure 4: Histopathologic changes in the cochlea 30 min after acetic acid (pH 5.0) treatment. The histopathology was performed in a less mature animal (body weight 200 g). No significant pathology was observed. The cross section of the cochlea is at the basal turn. (Magnification×200).

Conclusions

The less mature animal group was more vulnerable to topically applied acetic acid than the mature animal group. From these data, we hypothesize that differences in ototoxicity may exist between adults and pediatric patients. Ear drops are frequently used for the treatment of intractable ear discharge such as otitis media and otomycosis. In conclusion, we advocate more caution when prescribing certain types of ear drops to pediatric compared to adult patients.

References

1. Yamano T, Morizono T, Shiraishi K, Miyagi M, Imamura A, et al. (2007) Safety of ofloxacin (OFLX) and fosfomycin sodium (FOM) ear drops. Int J Pediatr Otorhinolaryngol 71: 979-983.

2. Ichibangase T, Yamano T, Miyagi M, Nakagawa T, Morizono T (2011) Ototoxicity of Povidone-Iodine applied to the middle ear cavity of guinea pigs. Int J Pediatr Otorhinolaryngol 75: 1078-1081.

3. Sugamura M, Yamano T, Higuchi H, Takase H, Yoshimura H, et al. (2012) Ototoxicity of Burow solution on the guinea pig cochlea. Am J Otolaryngol 33: 595-599.

4. Higuchi H, Yamano T, Takase H, Yoshimura H, Nakagawa T, et al. (2014) Ototoxicity of gentian violet on the guinea pig cochlea. Otol Neurotol 35: 743-747.

5. Yamano T, Sugamura M, Ueno T, Higuchi H, Nakagawa T, et al. (2007) Ototoxicity of Acetic Acid. Association for Reseach in Otolaryngology Abstracts of the thirtieth annual midwinter reseach meeting P86.

6. Yamano T, Sugamura M, Ueno T, Higuchi H, Nakagawa T, et al. (2008) Long-Term Effects of the Cochlear Function in the Guinea Pig. Association for Reseach in Otolaryngology. Abstracts of the thirtieth annual midwinter reseach meeting P87.

7. Prieve BA, Yanz JL (1984) Age-dependent changes in susceptibility to ototoxic hearing loss. Acta Otolaryngol 98: 428-438.

8. Morizono T, Sikora MA (1982) The ototoxicity of topically applied povidone-iodine preparations. Arch Otolaryngol 108: 210-213.

9. Morizono T (1990) Toxicity of ototopical drugs: animal modeling. Ann Otol Rhinol Laryngol Suppl 148: 42-45.

10. Ikeda K, Morizono T, Juhn SK (1991) Cochleotoxicity of otic drops in the chinchilla: comparative study of Bestron and Cortisporin. Am J Otol 12: 429-434.

11. Nomura Y (1984) Otological significance of the round window. Adv Otorhinolaryngol 33: 1-162.

12. Ikeda K, Sakagami M, Morizono T, Juhn SK (1990) Permeability of the round window membrane to middle-sized molecules in purulent otitis media. Arch Otolaryngol Head Neck Surg 116: 57-60.

13. Ikeda K, Morizono T (1990) Round window membrane permeability during experimental purulent ctitis media: altered Cortisporin ototoxicity. Ann Otol Rhinol Laryngol Suppl. 148: 46-48.

14. Sahni RS, Paparella MM, Schachern PA, Goycoolea MV, Le CT (1987) Thickness of the human round window membrane in different forms of otitis media. Arch Otolaryngol Head Neck Surg 113: 630-634.

8

Dymista© Nasal Spray with Multifocal Analysis of its Impact on the Rhinitis Disease Experience

Amtul Salam Sami[1] and Nida Ahmed[2]

[1]ENT and Allergy Department, Royal National Throat, Nose and Ear Hospital, University College London Hospitals, London, UK

[2]King's College London School of Medicine at Guy's, King's College and St Thomas' Hospitals, London, UK

*Corresponding author: Dr. Amtul Salam Sami, 1 Cow Leaze, E6 6WX, ENT and Allergy Department, Nose and Ear Hospital, University College London Hospitals, London, UK; E-mail: amtul_salam@hotmail.com

Abstract

Background: Rhinitis is a prevalent condition both in primary care and in specialist centres. It has been shown to significantly impact on quality of life. Treatment is often best managed on combined therapies. Dymista© nasal spray is filling a niche for an 'all in one' treatment of allergic rhinitis.

Method: The MSNOT-20 is a valid disease specific quality of life instrument for rhinitis and rhinosinusitis and it was used to evaluate the symptomatic response to treatment with Dymista nasal spray.

Results: Dymista has been shown to improve all domains of the patient experience of rhinitis and rhinosinusitis with positive feedback by both patients and prescribing physicians.

Conclusion: Dymista is effective at improving patient symptomatology and improves quality of life. These positive results have opened up further avenues for research to explore its efficiency and place as mode of treatment.

Background

Rhinitis means inflammation of the nasal mucous membrane and often precedes sinusitis (inflammation of the lining of the paranasal sinuses), it is rare for sinusitis to occur without coexisting rhinitis and as such the most appropriate term for both is rhinosinusitis [1,2].

The MSNOT-20 questionnaire is a valid, disease specific quality of life instrument for Rhinitis/Rhinosinusitis (R/RS). The MSNOT-20 questionnaire has been shown to identify and discriminate between R/RS and non-disease and can evaluate the effect of treatment on symptomatology, based on severity scores, and on quality of life domains [3]. The MSNOT-20 consists of three sections; section one comprises of demographic details, section two is the disease specific section and section three is the quality of life section. The MSYP Questionnaire (MSYPQ), based on the MSNOT-20, is the equivalent tool to be used in young people (11-16 years old) and has proven to be able to identify and discriminate between R/RS and non-disease and to quantify severity [4-6]. This project shall use the MSNOT-20 to identify disease; it is validated for this condition and is disease specific as well as being technically quick and appropriate for the busy clinical setting.

Rhinitis affects the quality of life of sufferers and leads to deterioration in daily functioning related to study, work or profession. It is important to deal with the issues related to the disease and treat the cause in order to avoid physical, social and emotional issues which will help to optimize the efficiency and productivity of the educational and professional environment [7].

The MSNOT-20 questionnaire assesses symptomatology, which can be grouped into 7 different subgroups (Table 1), each one assessing a different domain affected by R/RS including paranasal, social and sleep domains [4].

Subgroup	Questions within this sub group
Nasal	1, 2, 3, 19
Paranasal	5, 6,7,8,9, 10
Sinus	5, 6, 10
Ear	7, 8, 9
Sleep	11, 12, 13, 14
Social	15, 16, 17
Emotional	18, 20

Table 1: Breakdown of sub groups from section 2, MSNOT-20

Rhinitis and rhinosinusitis are some of the most frequent diseases in the population [1-8]. A large scale epidemiological study carried out in Farnborough, UK in 2002 quoted the prevalence of R/RS at 30% [4], which is slightly higher than a postal survey in the UK in 1991 which reported the prevalence of all forms of rhinitis to be 24%[9]. Seasonal allergic rhinitis has been shown to account for 16% in studies of 15-24 year olds [10,11].

The British Society of Allergy and Clinical Immunology (BSACI) have put forward an algorithm for treatment of Rhinitis which takes into account the symptoms and its severity; this has been adapted and is shown in Figure [12]. A brief summary is such that mild cases would warrant oral or topical non-sedating anti-histamines used regularly with moderate to severe illness requiring additional intranasal corticosteroids. Further management would require a review of patient compliance, any dosage adjustments and even a modification of treatment dependent on symptomatology.

According to these guidelines, as above, and hence in clinical practice nasal steroids are frequently used as treatment for patients with nasal and sinus symptoms. Spraying steroids directly into the nose optimizes medication delivery to its target site, in this case the nasal mucosa, to maximize the wanted therapeutic effect; reducing inflammation which may be caused by an allergy or an infection [7,13]. There are many different nasal sprays available in the market, from over the counter to prescription only nasal sprays however most patients need to use the nasal spray for three to four days before they begin to notice any benefit. Multiple systematic reviews have proven intranasal corticosteroids to be effective at improving symptoms for allergic rhinitis [14,15] and it is currently endorsed by the BSACI guidelines for use in moderate to severe case (Figure 1).

Figure 1: BSACI algorithm for the treatment of Rhinitis

Antihistamine nasal sprays are also used for nasal and sinus symptoms, they have been shown to improve rhinitic symptoms and quality of life [16]. Their function is to reduce swelling and relieve congestion by blocking the allergic cascade triggered by histamine. Effectiveness of these medications varies between individuals [17,18] such that where antihistamine may effectively relieve nasal and sinus symptoms in one patient it may prove not as effective in another. Antihistamines can be used either alone or in combination with steroid based nasal sprays. One study reported combination treatment (an antihistamine agent and a steroid agent) as being more efficacious in improving nasal symptoms than steroid, antihistamine and placebo treatment alone [19]. Combination therapy is also a strategy preferred, and more commonly used, by general practitioners [20]. Dymista nasal spray is a combination of azelastine hydrochloride (an antihistamine) and fluticasone propionate (a steroid agent) which will be assessed in this study.

The primary aim of this study was to assess the effect of Dymista nasal spray on patients suffering from rhinitis/rhinosinusitis symptomatology with a detailed analysis on effects in different symptom subgroups. Secondary aims are to look into the patient experience when using this medication.

Method

Dymista nasal spray was used in this study which evaluated the response of rhinitis/rhinosinusitis sufferers' symptomatology to this medication. Section two of MSNOT-20 (Appendix 1) was used to assess patient symptomatology and symptom severity before treatment (values recorded when they first presented to clinic) and after treatment (the questionnaire was completed after 4 weeks of taking the medication). Treatment prescribed is defined as using the Dymista nasal spray at the recommended dose (see Dysmita information leaflet for more details). This project was carried out during the pollen season.

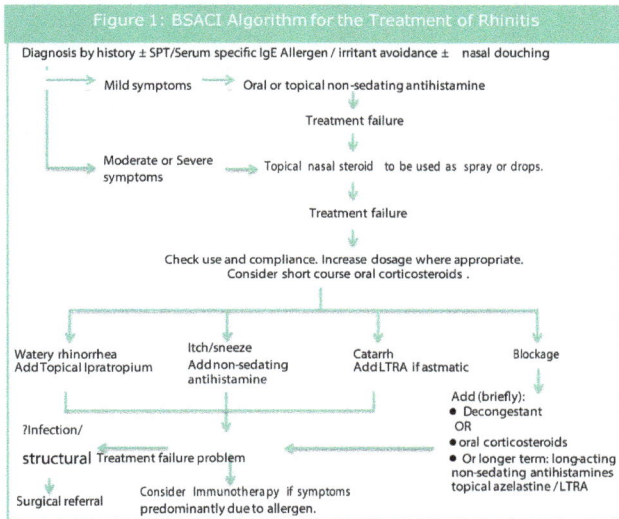

Appendix 1: Section 2 of MSOT-20

Patients considered for inclusion in this project were patients referred from general practice for assessment and treatment of their nasal and sinus symptoms as they were not responding to primary care treatment. Failure of primary care treatment is based upon BSACI treatment guidelines and equates to no significant response of symptomatology to oral or topical non-sedating anti-histamines used regularly then to additional intranasal corticosteroids. Such patients were assessed through history taking, clinical examination, skin prick test and Nasal Inspiratory Peak Flow (NIPF) at their first visit. The severity of the illness was quantified through the completion of section 2, MSNOT-20 which uses a Likert scale to represent increasing severity on a scale of 0-5, with 0 denoting no problem and 5 denoting that the symptom severity is as bad as it can be. Symptom severity was rechecked after four weeks of having started the treatment by, again, filling out section 2, MSNOT-20.

History taking and clinical analysis were used to determine suitability for involvement into the study and the data analysis presented in this study includes skin prick test results, nasal inspiratory peak flow results and data collected from section 2 of MSNOT-20 with a breakdown of symptomatology by grouping symptoms related to a particular pathology. These subgroups allow us to see how treatment affects each domain and are classified in Table 1. The overall result from the questionnaire was then analyzed for statistical significance.

Results

In total, data from 26 patients were found suitable for this research project. This study was initially planned to be larger however administrative and managerial restrictions limited the overall number of patients enrolled onto the study.

Allergy status and Nasal Inspiratory Peak Flow

Tables 2, 3 and 4 show the results of the skin prick test, common allergens and nasal inspiratory peak flow values, respectively.

Subgroup	Questions within this sub group
Nasal	1, 2, 3, 19
Paranasal	5, 6,7,8,9, 10
Sinus	5, 6, 10
Ear	7, 8, 9
Sleep	11, 12, 13, 14
Social	15, 16, 17
Emotional	18, 20

Table 2: Skin Prick Test results

HDM	MGP	ALTERNIA	MTP	ASPERGILLUS	CAT	DOG	BIRCH POLLEN
15	16	2	4	1	6	6	5

Table 3: The allergens patients are sensitive to; HMD= House Dust Mite, MGP= Mixed Grass Pollen, MTP=Mixed Tree Pollen.

NIPF	n
Below 50	4
50-100	17
100-150	4
150-200	1

Table 4: Nasal Inspiratory Peak Flow values

Symptoms subgroup analysis

This data has been graphically represented [Graph 1-9] to show the differences in symptom severity before and after treatment with Dymista. Each sub group is individually represented, with 'n' signifying each individual patient and the MSNOT-20 signifying the severity of disease. The score is calculated using the quantitative severity (on the 0-5 scale, see above) as chosen by the patient on their completed section 2, MSNOT-20.

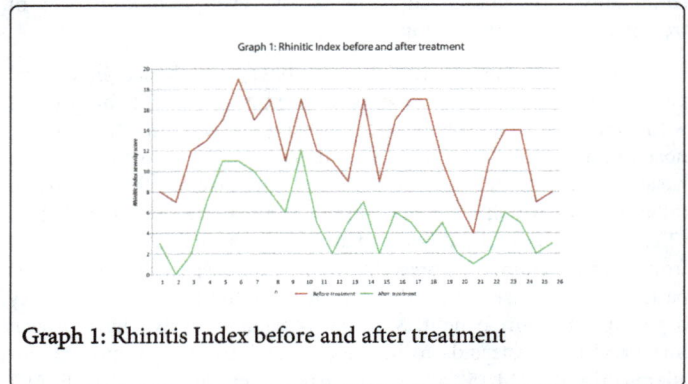

Graph 1: Rhinitis Index before and after treatment

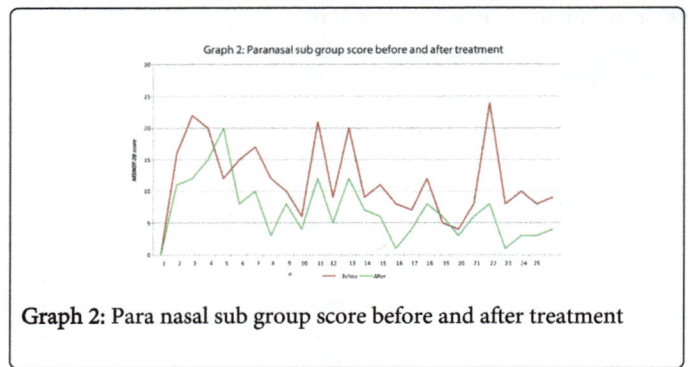

Graph 2: Para nasal sub group score before and after treatment

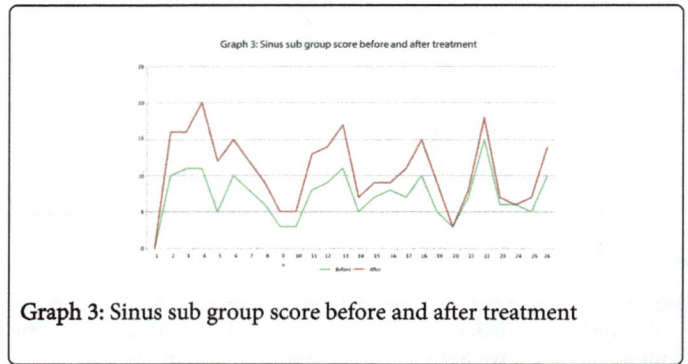

Graph 3: Sinus sub group score before and after treatment

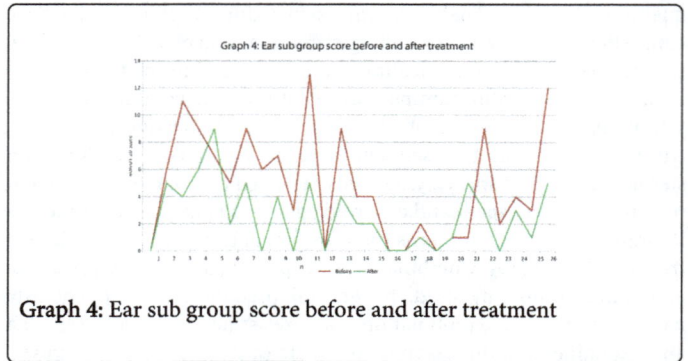

Graph 4: Ear sub group score before and after treatment

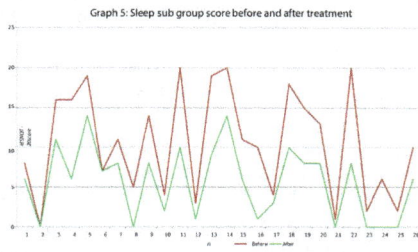

Graph 5: Sleep sub group score before and after treatment

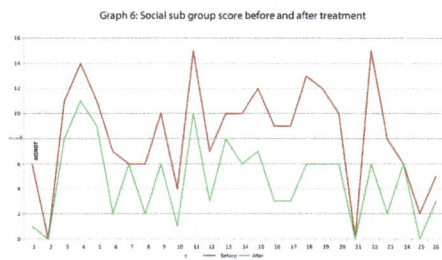

Graph 6: Social sub group score before and after treatment

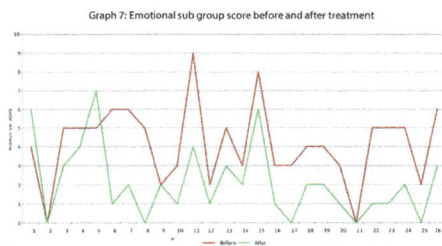

Graph 7: Emotional sub group score before and after treatment

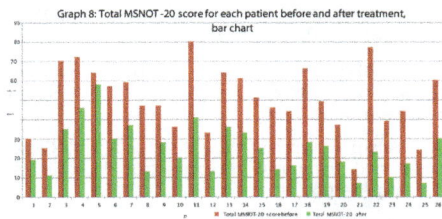

Graph 8: Total MSNOT-20 score for each patient before and after treatment.

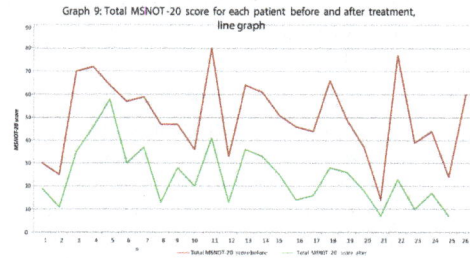

Graph 9: Total MSNOT-20 score for each patient before and after treatment.

The Nasal subgroup score was analysed and is represented by a value called the 'Rhinitic index' (Graph 1), this value has been shown to be a good representative of symptoms associated with R/RS [3].

Overall MSNOT-20 score analysis

Graphs eight and nine show the total MSNOT-20 score (a result of the responses to all questions irrespective of sub group) before treatment with direct comparison to post treatment use score, this highlights the impact of treatment on patient symptomatology as a whole.

Statistical analysis

The statistical significance of change in symptomatology post treatment was calculated for each subgroup and the total MSNOT-20 score (this score was calculated by combining the data from each of the 20 items in Section 2 of the MSNOT-20). The statistical significance was calculated using Students T Test with the p value shown in Table 5.

Discussion

This study aimed to see the impact of the Dymista nasal spray on symptoms and symptom severity, as quantified by the validated disease specific quality of life questionnaire, MSNOT-20. This study further proved that the MSNOT-20 is a sensitive tool when analysing nasal and sinus disease and sensitive to changes in symptomatology following treatment.

This study was limited in number due to administrative and managerial issues; as such this shall be considered a pilot study with a larger project to be carried out in the future. These limitations also restricted the use of a control and comparison group. Having identified that Dymista has a positive impact on symptomatology and the patient experience (also see below) this opens the door to further projects which, on a larger scale, can use a greater sample with direct comparison to alternative treatment arms.

The majority of patients in this study had an allergic rhinitis with 73% of patients having a positive skin prick test [Table 2]. The commonest allergies [Table 3] were to house dust mite and mixed grass pollen. This is significant as the project was carried out during the pollen season and so represented the effect of the medication with patients at their symptomatic peak.

In this pilot project we did not use a positive skin prick test as an inclusion criterion as we wanted to first gauge the response of symptoms related to R/RS to the medication and the patient experience. For future studies, as the majority of our patients suffered from allergic rhinitis, consideration can be given to using the skin prick test as such a criterion.

The Nasal Inspiratory Peak Flow (NIPF), a measure of nasal airway patency which is decreased by nasal obstruction, was less than normal in 15% of patients. It was not possible to repeat the NIPF at the 4 weeks symptom severity check due to issues with appointment allocations within the 4 week timeframe, the symptom check was unaffected by such problems as the questionnaire could be submitted or posted to the department within the 4 weeks. The NIPF has been shown to be an applicable tool to be used in monitoring response to treatment in allergic rhinitis patients [21] and this can be considered for future projects.

Analysis of all 7 subgroups [defined in Table 1, represented in Graphs 1-7] showed that there is a significant improvement in symptomatology in each subgroup after using Dymista. The greatest benefit was seen in the nasal sub group (Graph 1, named rhinitis index) showing patients found greatest improvements in these symptoms. This was followed by improvement in sleep scores [Graph 5], closely followed by the positive impact in the paranasal subgroup [Graph 2].

There was a statistically significant decrease in symptom severity in all subgroups, including the quality of life domains [Graph 1-7], and in the overall MSNOT-20 score [Graph 8 and 9]. These were all highly significant as all the calculated p values were equal to or lower than 0.01 [21] [Table 5].

Patient comments

Patients who used Dymista combination nasal spray (as opposed to the standard two individual sprays co-prescribed) found the combination spray more convenient and more effective to use. The below are a few remarks made by some patients, reproduced with permission:

"Within three days of using Dymista nasal spray I started noticing a difference"

"One bottle is really convenient to use, not a hassle at all!"

"Cheaper to buy one than two sprays".

"Dymista nasal spray is more effective than all the other nasal sprays up until now"

Conclusion

This project reconfirms that the disease specific section of the MSNOT-20 is a sensitive instrument which can assess the changes in patients' symptoms. This study also concludes that Dymista nasal spray can help improve the patients' symptoms in all domains impacted by rhinitis and rhinosinusitis. The overall symptom burden and symptom severity is reduced and patients find this a satisfactory treatment method in terms of convenience and efficiency.

References

1. Lanza DC, Kennedy DW (1997) Adult rhinosinusitis defined. Otolaryngol Head Neck Surg 117: S1-7.

2. Fokkens W1, Lund V, Mullol J; European Position Paper on Rhinosinusitis and Nasal Polyps group (2007) European position paper on rhinosinusitis and nasal polyps 2007. Rhinol Suppl : 1-136.

3. Sami A (2010) Epidemiology of Rhinitis in secondary school children using MSYPQ and comparison with Modified SNOT-20 used in adult community based survey. European Academy of Allergy and Clinical Immunology.

4. Sami AS, Scadding GK, Amjad M, Malik M (2013) "Rhinitis, sinusitis and ocular disease€"2091. The MSYPQ: repeatability and applicability to rhinitis/rhinosinusitis." The World Allergy Organization Journal 6: 169.

5. Sami, A; Scadding, G (2014) Rhinosinusitis in Secondary School Children-Part 1: Pilot of MSNOT-20 Young Persons Questionnaire (MSYPQ). Rhinology 52: 215.

6. Sami A, Scadding, G. (2014) Rhinosinusitis in Secondary School Children-Part 2: Main project analysis of MSNOT-20 Young Persons Questionnaire (MSYPQ). Rhinology 52: 225.

7. Sami A. Scadding G (2013) Management of Allergic Rhinitis in schools. British Journal of School Nursing 8: 119-123.

8. Ghouri N1, Hippisley-Cox J, Newton J, Sheikh A (2008) Trends in the epidemiology and prescribing of medication for allergic rhinitis in England. J R Soc Med 101: 466-472.

9. Sibbald B1, Rink E (1991) Epidemiology of seasonal and perennial rhinitis: clinical presentation and medical history. Thorax 46: 895-901.

10. Strachan DP (1995) Epidemiology of hay fever: towards a community diagnosis. Clin Exp Allergy 25: 296-303.

11. Wüthrich B (1989) Epidemiology of the allergic diseases: are they really on the increase? Int Arch Allergy Appl Immunol 90 Suppl 1: 3-10.

12. Scadding GK1, Durham SR, Mirakian R, Jones NS, Leech SC, et al. (2008) BSACI guidelines for the management of allergic and non-allergic rhinitis. Clin Exp Allergy 38: 19-42.

13. Masayuki Karaki, Kosuke Akiyama, Nozomu Mori (2001) Efficacy of intranasal steroid spray (mometasone furoate) on treatment of patients with seasonal allergic rhinitis: Comparison with oral corticosteroids. Department of Otorhinolaryngology Head and Neck Surgery, Faculty of Medicine, Kagawa University, Japan. Ann Allergy Asthma Immunol 86: 28-35.

14. Weiner J.M, Abramson M.J and Puy R.M (1998) Intranasal corticosteroids versus oral H1 receptor antagonists in allergic rhinitis: systematic review of randomised controlled trials. British Medical Journal 317: 1624-1629.

15. Yanez A. and Rodrigo G.J (2002) Intranasal corticosteroids versus topical H1 receptor antagonists for the treatment of allergic rhinitis: a systematic review with meta-analysis. Annals of Allergy, Asthma & Immunology 89: 479-484.

16. Sheikh A1, Singh Panesar S, Dhami S, Salvilla S (2007) Seasonal allergic rhinitis in adolescents and adults. Clin Evid (Online) 2007.

17. Golden SJ, Craig TJ (1999) Efficacy and safety of azelastine nasal spray for the treatment of allergic rhinitis.PennState University College of Medicine, Hershey Medical Center, Hershey, Pa. 17033-0850, USA.J Am Osteopath assoc 99: 7S.

18. Banov CH, Lieberman P (1999) Vasomotor Rhinitis Study Groups. Efficacy of azelastine nasal spray in the treatment of vasomotor (perennial nonallergic) rhinitis. J Am Osteopath Assoc. 86: 28-35.

19. Wolthers OD (2013) New patents of fixed combinations of nasal antihistamines and corticosteroids in allergic rhinitis. Recent Pat Inflamm Allergy Drug Discov 7: 223-228.

20. Navarro A1, Valero A, Rosales MJ, Mullol J (2011) Clinical use of oral antihistamines and intranasal corticosteroids in patients with allergic rhinitis. J Investig Allergol Clin Immunol 21: 363-369.

21. de Souza Campos Fernandes S, Ribeiro de Andrade C, da Cunha Ibiapina C (2014) Application of Peak Nasal Inspiratory Flow reference values in the treatment of allergic rhinitis. Rhinology 52: 133-136.

22. Harris M, Taylor G (2008) Medical statistics made easy, 2th edition. Oxfordshire: Scion·

9

Effectiveness of Second-Generation Antihistamine for the Treatment of Morning Symptoms Observed in Patients with Perennial Allergic Rhinitis: Comparison Study of Bepotastine Besilate versus Olopatadine Hydrochloride

Terumichi Fujikura[1,2]* **and Kimihiro Okubo**[1]

[1]*Department of Otorhinolaryngology, Nippon Medical School, Japan*

[2]*Department of Otolaryngology, Tokyo Woman's Medical University Medical Center East, Japan*

*Corresponding author: Terumichi Fujikura, Department of Otorhinolaryngology, Nippon Medical School, 1-1-5, Sendagi Bunkyo-ku, Tokyo 113-8603, Japan; E-mail: teru-fujik@nms.ac.jp

Abstract

Objective: The aim of the present study was to examine circadian rhythm-based treatment strategies with the intension of improving the pharmacotherapy for morning symptoms with perennial allergic rhinitis. We investigated the effects of two second generation antihistamines, with different pharmacokinetic parameters, bepotastine besilate and olopatadine hydrochloride, for the treatment of morning symptoms.

Methods: Twenty-four subjects with perennial allergic rhinitis were recruited for this study. They were randomly allocated to either a bepotastine group (n=10) or an olopatadine group (n=14). During the 1-hour period after waking up in the morning, the patients counted and recorded the number of sneezes and nose blowing. PNIF was also measured. The study participants took the allocated medicine twice a day. They continued recording their nasal symptoms and PNIF after awakening for 10 to 14 days.

Results: In both group, taking bepotastine and olopatadine, the mean sneezing count and the mean nose blowing count were well suppressed. However, a significant change in the nasal congestion score was not observed throughout the study. Especially in olopatadine group, PNIF increased from day 2 onward and a significant increase was observed for the following 10 days.

Conclusion: The worsening of nasal symptoms after awakening that is associated with perennial allergic rhinitis has a significant impact on the quality of life of patients. Two second-generation antihistamines, bepotastine besilate and olopatadine hydrochloride, were effective for the treatment of these morning symptoms. The measurement of Peak Nasal Inspiratory Flow (PNIF) value might lead to a favorable self-evaluation of nasal symptom and treatment effects. Some guidance regarding the taking of medicine from Powered by Editorial Manager® and ProduXion Manager® from Aries Systems Corporation the viewpoint of chronotherapy might improve the satisfaction of patients with the results of pharmacotherapy.

Keywords: Gastrointestinal tract; Antihistamine; Pharmacotherapy

Introduction

Chronobiology is the science of biological rhythms and the bioclocks that drive them. Circadian rhythms influence disease symptomatology and affect the pharmacokinetics and pharmacodynamics of many drug classes. Therefore, these phenomena sometimes have important implications for the treatment of allergic rhinitis. The circadian rhythms that influence the gastrointestinal tract, liver, and kidney affect the absorption, distribution, and elimination of medications [1-4]. Thus, the effects of medications can differ depending on whether they are administered during the evening or morning [5].

Bronchial asthma tends to worsen or to occur mainly at night. The chronobiology and chronotherapy of asthma are important subjects of investigation. Circadian rhythms influencing the autonomic nervous system, endocrine function, and airway inflammation can contribute to the pathogenesis of bronchial asthma [6,7]. The symptoms of allergic rhinitis are also affected by these phenomena and other circadian functions [8]. In patients with allergic rhinitis, a worsening of nasal symptoms after waking up is often observed [9]. This phenomenon is known as a "morning attack". In allergic rhinitis, the intensities of nasal congestion, rhinorrhea, and sneezing are greatest early in the morning in approximately 70% of patients [3]. One or more of the following factors may contribute to the occurrence of maximum nasal congestion in the morning: nasal congestion is worse when the subject is in a recumbent position; secretions accumulate overnight; allergen exposure to mites, mold, or dander may occur while sleeping; cortisol levels are lowest at night (increasing the levels of inflammatory mediators); and autonomic nervous system activity at night promotes vagal tone, favoring vasodilatation [4,8].

The aim of the present study was to examine circadian rhythm-based treatment strategies with the intention of improving pharmacotherapy for allergic rhinitis. In the present study, we focused on the treatment of morning symptoms. We investigated the effects of two second-generation antihistamines, with different pharmacokinetic parameters, bepotastine besilate and olopatadine hydrochloride, for the treatment of morning symptoms.

Method

Study subjects

Twenty-four subjects were recruited for this study. All the subjects were patients with perennial allergic rhinitis associated with a house dust mite allergy (19 women, 5 men; 32 ± 5 years old). Some of the patients had seasonal Japanese cedar pollinosis, but this study was not performed during the season for pollinosis. All the patients with allergic rhinitis had tested positive for mite nasal allergy, as diagnosed based on a clinical history of moderate to severe rhinosinusitis, a rhinoscopic examination, a nasal smear for eosinophilia, and an intradermal test or the determination of specific IgE antibodies using a capsulated hydrophobic carrier polymer radioallergosorbent test (CAP-RAST). The inclusion criteria for allergic rhinitis were a positive CAP-RAST result (score of 2 or greater) or a positive skin prick test (wheal >5 mm) for house dust or mites. The protocol was approved by the ethics committees of Tokyo Woman's Medical University and the Nippon Medical School, Musashikosugi Hospital. Written informed consent was obtained from each of the participating patients before the start of the study.

Study design

A 2-week washout period was scheduled before the present study during which none of the subjects received anti-allergic medicines, such as antihistamines or intra-nasal corticosteroids. During the 1-hour period after waking up in the morning, the patients counted and recorded the number of sneezes and the number of times they blowed their noses using a self-check sheet. Nasal congestion was evaluated using a 5-point scale (0-4), according to the classification of symptom severity used by the Japanese guidelines for allergic rhinitis [10]. The Peak Nasal Inspiratory Flow (PNIF) was also measured using a portable inspiratory flow meter (In-checkTM; Clement Clarke International Limited, Harlow, UK) with an anesthetic mask for the evaluation of nasal congestion (Figure 1).

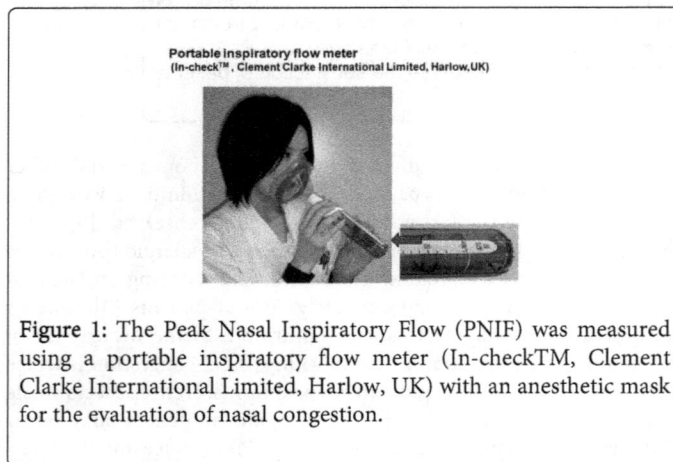

Figure 1: The Peak Nasal Inspiratory Flow (PNIF) was measured using a portable inspiratory flow meter (In-checkTM, Clement Clarke International Limited, Harlow, UK) with an anesthetic mask for the evaluation of nasal congestion.

The PNIF was measured while the subject was in a seated position. A good seal was ensured, and each of the patients was instructed to make a maximal inspiratory effort with his or her mouth closed. The best result of three attempts was used after appropriate training had been performed. Three days before the start of treatment, the subjects were asked to begin recording their nasal symptoms and PNIF values during the 1-hour period after awakening. The averages of these counts and data obtained during the 3-day period were used as control values.

We conducted this clinical study to evaluate the inhibitory effects of two second-generation anti-histamines, bepotastine besilate (10 mg) and olopatadine hydrochloride (5 mg), on the morning nasal symptoms of patients with allergic rhinitis. The study participants took the allocated medicine twice a day (after breakfast and before bed). They continued recording their nasal symptoms and PNIF after awakening for 10 to 14 days. Twenty-four subjects who provided their informed consent were randomly allocated to either a bepotastine group (B group; n=10) or an olopatadine group (O group; n=14).

Statistical analysis

Data were expressed as the mean ± standard error of the mean. The nasal symptoms and PNIF values at each measurement point were compared with those observed before drug administration. The Wilcoxon signed-rank test was used for the statistical analysis. Differences with P values of less than 0.05 were considered significant.

Results

The average compliance rate was approximately 92%.

A) Nasal symptoms during 1 hour after awakening

1) Sneezing

The mean ± SEM sneezing count before the study was 1.43 ± 0.45 for group B and 2.64 ± 1.00 for group O. In group B, the mean sneezing count was significantly lower on day 3, 7, 10, and 13. In group O, it was significantly lower on day 2 and was well suppressed for the following 10 days (Figure 2).

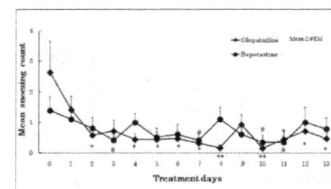

Figure 2: Changes of the mean ± SEM sneezing count throughout the study. They were followed during 2 weeks using second-generation antihistamines. Especially in group O (olopatadine hydrochloride), it was well suppressed.

*p<0.05 Group O vs before administration

**p<0.01 Group O vs before administration

#p<0.05 Group B (bepotastine besilate) vs before administration

2) Rhinorrhea

The mean nose blowing count before the study was 2.30 ± 0.5 for group B and 2.71 ± 0.45 for group O. In group B, the mean nose blowing count was significantly lower on day 2. Thereafter, the count varied day by day, but it was reduced on day 11 and day 14. In group

O, it was significantly lower from day 2 onwards, and this symptom was well suppressed for the following 10 days (Figure 3).

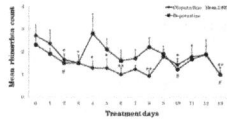

Figure 3: Changes of the mean nose blowing count throughout the study. Especially in group O, it was well suppressed.

*p<0.05 Group O vs before administration

**p<0.01 Group O vs before administration

#p<0.05 Group B vs before administration

3) Nasal congestion

The mean nasal congestion scores using a 5-point scale before the study were 1.70 ± 0.26 in group B and 1.86 ± 0.21 in group O. In both groups, a significant change in the nasal congestion score was not observed throughout the study (Figure 4).

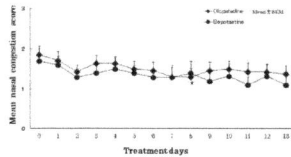

Figure 4: Changes of the mean nasal congestion score throughout the study

In comparison with other scores, a significant change was not observed in both groups.

*p<0.05 Group O vs before administration

B) PNIF measured within 1 hour after awakening

The mean ± SEM of the PNIF value measured before the study was 73.5 ± 3.80 for group B group and 72.9 ± 7.00 for group O. In group B, the PNIF increased during the study, but the change was statistically significant only on day 11. In group O, the PNIF increased from day 2 onwards, and a significant increase was observed for the following 10 days (Figure 5).

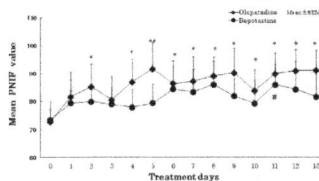

Figure 5: Changes in the mean ± SEM value of PNIF throughout the study

Especially in group O, significant increase of PNIF was observed.

*p<0.05 Group O vs before administration

**p<0.01 Group O vs before administration

#p<0.05 Group B vs before administration

Discussion

The maximum drug concentration time (Tmax) and the half-life period (t 1/2) of bepotastine besilate were 1.2 and 2.4 hours, respectively, while the Tmax and t 1/2 of olopatadine hydrochloride were 1.0 and 8.8 hours, respectively. We hypothesized that a medicine with a long t 1/2 and a short Tmax might be useful for controlling the morning symptoms of allergic rhinitis if it was taken before bed and after breakfast. The results of the present study indicated that the second-generation antihistamines bepotastine and olopatadine were useful for relieving the morning symptoms of allergic rhinitis. Especially, in olopatadine group, PNIF increased from day 2 onward and a significant increase was observed for the following 10 days. The t 1/2 of olopatadine is 8.8 hours, which is longer than that of bepotastine. Therefore, the effects of olopatadine taken the night before were more likely to persist and be more prominent than those of bepotastine. On the other hand, morning dosing with a quick-acting medicine can control morning suffering. The Tmax of these two medicines is 1.0 to 1.2 hours. Thus, to some extent, these medicines can be expected to act quickly from a clinical perspective. Although anti-leukotrienes are also useful for the treatment of allergic rhinitis, their pharmacokinetic parameters are different from anti-histamines. The Tmax and the t 1/2 of montelukast sodium are 3.9 and 4.6 hours, respectively, while the Tmax and t 1/2 of pranlukast hydrate are 5.2 and 1.2 hours, respectively. We hypothesized that their Tmax is too long to control the morning symptoms of allergic rhinitis if it was taken after breakfast. The t 1/2 of montelukast sodium is 4.6 hours and the effects of montelukast taken the night before may persist until next morning. The comparison study using anti-leukotriene is our concern.

In this study, we recruited patients who worked regular hours at the same workplace. Many of them were staff members at our hospital and were women. Therefore the sex ratio was not well balanced in this study (5 men and 19 women). Morning attacks of allergic rhinitis are thought to occur regardless of sex or age [11]. Although the number of participants was not very large, we analyzed the subjects regardless of these patient characteristics.

Sneezing and rhinorrhea decreased significantly 2 days after the start of treatment. Concerning nasal congestion, we used a 5-point scale for evaluation, but we could not detect any significant changes, probably because this evaluation was performed during the first hour after awakening. According to the Japanese guidelines for allergic rhinitis, the degree of nasal congestion should be evaluated according to the presence or absence of mouth breathing throughout the day, and an evaluation performed within a 1-hour period, as in the present study, might not be appropriate [10]. All the patients selected 1 point or 2 points to represent their daily nasal congestion, but we could not detect any significant changes.

As this result was anticipated, we also used the PNIF to evaluate nasal congestion, and this method seemed suitable for our purposes. The peak expiratory flow is often used as a measure in the management of lower airway diseases, such as bronchial asthma. On the other hand, the PNIF is not broadly used in clinical fields for diseases of the upper airways. The clinical use of PNIF for the evaluation of nasal congestion was recommended in ARIA, and some studies have demonstrated the usefulness of PNIF [12-14]. In the present study, we used a portable inspiratory flow meter (IncheckTM) originally used for the management of bronchial asthma. Using the facemask attached to this device, it can be adapted for the evaluation of nasal congestion. PNIF can be used to evaluate nasal congestion objectively and is useful for the self-evaluation of nasal congestion. Moreover, the results of the self-evaluation encouraged the subjects to continue their treatments. We concluded that PNIF is a useful tool for evaluating the therapeutic effects of treatment for allergic rhinitis.

At the beginning of this study, we performed a medical interview and confirmed that the patients' morning nasal symptoms had worsened. However, none of the subjects had previously heard of a doctor mentioning the "morning attack" phenomenon. This study dealt with perennial allergic rhinitis, but many patients also suffer from morning attacks of seasonal allergic rhinitis in their daily lives [9]. When second-generation antihistamines are used daily, we usually recommend that patients take them after breakfast or before bed and do not clearly explain the difference in the clinical effects of these strategies. Chronotherapy should be performed on a case-by-case basis after considering the Tmax of the medicine and the patient's lifestyle and situation.

A previous study examining chronotherapy using the antihistamine meqitazine has been reported [5]. Meqitazine (7.5 mg) was more useful when administered once after supper for the management of morning attacks of perennial allergic rhinitis. Bepotastine besilate and olopatadine hydrochloride are typically administrated twice daily, but considering their Tmax and T1/2 values, they are suitable for managing morning attacks and are effective against nasal congestion. While our study examined chronotherapy using antihistamines, it is important to note that the medicines were administered twice daily, and the study was not a comparison of the effects of these medicines when administered according to an evening versus morning dosing schedule. Thus, strict chronotherapeutic comparisons and assessments cannot be made.

The results of a survey of 770 patients showed that morning attacks occur in 66% of perennial allergic patients and 56% of seasonal allergic rhinitis patients [9]. Another study, which investigated 756 patients with perennial allergic rhinitis, demonstrated that sneezing, rhinorrhea, and nasal congestion were most severe after awakening [11]. In the present study, it was impossible to ask the participants to record their nasal symptoms for 24 hours because of their jobs. Therefore, our study investigated only morning symptoms, and not morning attacks in the strictest definition; nevertheless, the goal of our study was achieved.

In recent years, the relationship between allergic rhinitis and sleep disturbance has become a concern [15]. Treatments with intra-nasal corticosteroids and/or leukotriene receptor antagonists reduce nighttime nasal congestion and, as a result, improve the quality of sleep [16-18]. First-generation antihistamines are not effective for nasal congestion and worsen daytime somnolence [19]. On the other hand, second-generation antihistamines have been shown to relieve nasal congestion. However, the nighttime effects of second-generation antihistamines have not been fully investigated [4,20]. Although sleep disturbance itself and daytime symptoms were not evaluated in our study, chronotherapeutic dosing should contribute to the alleviation of nasal congestion during sleeping.

An Internet survey in Japanese regarding seasonal allergic rhinitis reported that only 35% of patients were satisfied with the first antihistamine that was prescribed to them [21]. Until now, chronotherapy for allergic rhinitis has not been widely considered. Some guidance regarding the taking of medicine from the viewpoint of chronotherapy could improve the satisfaction of patients with pharmacotherapy. The measurement of PNIF values might also lead to a favorable self-evaluation of nasal symptoms and treatment effects. Suggestions regarding chronotherapy and self-evaluations could greatly improve the satisfaction of patients with the results of therapy.

Conclusions

The worsening of nasal symptoms after awakening that is associated with perennial allergic rhinitis has a significant impact on the quality of life of patients. Two second-generation antihistamines, bepotastine besilate and olopatadine hydrochloride, were effective for the treatment of these morning symptoms. The evaluation of nasal congestion using subjective scores is not appropriate for short observation periods, such as 1 hour. The PNIF was useful for self-evaluations of nasal congestion and the effects of therapy. Some guidance regarding the taking of medicine from the viewpoint of chronotherapy might improve the satisfaction of patients with the results of pharmacotherapy.

References

1. Reinberg A, Smolensky MH (1982) Circadian changes of drug disposition in man. Clin Pharmacokinet 7: 401-420.
2. Vener KJ, Moore JG (1988) Chronobiologic properties of the alimentary canal affecting xenobiotic absorption. Annu Rev Chronopharmacol 4: 257-281.
3. Smolensky MH, Reinberg A, Labrecque G (1995) Twenty-four hour pattern in symptom intensity of viral and allergic rhinitis: treatment implications. J Allergy Clin Immunol 95: 1084-1096.
4. Storms WW (2004) Pharmacologic approaches to daytime and nighttime symptoms of allergic rhinitis. J Allergy Clin Immunol 114: S146-153.
5. Reinberg A, Gervais P, Ugolini C, Del Cerro L, Ricakova-Rocher A, et al. (1986) A multicentric chronotherapeutic study of mequitazine in allergic rhinitis. Ann Rev Chronopharmacol 3: 441-444.
6. Martin RJ (1993) Characteristics and mechanisms of nocturnal asthma. Allergy Proc 14: 1-4.
7. Martin RJ (1993) Nocturnal asthma: circadian rhythms and therapeutic interventions. Am Rev Respir Dis 147: S25-28.
8. Meltzer EO (2002) Dose rhinitis compromise night-time sleep and daytime productivity? Clin Exp Allergy Rev 2:67-72.
9. Binder E, Holopainen E, Malmberg H, Salo O (1982) Anamnestic data in allergic rhinitis. Allergy 37: 389-396.
10. Okubo K, Kurono Y, Fujieda S, Ogino S, Uchio E, et al. (2011) Japanese guideline for allergic rhinitis. Allergol Int 60: 171-189.
11. Reinberg A, Gervais P, Levi F, Smolensky M, Del Cerro L, et al. (1988) Circadian and circannual rhythms of allergic rhinitis: an epidemiologic study involving chronobiologic methods. J Allergy Clin Immunol 81: 51-62.
12. Bousquet J, Van Cauwenberge P, Khaltaev N; Aria Workshop Group; World Health Organization (2001) Allergic rhinitis and its impact on asthma. J Allergy Clin Immunol 108: S147-334.
13. Ottaviano G, Scadding GK, Coles S, Lund VJ (2006) Peak nasal inspiratory flow; normal range in adult population. Rhinology 44: 32-35.
14. Starling-Schwanz R, Peake HL, Salome CM, Toelle BG, Ng KW, et al.(2005) Repeatability of peak nasal inspiratory flow measurements and utility for assessing the severity of rhinitis. Allergy 60: 795-800.
15. Lunn M, Craig T (2011) Rhinitis and sleep. Sleep Med Rev 15: 293-299.

16. Davies MJ, Fisher LH, Chegini S, Craig TJ (2006) A practical approach to allergic rhinitis and sleep disturbance management. Allergy Asthma Proc 27: 224-230.

17. Craig TJ, Mende C, Hughes K, Kakumanu S, Lehman EB, et al. (2003) The effect of topical nasal fluticasone on objective sleep testing and the symptoms of rhinitis, sleep, and daytime somnolence in perennial allergic rhinitis. Allergy Asthma Proc 24: 53-58.

18. Hara H, Sugahara K, Hashimoto M, Mikuria T, Tahara S, et al. (2014) Effectiveness of the leukotriene receptor antagonist pranlucast hydrate for the treatment of sleep disorder in patients with perennial allergic rhinitis. Acta Oto-Laryngologica 134: 307-313.

19. Hindmarch I, Shamsi Z (1999) Antihistamines: models to assess sedative properties, assessment of sedation, safety and other side-effects. Clin Exp Allergy 29 Suppl 3: 133-142.

20. Hara H, Sugahara K, Mikuriya T, Hashimoto M, Tahara S, et al. (2013) The effectiveness of epinastine hydrochloride for pediatric sleep breathing related symptoms caused by huperesthetic noninfectious rhinitis. Otolaryngology 4: 150.

21. Konno A, Kubo N (2008) Evaluation of patient satisfaction with treatment of Japanese cedar pollinosis using 2nd generation antihistamine. (in Japanese) Prog Med 28: 2285-2296.

10

Efficacy of Muscle Relaxants in Routine Treatment Protocol of OSMF

Aparna Upadhye Chavan* and Gajanan Namdeorao Chavan

Department of Anesthesia, Jawaharlal Nehru Medical College, Maharashtra, India

*Corresponding author: Gajanan Namdeorao Chavan, Associate Professor, Department of Anesthesia, Jawaharlal Nehru Medical College, Sawangi Meghe, Wardha, Maharashtra, India; E-mail: gcgcny@gmail.com

Abstract

Oral submucous fibrosis is a chronic disorder presenting with the plaguing symptoms of burning sensation in mouth, intolerance to spicy food and progressive trismus. OSMF is insidious in onset characterized by fibrosis of the lining mucosa of the upper digestive tract involving the oral cavity, oropharynx and hypopharynx and the upper third of oesophagus. The fibrosis involves the lamina propria and the submucosa and may extend into the underlying musculature resulting in the deposition of dense fibrous bands, resulting in limited mouth opening. It is widely prevalent in all age groups and across all socioeconomic strata in India. OSMF is etiologically related to chewing of areca nut [betel nut] and its commercial products, a habit prevalent in India and South-East Asia. This increaing prevalence is not only our concern but its treatment challenges is also our concern. Though a benign disease, the frequency of malignant change in patients with OSMF ranges from 3% to 6%. We have various established treatment modalities available, medical and surgical both. But the results vary. Hence after understanding its etiopathogenesis and reviewing various treatment modalities, we planned to carry out the study to find out the efficacy of muscle relaxants to treat OSMF.

Keywords: Oral submucous fibrosis; Epidemilogical trends; Muscle relaxants

Introduction

Oral submucous fibrosis is a chronic disorder presenting with the plaguing symptoms of burning sensation in mouth, intolerance to spicy food and progressive trismus. OSMF is insidious in onset characterized by fibrosis of the lining mucosa of the upper digestive tract involving the oral cavity, oropharynx and hypopharynx and the upper third of oesophagus. The fibrosis involves the lamina propria and the submucosa and may extend into the underlying musculature resulting in the deposition of dense fibrous bands, resulting in limited mouth opening [1]. It is widely prevalent in all age groups and across all socioeconomic strata in India. OSMF is etiologically related to chewing of areca nut [betel nut] and its commercial products, a habit prevalent in India and South-East Asia [2].

This increasing prevalence is not only our concern but its treatment challenges is also our concern. Though a benign disease, the frequency of malignant change in patients with OSMF ranges from 3% to 6% [3]. We have various established treatment modalities available, medical and surgical both. But the results vary. Rooban et al. [4], in their light microscopic study of OSF revealed varying degrees of alterations involving the muscle fibres as the disease progresses.

Trismus could not only due to muscle fibrosis but also due to inflammatory spasm. This spasm could be relieved by muscle relaxant [5]. Hence after understanding its etiopathogenesis and reviewing various treatment modalities, we planned to carry out the study to find out the efficacy of muscle relaxants to treat OSMF [6].

Aims and Objectives

To study the efficacy of muscle relaxants [chlorzoxazone] in the routine treatment protocol of OSMF.

To study the epidemiological trends in the patients with oral submucous fibrosis in our region.

Materials and Methods

The present study was conducted on 40 patients with OSMF, attending as outpatients in the department of ENT, JNMC, Sawangi [Meghe], Maharashtra, after getting approval from Institutional ethical committee. At the beginning of the study, the mouth opening [interincisonal distance of maxillary and mandibular incisors at maximum possible mouth opening] was measured with the help of vernier calipers and graded as follows [6].

Grade 1 [>40 mm], Grade 2 [20–39 mm], Grade 3 [<19 mm].

Inclusion criteria:

Patients of OSMF with grade II and III.

Patients coming for regular follow up.

Extension criteria:

OSMF patients with grade I disease.

Patients who lost follow up.

Patients with trismus other than OSMF.

These 40 patients were randomly divided into two groups. 20 patients of these underwent the routine treatment protocol of weekly injection of hyaluronidase with hydrocortisone and antioxidant capsules with added lycopene for 1 month. This group was labelled as control group.

The remaining 20 patients, in addition to the routine injections and antioxidants, were given skeletal muscle relaxants like chlorzoxazone. This group was labelled as case group.

This measurement was repeated after the study period of 1 month.

Data analysis

The required data was collected and analyzed by using unpaired t-test.

Observations

Sex distribution

Among 40 patients, only 3 patients were females. Amongst these 3 females, only 1 female had habit of chewing tobacco and commercial preparation of areca nut. This explains that apart from areca nuts, there are some other factors contributing to OSMF. Nutritional deficiency or immunological factor can be attributed to cause OSMF. These findings have been shown in Table 1.

Group	Males	Females	Total
Case	18	2	20
Control	19	1	20

Table 1: Sex distribution.

Age distribution

Usually OSMF is prevalent in age group of 20 to 40 years. In our study group, 31 patients [77.5%] were in 20 to 40 years of age group. The youngest patient in this study was 8 years old male child. He did not have any habits related to areca nut or tobacco chewing.

This explains that apart from habits, nutrition, autoimmune factors and genetics also may play role in causation of disease. The other two male patients, who were 14 and 16 years old, had positive history of commercial preparation of areca nut and kharra. Kharra, which is different from ghutka, is locally made preparation of tobacco, areca nut, lime and masala.

Group	1-10 yrs	11-20 yrs	21-30	31-40	Above 40	Total
Case	1	4	10	5	0	20
Control	0	3	10	6	1	20

Table 2: Age wise distribution of patients.

Amongst 40 patients, 37 patients [92.5%] had positive history of chewing areca nut in one form or the other. This explains the strong association of areca nut and OSMF. The following Table 2 shows the age wise distribution of the patients.

After one month study, Mouth Opening [MO] was measured with vernier callipers and the findings observed are shown in Table 3.

The Table 4 shows the mouth opening noted in control group before and after the treatment.

S. No.	MO before treatment	MO after treatment	Overall improvement
1	25	40	15
2	23	38	15
3	26	38	12
4	22	39	17
5	21	40	19
6	25	39	14
7	27	39	12
8	28	38	10
9	25	38	13
10	22	39	17
11	14	23	9
12	15	23	8
13	18	24	6
14	16	22	6
15	16	23	7
16	17	21	5
17	15	24	9
18	15	19	4
19	19	24	5
20	16	24	8

Table 3: Mouth opening [MO] noted in tests subjects.

S. No.	MO before treatment	MO after treatment	Overall improvement
1	29	35	4
2	23	27	4
3	24	31	7
4	21	29	8
5	24	26	2
6	25	24	1
7	20	25	5
8	25	26	1
9	27	24	3
10	26	22	4
11	19	24	5
12	14	18	4
13	16	24	8

14	15	16	1
15	19	18	Progression
16	18	20	2
17	15	18	3
18	14	17	Progression
19	16	19	3
20	14	16	2

Table 4: Mouth opening [MO] noted in control subjects.

In two cases, amongst the control group, we noticed the progression of disease. They came for regular treatment and follow up. Though they had stopped commercial preparations and tobacco, they continued with chewing plain areca nut.

From above observations, following overall improvement in mouth opening after the treatment was noted this has been tabulated in Table 5.

Group [Control]	Overall improvement [control]	Overall improvement [cases]
Grade 2	5.8	14.4
Grade 3	3	6

Table 5: Average overall improvement in mouth opening [in mm].

In our study, we found that group II [case] and group II [control] has significant difference in mean value [t=7.549, P=0.00], this means that the improvement in group II [cases] is significantly more than group II [controls]. This means that patients were benefitted with muscle relaxants.

Group III [case] and group III [control] has significant difference in mean value [t=3.72, P=0.001], this means that the improvement in case- grade III is significantly more than controls. This again proves the efficacy of muscle relaxants, when added to the routine treatment protocol.

The improvement in grade III cases is significantly higher than grade III controls.

Discussion

OSMF was mentioned by Sushrutha [2500-3000 BC] as Vidari in ancient Indian literature. Later In modern literature it was described by Schwartz in 1952. Since then enormous research is going on to study its etiopathogenesis, epidemiological trends, clinical features, treatment, etc.

Even today, in spite of so much of research, OSMF poses a challenge in various aspects.

OSMF is etiologically related to chewing of areca nut [betel nut] and its commercial products, a habit prevalent in India and South-East Asia. This habit is not only popular in urban population but also becoming popular among rural adolescents too. The increased prevalence of OSMF in the last two decades or so corresponds with the increased processing and commercialization of areca nut products, like ghutka, kharra, masala supari, etc. It is a chronic disorder characterized by fibrosis of the lining mucosa of the upper digestive tract involving the oral cavity, oro- and hypopharynx and the upper third of oesophagus. The fibrosis involves the lamina propria and the submucosa and may extend into the underlying musculature resulting in the deposition of dense fibrous bands, resulting in limited mouth opening. It also results from increased production of collagen by fibroblasts. In addition to this there is decreased breakdown leading to accumulation of excessive amount of collagen. The pre-cancerous nature was first described by Paymaster in 1956 that was later confirmed by various studies. A malignant transformation rate was shown to be in the range of 7 to 13% and a transformation rate of 4.5% was reported by Murti et al. [7]. Previous data indicated that the prevalence of OSMF was in the range of 0.03% to 3.2%. The prevalence of OSMF was 6.3% was mentioned by Nitin et al. [8]. The incidence is progressively increasing owing to the excessive usage of areca nut among various groups of population. Oral submucous fibrosis is widely prevalent in all age groups and across all socioeconomic strata in India. Younger generations in India are getting attracted to the advent of attractive

The main problems plaguing the patients with OSF are the burning sensation and progressive trismus which impedes normal function. The treatment should aim at alleviating the symptoms as well as try to stop the progression of fibrosis. But, whatever the treatment method may be, the first step of preventive measure should be in discontinuation of habit, which can be encouraged through education, counselling and advocacy [9,10]. This was the first challenge in our study. Patients needed very intense and continuous motivation to quit the habit and come for treatment and follow up.

In spite of increasing prevalence, there are no known effective treatments for OSF till date. The treatment modalities which are currently being used can be broadly divided into three main categories, viz.: Medical therapy, surgical therapy and physiotherapy [11,12].

When literature was reviewed for various treatment modalities, we came across the study regarding use of muscle relaxants. After studying various literature and researches regarding pathophysiology of OSMF, we decided to find out the efficacy of muscle relaxants in the routine protocol of treatment of oral submucosal fibrosis which we thought will probably help us to alleviate the symptom of trismus.

In our study, we found that muscle relaxants were effective in treating OSMS, if they were added to routine treatment protocol. In fact they were more effective in grade II cases rather than grade III cases. This means that if muscle relaxants are added at early stage of the disease, patient will be benefitted more. Probably in grade II cases muscles relaxants helps to relieve muscle spasm caused by the inflammation facilitating mouth opening. The major drawback of this study was none of the patient consented for biopsy, whatever hard we tried to convince. So we could not study the histopathological changes occurring before study and after study. Medications works better with discontinuation of the habit. This explains the role of areca nut in etiopathogenesis of OSMF. Severe cases of trismus may need surgical intervention to break the extensive and tough fibrous bands. Thus patient counselling; motivation and education to quit habit, forms the important part of the treatment [13]. Apart from ghutka, we across new and locally made preparation of beetle nut and tobacco called " kharra" in Maharashtra which is found to be equally hazardous. We would like to continue our research further with stem cell therapy [14].

References

1. Rajendran R (1994) Oral submucous fibrosis: Etiology, pathogenesis, and future research. Bull World Health Organ 72: 985-996.

2. Pillai R, Balaram P, Reddiar KS (1992) Pathogenesis of oral submucous fibrosis. Relationship to risk factors associated with oral cancer. Cancer 69: 2011-2020.

3. Fareedi MA, Prasant MC, Ashok P, Vinit A, Safiya T, et al. (2012) Oral submucous fibrosis: Medical management. Global Journal of Medicine and Public Health 1: 1-8.

4. Rooban T, Saraswathi TR, Al Zainab FH, Devi U, Eligabeth J, et al. (2005) A light microscopic study of fibrosis involving muscle in oral submucous fibrosis. Indian J Dent Res 16: 131-134.

5. Chou R, Peterson K, Helfand M (2004) Comparative efficacy and safety of skeletal muscle relaxants for spasticity and musculoskeletal conditions: a systematic review. J Pain Symptom Manage 28: 140-175.

6. Sunil SN, Mohan VJ, Arunprabhu G (2011) Benefit of Using Muscle Relaxants in the Routine Treatment Protocol of Oral Submucosal Fibrosis: A Pilot Study Indian J Otolaryngol Head Neck Surg 63: 317-320.

7. Murti PR, Bhonsle RB, Pindborg JJ, Daftary DK, Gupta PC, et al. (1985) Malignant transformation rate in oral submucous fibrosis over a 17 year period. Community Dent Oral Epidemiol 13: 340-341.

8. Nitin KN, Aravinda, Manu D, Siddharth G, Satheesha R, et al. (2014) Prevalence of oral submucous fibrosis among habitual gutkha and areca nut chewers in Moradabad district. Oral Biol Craniofac Res 4: 8-13.

9. Lai DR, Chen HR, Lin LM, Huang YL, Tsai CC (1995) Clinical evaluation of different treatment methods for oral submucous fibrosis. A 10 year experience with 150 cases. J Oral Pathol Med 24: 402-406.

10. Bhonsle RB, Murti PR, Daftary DK, Gupta PC, Mehta FS, et al. (1987) Regional variations in oral submucous fibrosis in India. Community dent. oral epidemiol 15: 225-229.

11. Borle RM, Borle SR (1991). Management of oral submucous fibrosis: a conservative approach. J Oral Maxillofac Surg 49: 788-791.

12. Ranganathan K, Devi MU, Joshua E, Kirankumar K, Saraswathi TR (2004) Oral submucous fibrosis: a case control study in Chennai, South India. J Oral Pathol Med 33: 274-277.

13. Hebbar PB, Sheshaprasad R, Gurudath S, Pai A, Sujatha D (2014) Oral submucous fibrosis in India: Are we progressing? Indian J Cancer 51: 222-226.

14. Suma GN, Madhu PA, Manisha L (2015) Stem cell therapy: A novel treatment approach for oral mucosal lesions. J Pharm Bioallied Sci 7: 2-8.

11

Epistaxis Related to Internal Carotid Artery Cavernous Sinus Aneurysm

Bibek Gyanwali, Hongquan Wu, Meichan Zhu and Anzhou Tang*

Department of Otolaryngology-Head and Neck Surgery, First affiliated Hospital of Guangxi Medical University, Nanning Guangxi, People's Republic of China

Abstract

Background: Nasal bleeding is one of the most common clinical presentation in the Otolaryngology Department. Epistaxis related to internal carotid artery aneurysm is a rare cause of epistaxis. In this case we report a case of recurrent epistaxis for more than 7 months in a previously healthy Chinese man.

Case report: Patient complained recurrent nasal bleeding for seven months without any inducing factors, with no history of trauma to the nose, congestive heart failure, diabetes mellitus, hypertension and other diseases. Head and neck computed tomography revealed left maxillary sinus, sphenoid sinus and the right frontal sinus inflammation and nasal septum deviation to the right. Head and neck angiography revealed left internal carotid artery cavernous sinus aneurysm.

Conclusion: Epistaxis related to internal carotid artery aneurysm is quite rare but it is important to consider aneurysms in the etiology of epistaxis. Which may be fatal if the cause of nasal bleeding cannot be identified. We managed our patiently conservatively using nasal packing, hemostatic, anti-inflammatory drugs. The aneurysm was managed by using stent.

Keywords: Epistaxis; Sphenoid sinus; Internal carotid artery; Cavernous sinus; Aneurysm

Introduction

Epistaxis is simply known as nose bleeding, presented as hemorrhage from the nasal cavity which is noticed when blood flows out through nostrils. Nasal bleeding may occur due to nasal cavity and sinus disease, nasopharyngeal lesions, cavernous sinus lesions, rupture of artery and false aneurysm, some systemic diseases can also cause nasal bleeding. We describe an uncommon cause of epistaxis in this report and discuss the imaging findings, treatment course of our patient.

Case Report

A previously healthy 71-year old Chinese man was admitted in our department for recurrent epistaxis. He complained of recurrent left nasal bleeding for seven months without any inducing factors, amount of blood loss about 400 ml, the bleeding was fresh blood. After pressing the nasal cavity by fingers bleeding stopped. One month before the admission patient again suffered from left nasal bleeding, fresh blood, continuous bleeding, amount of blood loss was about 600 ml, accompanied by dizziness, nausea, thirst, sweating. Patient sought medical consultation went to local hospital diagnosed as Epistaxis. Patient underwent endoscopic guided nasal packing. When the nasal packing was removed after 7 days, epistaxis still continued, mainly from left nostril. For the better diagnosis and treatment patient came to our hospital diagnosed as EPISTAXIS and admitted to our department. Since the onset of illness patient has no history of coma and loss of consciousness, no fever, no head and face pain and no visual changes, no nasal itching, sneezing, purulent nasal discharge and other symptoms. No history of nasal bone trauma and fracture. The general mental state, sleep and appetite are normal, no significant changes in body weight. No other surgical and medical history revealed by patient. Physical examination revealed no external nose deformity slightly nasal mucosa edema, bilateral nasal turbinates, concha olfactory groove, nasopharyngeal structures were seemed to be normal, no any continuous bleeding spot and old bleeding lesion was seen. Blood test showed slight anemia (103. 00 g/l) and elevated white cell count (14. 40*10~9/L). The Patient tested negative for all bleeding disorder examinations.

Urgent Head and neck Computed Tomography (CT) revealed Left maxillary sinus, sphenoid sinus and the right frontal sinus inflammation and nasal septum deviation towards right. The patient was treated with hemostatic, anti-inflammatory drugs and other symptomatic treatment. On the 3rd and 4th day of admission patient again suffered from nasal bleeding, the amount of bleeding was about 5-6 ml, after applying pressure for about 1 minute bleeding stopped itself. At that time anterior and posterior rhinoscope reveal no active bleeding lession, no any further medical intervention was taken and continued previous medication. On 7th day of admission patient suffered from massive epistaxix, under the guidance of nasopharyngeal endoscope nasal cavity and nasopharynx was explored, saw bleeding from left side olfactory grove (Figures 1 and 2), anterior and posterior nasal packing was done and was able to control bleeding. 3 days after nasal packing patient removed the packing himself, but patient still conitnue to have slight nasal bleeding. Head and neck angiography was done in order to find the condition of blood vessels in that region. Angiography revealed internal carotid artery cavernous sinus segment aneurysm (Figures 3 and 4). Patient was transferred to the departent of neurosurgery and underwent Digital substraction angiography and stent surgery. The patient had no further episodes of nasal bleeding and other complications.

*Corresponding author: Anzhou Tang, Department of Otolaryngology-Head and Neck Surgery, First affiliated Hospital of Guangxi Medical University, 22# Shuangyong Road, Nanning Guangxi, People's Republic of China, 530021; E-mail: tazgxmu@163. com

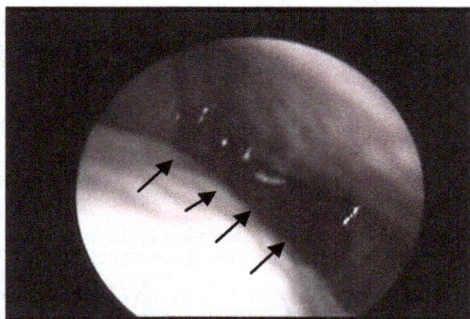

Figure 1: Left Olfactory Groove Bleeding (Nasopharyngeal Endoscopy).

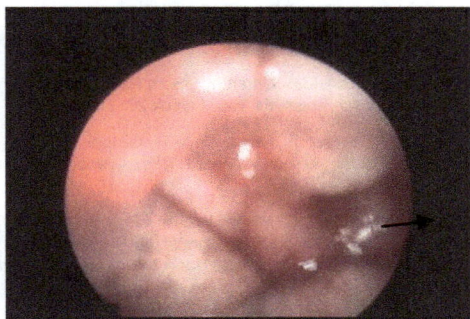

Figure 2: Left Olfactory Groove Bleeding (Nasopharyngeal Endoscopy).

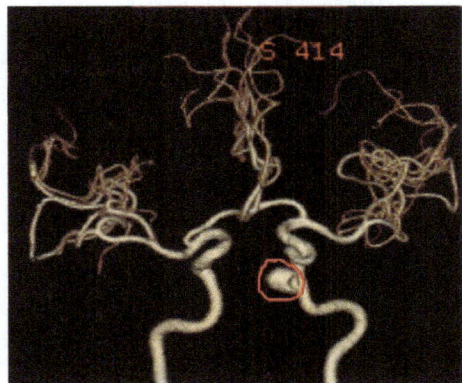

Figure 3: Left Internal Carotid artery Cavernous sinus aneurysm. (Head and Neck Angiography).

Discussion

Patient had been suffering from recurrent epistaxix for 7 months . Inspite of medical and surgical intervention was not been able to control bleeding . Nasal bleeding is a common medical problem, the cause of nasal bleeding may be local cause (trauma, inflammation, nasal septum disease, tumor, foreign bodies, etc.) or systemic cause(cardiovascular disease, blood diseases, acute febrile diseases and severe nutritional disorders and vitamin deficiency, drug poisoning, endocrine disorders, vascular dilatation disease, liver and kidney chronic disease. In 90% of case bleeding occur from little's area [1]. Children have mild anterior nasal bleeding while elderly have profuse posterior nasal bleeding. Bleeding site may be (1) above the level of middle turbinate

from anterior and posterior ethmoidal branches of ophthalmic artery (branch of internal carotid artery). (2) Below the level of middle turbinate from sphenopalatine branch of maxillary artery (branch of external carotid artery). (3) Some time bleeding site may be hidden in middle and inferior turbinates [2]. Approximately 60% of population suffer nasal bleeding, about 6% require formal medical intervention, of those episode of epistaxis 10% can be serious and life threatening [3]. Males are affected more than female, but after the age of 50 both sexes are affected equally. Hypertension is the most common cause in the elderly population [2]. As increase in blood pressure the duration and the amount of nasal bleeding also increase. The elderly populations are more prone to nasal bleeding because their nasal mucosa tens to become dry and thin and the mucosal blood vessels are also not able to contract easily to control bleeding. In 90% of population nasal bleeding can be easily controlled, but under certain circumstances and in the presence of various undertaking conditions life itself may be at risk. Some time because of an inadequate history, the use of inappropriate or wrongly positioned packing, poor supervision after hemostasis, and the mistaken use of chemical cautery may leads to fatal complications and management will be stressful [4].

Cavernous carotid aneurysm is divided into mainly two types; traumatic and non-traumatic. Cavernous segment carotid artery aneurysm is a rare occurrence, represents less than 2% of all intracranial aneurysm [5]. Because of its close anatomical relationship with the sphenoid sinus as well as the nasal fossae in some cases may cause epistaxis. Non-traumatic carotid artery aneurysms are a rare cause of epistaxis [6]. The first case of epistaxis caused by intracranial aneurysm was published at a lecture at the Royal College of Surgeons of England by Dr. Beadles in 1907 [6]. Mass effect is the most common presentation for non-traumatic cavernous internal carotid artery aneurysms, with only 3% presenting with hemorrhage [7]. In those case which present with hemorrhage, severe, delayed, life-threatening, epistaxis often occurs after latent period, which sometimes make it very difficult to identify the relation between underlying cause and epistaxis [8]. Therefore early suspicion and detection is necessary for timely management. Goldenberg-Cohen et al. reported in 40 cavernous sinus aneurysms (27 women, 4 men), Mean age at diagnosis was 60. 4 years (range 25 to 86; median 64). The most common symptoms were diplopia (61%), headache (53%), and facial or orbital pain (32%). Fifteen patients (48%) were diagnosed after they developed cranial nerve pareses, four (13%) after they developed Carotid–Cavernous Sinus Fistulas (CCFs), and 12 (39%) by neuroimaging studies done for unrelated symptoms [9].

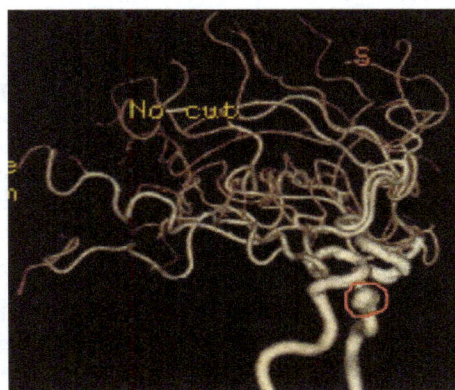

Figure 4: Left Internal Carotid artery Cavernous sinus aneurysm. (Head and Neck Angiography).

In another study conducted by Higashida, Halbach, Dowd, et al. in 87 patients, the most common presentation was mass effect (79%) rupture of aneurysm causing carotid –cavernous fistula (9%), trauma resulting to Cavernous pseudoaneurysm (8%) and hemorrhage (3%). Diplopia is secondary due to the compression of cranial nerves by aneurysm [10]. Variety of neurological deficits, related to vision, including diplopia from single or multiple oculomotor nerve pareses, decreased visual acuity from compressive or ischemic optic neuropathy, corneal and facial anesthesia or hyperesthesia from involvement of the trigeminal nerve, and facial pain may be related to cavernous carotid aneurysm. Like other intracranial aneurysms, these aneurysms can rupture, but this is a rare event and usually does not produce a subarachnoid or intracerebral haemorrhage. Instead, rupture of a Cavernous Carotid Aneurysm (CCA) usually causes a carotid–cavernous sinus fistula or, rarely, epistaxis [7].

The common cause of epistaxis; nasal perforation, nasal septum deviation, rhinitis, sinusitis, and upper respiratory tract infection, can be managed by nasal packing, or use of hemostatic agent or by chemical cautery or by use of a folley's catheter. That epistaxis which cannot be controlled by good nasal packing can be treated under endoscopic evaluation where nasal cavity is explored to indentify bleeding point and the bleeding vessels can be ligated. This commonly seen epistaxis has less risk of recurrence. Recurrent epistaxis other than cavernous carotid aneurysm may be due to congestive heart failure, diabetes mellitus, hypertension, and a history of anemia. Epistaxis related to cavernous carotid aneurysm is difficult to manage by nasal packing, even posterior packing is not sufficient to control bleeding, under certain circumstances and in the presence of various undertaking conditions life itself may be life threatening, so special attention and measures should be undertaken to manage such case of recurrent epistaxis. The clinical presentation of recurrent epistaxis which occurs in absence of any history of trauma and surgery may lead to miss diagnosis or delay the definitive diagnosis. The diagnosis of clinically suspected aneurysm causing nasal bleeding should be confirmed using ultrasonogrophy of neck with colored Doppler flow, CT imaging, CT angiography or Magnetic resonance inages, Angiography provides the most reliable and definitive diagnostic information and offers the opportunity of performing endovascular treatment [11]. High index of suspicion is required for the diagnosis of carotid cavernous aneurysm causing epistaxis and internal carotid artery angiography should be performed in those cases and when considering embolization [12]. Endovascular embolizations, clipping of aneurysm neck or ligation of internal carotid artery are few treatment options.

Conclusion

Although epistaxis is the most common clinical presentation in the department of Otolaryngology and the management of epistaxix is not very difficult, but some time management may be stressful for those epistaxis of unknown origin and recurrent episodes and may be fatal in case of massive bleeding. Aneurysm of the internal carotid artery is rarely mentioned as a cause of epistaxis. This condition is quite rare but it is important to consider aneurysms in the etiology of epistaxis because of their high mortality rate and since they require management quite different from that of epistaxis of other origins. We may consider the internal carotid artery aneurysm as the cause of epistaxis. Similar cases of epistaxis have been reported. Those are due to traumatic rupture of aneurysm or radiotherapy induced aneurysm. We described the rare cause of epistaxix which is related to non-traumatic cavernous carotid aneurysm in a healthy patient with no history of congestive

heart failure, diabetes mellitus, hypertension and other diseases and its management. As for otolaryngologist medical intervention and nasal packing are the management option. The stent placement is quick, safe, rapid and long term treatment of carotid artery aneurysm.

References

1. Jiakong W, Zhou L, Tang A (2010) Otolaryngology-Head and Neck Surgery, Beijing, People's Medical Publishing House 303-306.

2. Bansal M (2013) Disease of External Nose and Epistaxis. Disease of Ear, Nose and Throat, Jaypee Brothers Medical Publishers(P) Ltd. 289-297

3. Thomas A, Tami, James A, Marrell, Ballengera's (2009) Otorhinolaryngology Head and Neck Surgery, Shelton, People's Medical Publishing House 551-555.

4. Schreiner L (1976) Complications and errors in the management of nose bleeding (author's transl). Laryngol Rhinol Otol (Stuttg) 55: 257-263.

5. Handa J, Handa H (1976) Severe epistaxis caused by traumatic aneurysm of cavernous carotid artery. Surg Neurol 5: 241-243.

6. Beadles CF (1907) Aneurysm of larger cerebral arteries. Brain 30:285-336.

7. Chaboki H, Patel AB, Freifeld S, Urken ML, Som PM (2004) Cavernous carotid aneurysm presenting with epistaxis. Head Neck 26: 741-746.

8. Bavinzski G, Killer M, Knosp E, Ferraz-Leite H, Gruber A, et al. (1997) False aneurysms of the intracavernous carotid artery--report of 7 cases. Acta Neurochir (Wien) 139: 37-43.

9. Goldenberg-Cohen N, Curry C, Miller NR, Tamargo RJ, Murphy KPJ (2004) Long term visual and neurological prognosis in patients with treated and untreated cavernous sinus aneurysms. J Neurol Neurosurg Psychiatry 75: 863-867

10. Higashida RT, Halbach VV, Dowd C, Barnwell SL, Dormandy B, et al. (1990) Endovascular detachable balloon embolization therapy of cavernous carotid artery aneurysms: results in 87 cases. J Neurosurg 72: 857-863.

11. da Silva PS, Waisberg DR (2011) Internal carotid artery pseudoaneurysm with life-threatening epistaxis as a complication of deep neck space infection. Pediatr Emerg Care 27: 422-424.

12. Maldonado-Naranjo A, Varun R, Kshettry, Toth G (2013) Non-traumatic superior hypophyseal aneurysm associated with pseudoaneurysm presenting with massive epistaxis. Clinical Neurology and Neurosurgery 115: 2251-2253.

12

Giant Cell Reparative Granuloma Presenting as Cheek Swelling: Case Series of Four Patients

Minakshi Gulia* and Neelam Sood

Department of Pathology, Deen Dayal Upadhyaya Hospital, New Delhi, India

***Corresponding author:** Minakshi Gulia, Department of Pathology, Deen Dayal Upadhyaya Hospital, New Delhi, India; E-mail: mint.ucms@gmail.com

Abstract

Giant cell reparative granuloma is a clinically distinctive intraosseous proliferation most commonly arising in mandible and maxilla. It is classified under fibro inflammatory reactive-reparative lesion.

Histopathological features comprise of irregularly distributed multinucleated osteoclast like giant cells in a supporting fibrous stroma along with peripheral osteoid formation and stromal hemorrhage. All the four patients in this study had a characteristic clinicopathological presentation and immunohistochemistry.

Differential diagnosis from other giant cell lesions of the bone, especially Giant cell tumor, was pivotal since GCT has a tendency for recurrence and a rare ability to undergo sarcomatous transformation or metastasis. Postoperative follow up of all the patients was unremarkable and there was no recurrence.

Keywords: Giant cell reparative granuloma (GCRG); Giant cell tumor (GCT); Vimentin; CD68; Immunohistochemistry (IHC)

Introduction

Giant cell reparative granuloma, a pseudotumoral lesion, is a benign reactive intraosseous process most commonly arising in craniofacial skeleton and in small bones of the hand and feet and affects children and young adults [1]. Its origin could be triggered by trauma or inflammation. Histopathological examination shows giant cells arranged around hemorrhagic areas, stromal cells in storiform pattern and osteoid formation at the periphery [2]. In the present case reports Giant cell reparative granuloma in four patients is described focusing on the cytopathological and histopathological findings.

Case Report

First patient, a thirteen year old girl presented with pain and swelling in the right maxillary region since four months. On examination there was an ill-defined right cheek and nasolabial region swelling. Contrast Enhanced CT scan of the paranasal sinuses revealed relatively well defined homogenously enhancing cystic lesion on Right side in nasolabial region, suggestive of Nasolabial cyst (Figure 1). Second patient, 35 years old female presented with a fleshy mass in the Right maxillary antrum for past one year. The mass was gradually progressive and pushed the nasal bone medially (Figure 2). Another patient, 30 years old male, presented with a fleshy mass protruding from the alveolar ridge and it was gradually progressive (Figure 3). The fourth patient, 35 years old female had left maxillary swelling (Figure 4). The serum levels of calcium, phosphorous and alkaline phosphatase were normal in all four cases, with adequate renal function. Fine needle aspiration cytology was done.

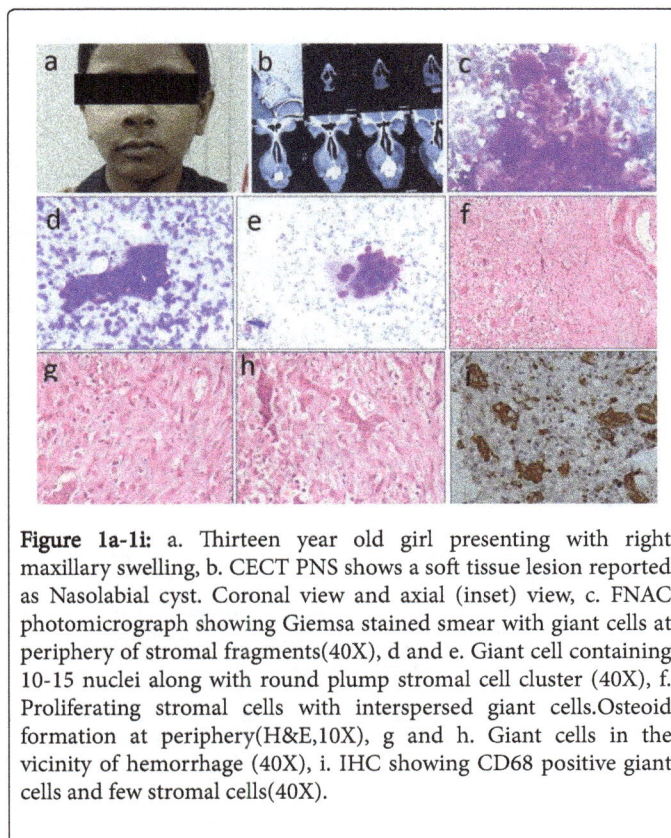

Figure 1a-1i: a. Thirteen year old girl presenting with right maxillary swelling, b. CECT PNS shows a soft tissue lesion reported as Nasolabial cyst. Coronal view and axial (inset) view, c. FNAC photomicrograph showing Giemsa stained smear with giant cells at periphery of stromal fragments(40X), d and e. Giant cell containing 10-15 nuclei along with round plump stromal cell cluster (40X), f. Proliferating stromal cells with interspersed giant cells.Osteoid formation at periphery(H&E,10X), g and h. Giant cells in the vicinity of hemorrhage (40X), i. IHC showing CD68 positive giant cells and few stromal cells(40X).

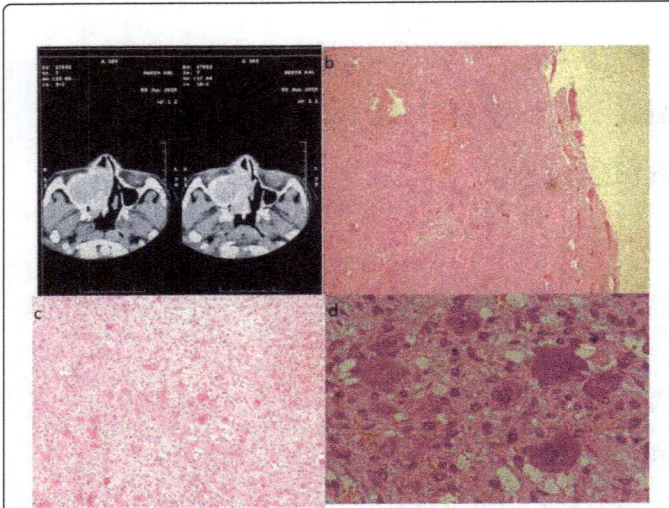

Figure 2a-2d: a. CECT(axial view) showing expansile maxillary lesion with peripheral bony rimming, b&c. Photomicrograph showing giant cells arranged around hemorrhagic areas and storiform pattern of stromal cell proliferation (H&E,10X), d.Haphazardly arranged giant cells in a hemorrhagic area (H&E, 40X).

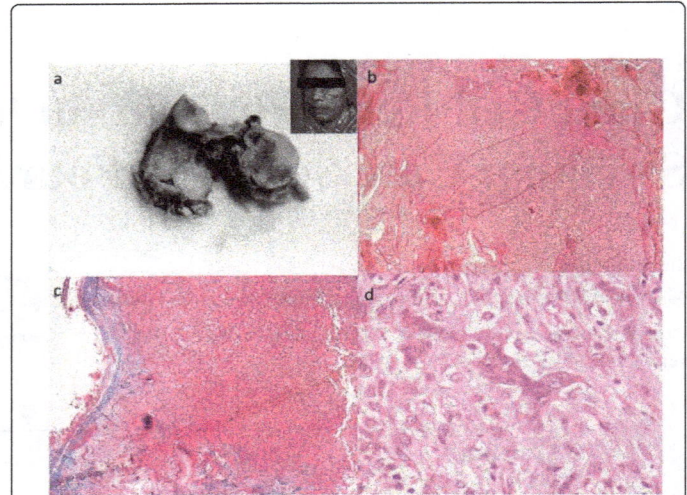

Figure 4a-4d: a. Gross specimen of circumscribed maxillary mass excised through external approach. Postoperative clinical picture of 35 years old female (inset), b. Photomicrograph showing stromal cell proliferation with interspersed giant cells, osteoid at the periphery (H&E,10X), c. Osteoid at the periphery stains blue with Trichrome staining (H&E,10X), d. Higher magnification of the above with areas of hemorrhage (H&E,40X).

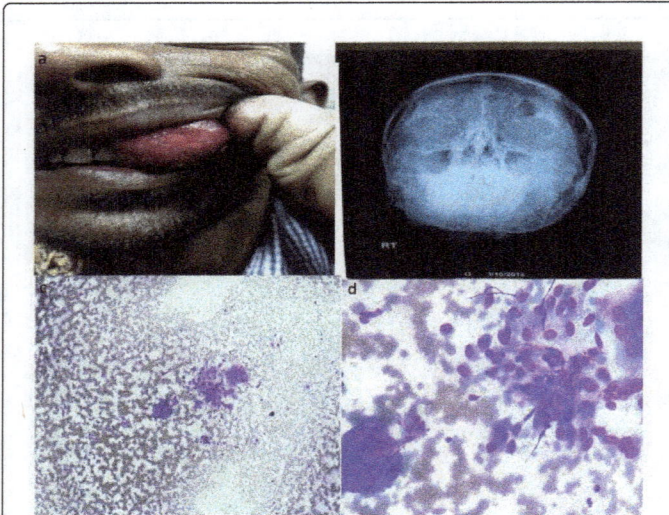

Figure 3a-3d: a. Thirty years old male with fleshy left alveolar mass, b. X Ray PNS showing a soft tissue lesion without bony involvement, c. FNAC microphotograph showing stromal cell cluster and multinucleated giant cells at the periphery(Giemsa, 10X), d. Higher magnification of the above (40X).

H and E and Giemsa stained FNA smears showed numerous giant cells (5-20 nuclei) having bland nuclear chromatin in a background of hemorrhage. Giant cells are located at the periphery of the stromal fragments. No mitotic activity was seen. FNAC was suggestive of a Giant cell lesion and possibility of Giant Cell Reparative Granuloma was considered. Excision was advised.

Excision was performed by Caldwell Luc's procedure in three patients and by open incision in the fourth patient. Histopathological examination of the excised specimens showed giant cells arranged around hemorrhagic areas, stromal cells in storiform pattern and osteoid formation at the periphery. IHC showed the stromal cells to be fibroblastic (or myofibroblastic) in origin and the Giant cells were positive for Vimentin and CD6. Features were suggestive of Giant Cell Reparative Granuloma in all of the four patients. The alveolar mass was classified as Peripheral giant cell reparative granuloma and the rest three were Central giant cell reparative granulomas [2-4].

Postoperative follow up of the fourth patient has been unremarkable for 20 years now. Five year follow up of the other patients too has been unremarkable.

Discussion

Giant cell reparative granuloma is a rare, benign reactive intraosseous lesion which represents a reactive process to intraosseous hemorrhage although a history of trauma is infrequent [1]. It was introduced into medical literature by Jaffe in 1953 and accounts for 1-7% of all benign lesions of the jaw and arises most often in the mandible and maxilla [3,5]. Cases have been reported in small bones of the hand & feet, sinuses, temporal bone, skull, spine, clavicle, tibia, humerus, ribs and femur. Children and young adults, predominantly females, are affected in the second and third decades of life. GCRG are further classified into two distinct clinical forms-the peripheral type, involving the gingiva and alveolar mucosa; and the central type which causes lytic destruction at the intraosseous level [4]. Although GCRG is described as a lytic lesion, the cortex usually remains intact. In the more aggressive type, cortical erosion and soft tissue expansion has been described.

Radiologically it presents as a solitary radiolucent expansive lesion with sharp margination. FNAC is suggestive of a giant cell rich lesion and histopathological examination of the excised specimen shows giant cells arranged around hemorrhagic areas with stromal cells in storiform pattern and periphery showing osteoid formation [6,7]. IHC findings suggest that the giant cells exhibit both osteoclastic and fibroblastic (or myofibroblastic) phenotype since they are positive for Vimentin as well as CD6 [8]. The mononuclear cells, however, are the major proliferative elements in the reparative granuloma and a subpopulation of these cells may represent precursors of the multinucleated giant cells [9].

Other Giant cell lesions of the bone should be considered in the differential diagnosis: Giant cell tumor (GCT), fibrous dysplasia, aneurysmal bone cyst, lesions of primary and secondary hyperparathyroidism (Brown tumor) and Cherubism [10].

The most important differential diagnosis for GCRG is that of GCT. GCT is distinctly unusual in the jaw and has a characteristic epiphyseal involvement in long bones. The giant cells are more regularly and uniformly distributed in GCT with a more uniformly ovoid stromal cell population, in which the nuclei are similar to those of the giant cells.

Fibrous dysplasia has a characteristic presence of Chinese figure like trabeculae of immature or woven bone within a proliferating fibroblastic stroma. Aneurysmal bone cyst shows large spaces filled by blood and is hence excluded. Brown tumor of Hyperparathyroidism is identical to GCRG but is ruled out on the basis of normal serum levels of calcium, phosphorous, alkaline phosphatase and adequate renal function. Cherubism, which is hereditary intraosseous fibrous swelling of the jaw, usually has bilateral presentation in a young individual with a hereditary autosomal dominant mode [10].

The accurate diagnosis of GCRG has considerable importance since it has relatively better prognosis and a surgery ranging from simple curettage to resection is usually curative. However, in cases of aggressive and extensive lesion, it must be completely excised because of high rate of recurrence after incomplete removal [8].

References

1. Liliana GO, Gonzalez ML, Santini-Araujo E (2015) Giant cell reparative granuloma. Tumors and Tumor-like lesions of Bone, Springer, pp: 793-800.

2. Whitaker, Bryan S, Waldron CA (1993) Central giant cell lesions of the jaws, a clinical, radiologic and histopathologic study. Oral Surgery, Oral Medicine, Oral Pathology 75: 199-208.

3. Kumar KAJ, S. Humayun, Kumar BP, and Rao JB (2011) Reparative giant cell granuloma of the maxilla. Ann Maxillofac Surg 1: 181-186.

4. Vasconcelos RG, Vasconcelos MG, Queiroz LMG (2013) Peripheral and central giant cell lesions: Etiology, origin of giant cells, diagnosis and treatment. Jornal Brasileiro de Patologia e Medicina Laboratorial 49: 446-452.

5. Schlorf RA, Koop SH (1977) Maxillary giant cell reparative granuloma. Laryngoscope 87: 10-17.

6. De Corso E, Politi M, Marchese MR, Pirronti T, Ricci R, et al. (2006) Advanced giant cell reparative granuloma of the mandible: Radiological features and surgical treatment. Acta Otorhinolaryngol Ital 26: 168-172.

7. Morris JM, Lane JI, Witte RJ, Thompson DM (2004) Giant cell reparative granuloma of the nasal cavity. AJNR Am J Neuroradiol 25: 1263-1265.

8. Seo ST, Kwon KR, Rha KS, Kim SH, Kim YM (2015) Pediatric aggressive giant cell granuloma of nasal cavity. Int J Surg Case Rep 16: 67-70.

9. Tian XF, Li TJ, Yu SF (2003) Giant cell granuloma of the temporal bone: A case report with immunohistochemical, enzyme histochemical and in vitro studies. Arch Pathol Lab Med 127: 1217-1220.

10. Pogrel AM (2012) The diagnosis and management of giant cell lesions of the jaws. Ann Maxillofac Surg 2: 102-106.

13

Guide Wire Augmented Nasofrontal Sinusotomy (GWANS)

Hamed Sajjadi*

Stanford University School of Medicine, San Jose, CA, USA

Abstract

Endoscopic frontal sinus surgery remains as a very challenging technique with potential for serious morbidity and even mortality. The close proximity of orbital contents, the cribriform plate and the anterior skull base pose serious challenges in performing this operation safely. The frontal recess anatomy is even more treacherous in recurrent cases and in diseased processes such as polyps and other tumors blocking the nasofrontal recess.

Guide Wire Augmented Nasofrontal Sinusotomy (GWANS) allows for real time surgical guidance allowing the surgeon to confidently dissect through diseased tissue knowing all along where the boundaries of the nasofrontal recess lies and thus avoid injuring vital structures. This is a new and adjunctive tool for augmenting the standard endoscopic nasofrontal sinusotomy technique.

Keywords: Endosocopic frontal sinus surgery; Minimally invasive frontal sinus surgery; Guide-wire assisted frontal sinus surgery; Balloon assisted frontal sinus surgery

Introduction

Since 1985 Functional Endoscopic Sinus Surgery (FESS) has become the gold standard in surgical management of intractable sinusitis in the United States [1-3]. Over 200,000 FESS cases are performed in the US on an annual basis, surgical success rates are reported as high as 98% for isolated maxillary disease and relatively lower success rates are reported for Ethmoid and sphenoid disease [4].

Frontal sinus recess is the most difficult area to dissect endoscopically, and the lowest success rates are quoted for the intractable frontal sinus disease [5-7]. Post-operative failure after frontal sinus surgery is often due to retained or residual diseased cells in the frontal recess [8]. This may be due to difficulty in surgical dissection and the surgeon's uncertainty of anatomical landmarks thus leaving disease behind.

Frontal sinus anatomy remains difficult and elusive, especially in recurrent disease and cases with polyps or other neoplasm in the frontal recess. Complicated frontal recess anatomy with potential risk of serious complications to the orbit or the brain, in combination with the surgeon's lack of anatomical confidence may lead to residual disease at the frontal recess.

Stereotactic Sinus Navigation has provided much improved surgical guidance, but it remains to be based on a pre-operative static CT scan and not real time imaging. However, ongoing surgical dissection can alter the observed anatomy on a real time basis and distort boundaries seen on a pre-operative navigational CT scan. It appears that computer guided sinus surgery may not necessarily improve clinical outcome, but it may reduce surgical complication rates [9,10].

In order to overcome the lack of real time data during computer assisted surgical dissection, other investigators have suggested the use of intra-operative volume controlled computed tomography scans. There seems to be a positive promise for this technique; however it is time consuming, cumbersome in the cramped operating rooms and very costly [11].

Guide Wire Augmented Nasofrontal Sinusotomy is a new and novel method that allows for a fast and relatively simple surgical guidance in a very difficult anatomy. It allows surgeon to clean disease process and widen the frontal recess with more confidence knowing where the recess is located and to avoid injuring adjacent vital structures. This method can be used on all difficult primary or revision frontal sinus cases where the nasofrontal recess anatomy is abnormal or is obscured by polyps, granulation tissue or scar tissue.

Method

Standard Endoscopic sinus surgery instruments were utilized. The fiberoptic Luma Guide wire assembly from the Acclarent Company of Menlo Park, California was used for all the cases in this study [12]. In all cases, the three dimensional LandMarx Navigation CT Scan, Stealth protocol, from Medtronic Company of Minneapolis, Minnesota were utilized [13].

The fiberoptic Luma guide wire is inserted under direct endoscopic visualization using a 45 degree Sinus Endoscope and a 70 degree frontal catheter guide. This can be accomplished in great majority of Polypoid and scarred recesses even where there is no visualization of an opening into the recess (Figures 1 and 2).

Operative room lights are dimmed to a minimum. Endoscopy light source is dimmed. Patient's forehead is scanned for the light reflection of the Luma guidewire (Figure 3). Once the location of the guide wire tip in the frontal sinus is confirmed via transillumination of the frontal sinus, a 7 by 24 ml frontal dilation balloon is inserted over the guide wire and inflated in the nasofrontal recess to 10 atmospheric pressure for one second (Figure 4) [13].

On all cases, once the forehead transillumination was confirmed, the navigational image guidance also confirmed the accurate positioning of the guide wire in the naso frontal recess.

The most important part of the GWANS technique is to carefully remove the balloon along with the catheter guide, but leaving the guide wire in place. In order to make sure the guide wire stays in place during

***Corresponding author:** Hamed Sajjadi, MD, FACS, FARS, Stanford University School of Medicine, San Jose, 2577 Samaritan Drive, #845, San Jose, CA 95124, USA; E-mail: Drsajjadi@earandsinus.com

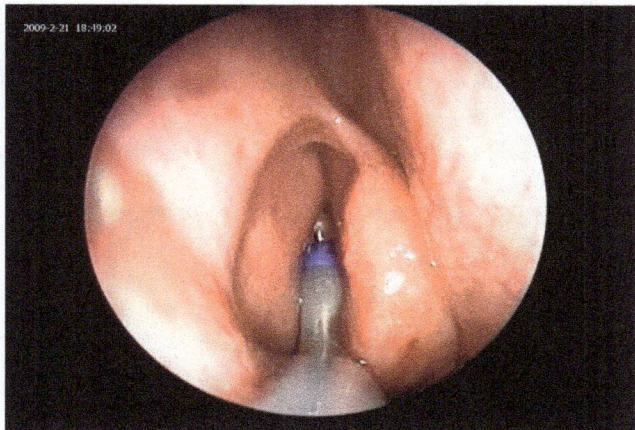

Figure 1: Angled Endoscopic view of the 70 degree catheter guide inserted in the nasofrontal recess in a cadaver.

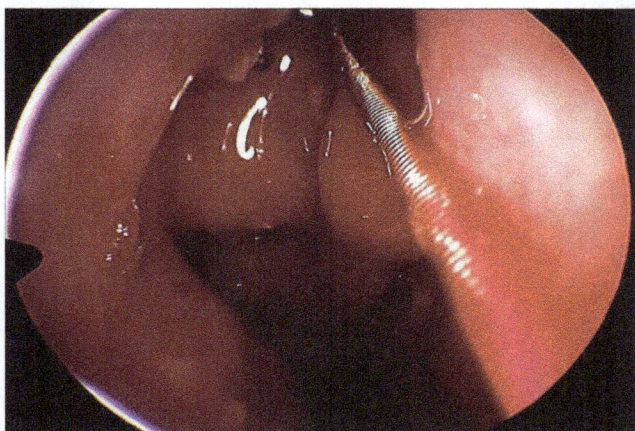

Figure 2: Angled Endoscopic view of the Fiberoptic Luma Guide wire in frontal recess in a patient full of polyps, prior to resection of the polyps.

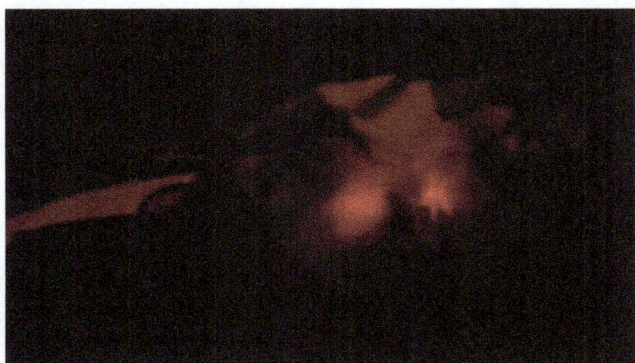

Figure 3: Transillumination of the light spot on the right forehead under subdued room lighting.

resection of the uncinate process, the agar nasi cells, polyps, obstructing frontal bony spurs/beak and granulation tissue thus enlarging the recess with full view of the guide wire at all times (Figures 5-7) [14,15].

Once the frontal recess is widely opened up, the Vortex Irrigation catheter from the Acclarent Company was inserted over the guide wire into the frontal sinus. Aspiration for culture and saline irrigation was then performed on all sinuses.

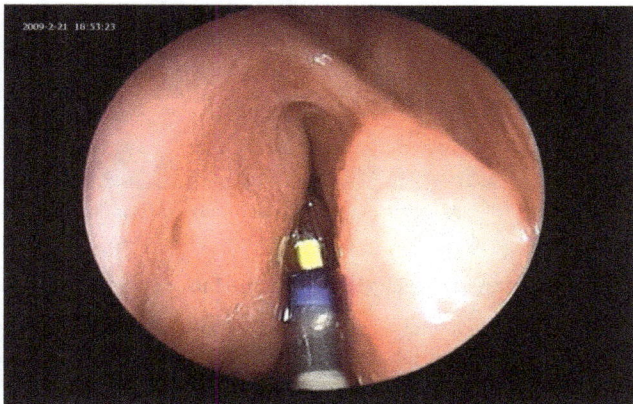

Figure 4: Large frontal sinus balloon being inflated in the nasofrontal recess.

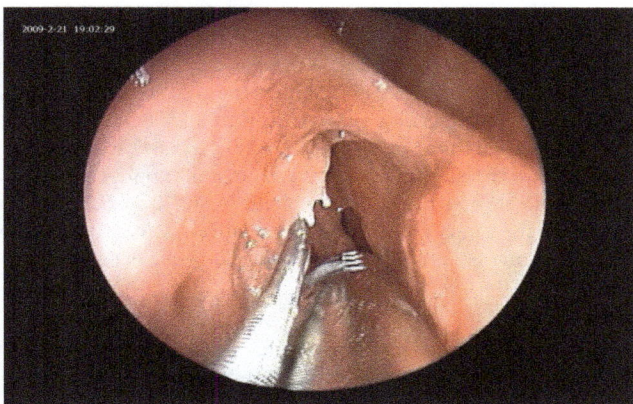

Figure 5: Removing the uncinate remnant with the microdebrider with the Fiberoptic Luma Guide wire in the recess.

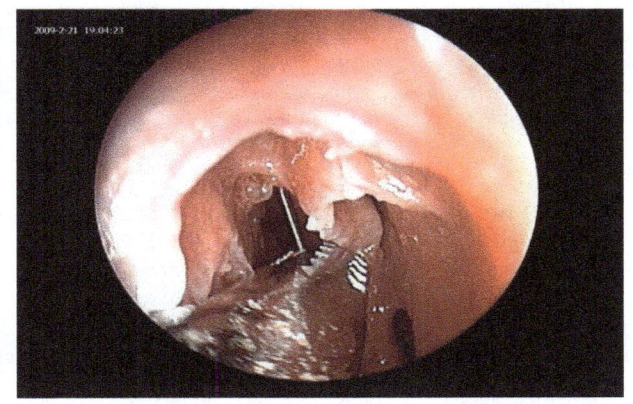

Figure 6: Removing the anterior nasofrontal bone with microdebrider with the Fiberoptic Luma Guide wire in the recess.

the dissection, the surgical assistant holds the guide wire in place and keeps the frontal sinus transillumination in the same spot on the forehead throughout the procedure.

With the guide wire left in the nasofrontal recess all the way into the frontal sinus, the surgeon then proceeds with the standard endoscopic

Even in these two initially unsuccessful Guide-Wire cases, once the recess was partially opened, the Guide wire was passed into the sinus and dissection of the bony disease continued around the Guide wire thus increasing the surgeon's confidence of the location of the recess into the frontal sinus at all times.

All frontal sinuses showed significant improvement in the degree of

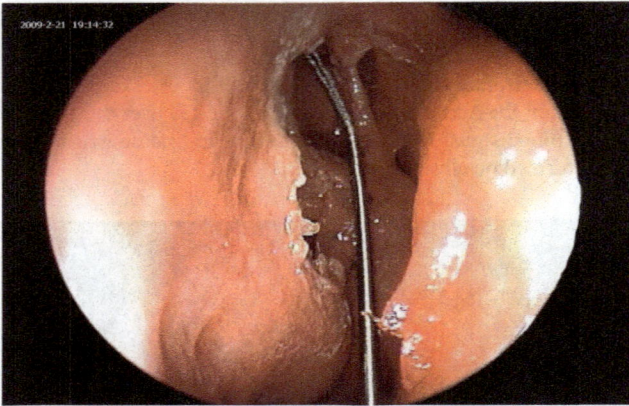

Figure 7: Guide wire in the recess after full dissection is done.

Guide wire's tensile strength test in the laboratory

The Fiberoptic Luma Guide wire was also tested for strength in the cadavers in the laboratory. The concern was that could the surgeon accidently cut the Guide wire during surgery using sharp instrumentations, such as the microdebrider, cutting forceps or scissors. The test was conducted in the cadaver laboratory to assess the Fiberoptic Luma Guide wire's tensile strength and resistance to fragmentation when faced with sharp cutting instruments. Multiple deliberate attempts to grab the wire with cutting forceps, even scissors, failed to transect the guide wire. Microdebrider and high-speed sinus drills also were unable to grab and transect the guide wire. After over 20 such deliberate attempts on a single wire, the Guide wire was bent and damaged but it still conducted light and did not transect. Multiple Luma Guide wires were tested in a similar fashion; none could be transected in vivo while staying in the nasofrontal recess. The laboratory data proved that the Luma Guide wire was relatively safe around cutting instruments, microdebrider (shaver) and drills (Figures 8-11).

Cases

Eighteen (18) patients with difficult, intractable frontal sinusitis were treated with this method over a 15 month period with a minimum of 3 month post-operative CT scan and office endoscopy. Thirty four (34) frontal sinuses were operated upon. Pre-operative CT Scans and infrared Image Guidance system was used on all patients. Only fiberoptic Luma Guide Wire was used. Fluoroscopy was not utilized. All patients were adults, age range of 36-67 years old. All cases were performed under general anesthesia using mild hypotension maintaining the systolic blood pressure around 90 mmHg. Intravenous antibiotic and Dexamethasone were used on all patients at the induction of general anesthesia (Table 1).

Results

In all but two cases out of thirty two sinuses, the frontal sinus recesses were successfully entered using the Fiberoptic Luma Guide wire. Once the guide wire was in place, standard endoscopic resection of the obstruction was performed for a wide open naso frontal recess in all cases. There were no complications. There was no entry into the orbit or the intracranial structures and no cases of Ethmoid artery violation.

The two unsuccessful Guide wire cases demonstrated complete bony stenosis where there was no detectable opening for the guide wire to pass, thus requiring standard frontal sinusotomy techniques [16-18].

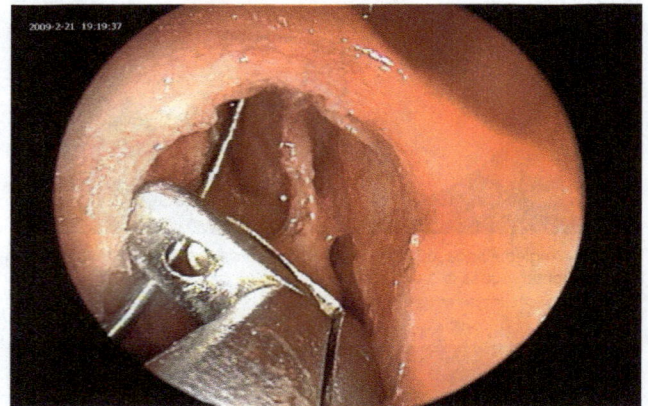

Figure 8: Attempt to cut the Fiberoptic Luma Guide wire in the lab with Cutting forceps.

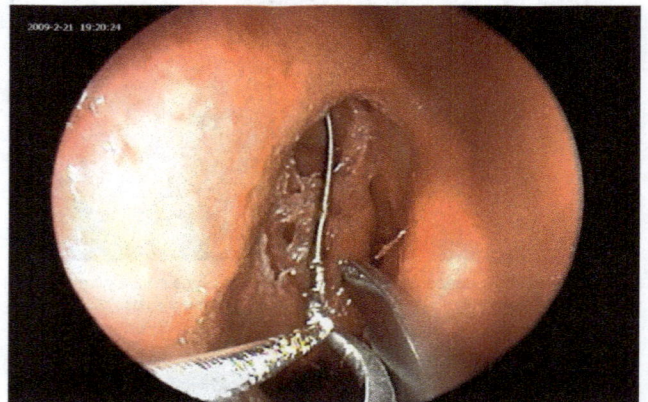

Figure 9: Attempt to cut the Fiberoptic Luma Guide wire in the lab with Endoscopic scissors.

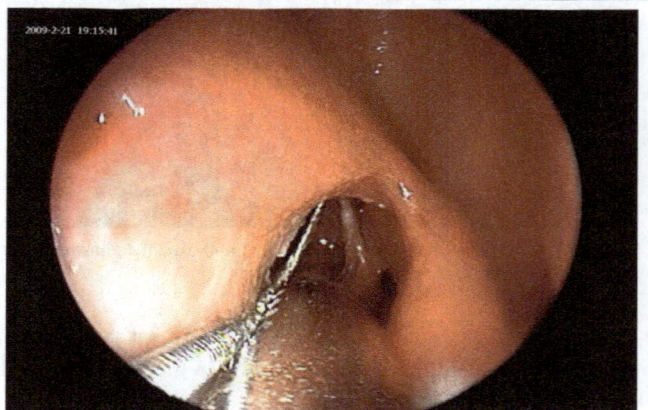

Figure 10: Attempt to cut the Fiberoptic Luma Guide Wire in the lab with Microdebrider.

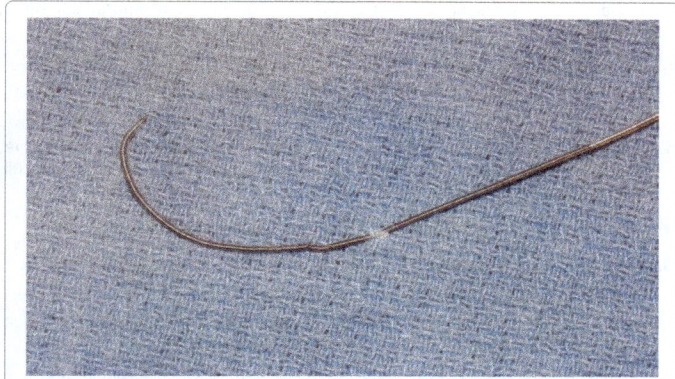

Figure 11: Damaged, but "intact" Fiberoptic Luma Guide Wire after 20 attempts in vivo to transect it with variety of sharp instruments.

Case No.	Age	Sex	Stage	Disease Status
1	52	M	Revision	Polyps, scar tissue
2	46	M	Revision	Polyps, bony narrowing
3	36	F	Primary	Polyps, small agger nasi
4	60	M	Revision	Polyps, Granulation tissue
5	62	F	Primary	Low uncinate, stenotic NFR
6	36	M	Revision	Polyps, scar tissue
7	40	M	Revision	Scar tissue, lateralized middle turbinate
8	49	F	Primary	Scar tissue, small agger nasi
9	49	M	Revision	Polyps, no middle turbinates, scar tissue
10	37	F	Primary	Polyps, granulation tissue
11	58	F	Revision	Polyps, scar tissue
12	34	M	Revision	Polyps, no landmarks, scarred uncinate
13	44	F	Primary	Polyps, granulation tissue
14	44	M	Revision	Inverted Papilloma in the frontal recess
15	49	M	Revision	Scar tissue, small agger nasi
16	54	M	Revision	Polyps, no landmarks, scarred uncinate
17	55	F	Revision	Polyps, granulation tissue
18	67	M	Revision	Polyps, granulation tissue

Table 1: Case distribution.

mucosal thickening on the post-operative CT Scans as compared to the pre-operative scans. Twenty Six sinuses (80%) showed relatively clear frontal sinuses with less than 3 mm mucosal thickening on the three month post-operative CT Scan. The remaining 20% showed significant reduction in the mucosal thickening. None of the pre-operatively opacified frontal sinuses remained opacified post-operatively thus demonstrating either partial or complete aeration of the frontal sinus (Table 2).

Discussion

Frontal sinus disease remains mostly a medical disease. Surgical intervention is best reserved for intractable and symptomatic frontal sinusitis [6]. Effective antibiotics and vigilant adjunctive remedies to improve sinus drainage have substantially reduced the need to perform frontal sinus surgery. Nevertheless, frontal sinus surgery remains a very challenging and difficult undertaking with potential for serious life-changing complications [19].

Abnormal frontal recess anatomy, with or without obstructing polyps or bony obstruction, can further complicate the surgical access into the frontal sinus and increase the risk of serious complications. As surgeons and healers, our primary job is to do no harm. Frontal sinus

surgery is designed to improve patients' quality of life, but it could lead to severe loss of function and morbidity.

Balloon dilation of the frontal recess has been shown to be an effective and safe method for intractable frontal sinus disease [20,21]. Long term frontal sinus outflow tract patency after balloon dilation of the frontal recess has been shown to be in the same range of the standard non-balloon surgical debridement of the frontal recess [22].

The Guide-Wire Augmented Nasofrontal Sinusotomy (GWANS) technique can be applied to uncomplicated primary as well as the difficult primary or the revision cases. However, in uncomplicated primary cases of intractable frontal sinusitis, straightforward guide wire balloon dilation without surgical debridement may suffice in the majority of cases. It is best to reserve GWANS for those difficult cases where the fiberoptic wire is unable to enter the frontal sinus on multiple attempts [7].

In difficult cases where the frontal recess is not overtly visible, the small 1 mm fiberoptic Luma Guide wire almost miraculously finds its way into the frontal sinus with a high degree of probability. Once the wire is in place the surgeon can then proceed with balloon dilation and subsequent standard endoscopic frontal sinusotomy [23,24].

The Guide-Wire Augmented Nasofrontal Sinusotomy (GWANS) as described hereby is utilized primarily in difficult cases where either scar tissue, polyps or granulation tissue with or without bony spurs are obstructing the nasofrontal recess thus necessitating a full nasofrontal sinusotomy. In such difficult cases, polyps or bony obstruction have to be physically removed, and balloon dilation alone may not be sufficient to assure long-term patency of the nasofrontal recess.

The Guide-wire and the subsequent balloon dilation provide a solid framework where standard endoscopic frontal sinusotomy can be accomplished with ease and the safety of knowing where exactly the pathway into the frontal sinus is located throughout every step of the procedure.

The Guide-wire Augmented Nasofrontal Sinusotomy significantly reduces the need to use navigational instruments during the case. For the purpose of this study navigational Image guidance was used in all

Case No. Score	Pre-op Right Score	Post-op Right LM	Pre-op Left Score	Post –op Left score
1	2	1	2	1
2	2	0	2	0
3	1	0	1	0
4	2	0	n/a	unilateral
5	1	0	1	0
6	2	1	2	0
7	2	0	1	1
8	1	0	1	0
9	2	0	2	0
10	1	0	1	0
11	2	0	n/a	unilateral
12	2	0	2	1
13	1	0	1	0
14	2	0	2	0
15	2	0	2	0
16	2	0	2	0
17	2	0	2	1
18	2	1	2	

Table 2: Pre-operative and Post-operative Lund-MacKay sinus CT Staging.

cases to confirm the location of the guide wire with the transillumination light reflex. On all cases, once the transillumination was confirmed, the navigational image guidance also confirmed the accurate positioning of the guide wire in the naso frontal recess. It is felt that with good transillumination, minimal to no navigational data is necessary in order to complete the Guide-Wire Augmented Nasofrontal Sinusotomy.

Keeping the guide wire in view during the dissection in the recess allows the surgeon real time surgical guidance to avoid injuring vital structures around the recess. This is accomplished by keeping the guide wire in the posterior plane of dissection and only removing obstructing tissues anterior to the guide wire. By keeping the dissection anterior to the guide wire, the more sensitive areas such as the Anterior Ethmoid artery and the skull base are mostly kept away from "harm".

In two out of 18 patients the nasofrontal recess could not be "intubated" with the guide wire, and a formal frontal recess drill out was needed. It is important to remember that Guide wires and Balloons are only surgical tools for getting the job done, and the surgeon needs to be well-versed on the difficult anatomy and be fully prepared to perform the standard nasofrontal surgical techniques as indicated should the guide wire fail to perform as expected.

It is important to remind ourselves that most of the time frontal sinusitis is not life threatening, but the surgical complications of frontal sinus surgery are definitely life threatening. Cerebrospinal fluid leaks, meningitis, brain abscess, brain hematomas, eye muscle injury, blindness and death are all potential complications of frontal sinus surgery.

It is the goal of this paper to present a relatively straight forward technique for improving the odds of obtaining a good frontal sinus pathway with significant reduction of uncertainty during surgical dissection. The risks of frontal sinus surgery remain with us no matter how we do this difficult operation, but this simple guide wire gives the surgeon a great deal of confidence as to the location of the recess during the surgical debridement of the recess.

The ultimate responsibility rests with the surgeon to master the anatomy and for accomplishing the desired task with the utmost precision and skill while utilizing all available means to insure patient safety and satisfactory outcome. Guide-Wire Augmented Nasofrontal Sinusotomy is one small step towards achieving this goal in frontal sinus surgery.

References

1. Messerklinger W (1985) Endoskipische diagnose and chirurgie der rezidivierenden sinusitis. In: Advances in Nose and Sinus Surgery, edited by Z. Krajina, Zagreb Universtity, Zagreb, Yugoslavia.

2. Stammberger H (1985) Endoscopic surgery for mycotic and chronic recurring sinusitis. Ann Otol Rhinol Laryngol Suppl 119: 1-11.

3. Stammberger H (1986) Endoscopic endonasal surgery--concepts in treatment of recurring rhinosinusitis. Part II. Surgical technique. Otolaryngol Head Neck Surg 94: 147-156.

4. Huang BY, Lloyd KM, DelGaudio JM, Jablonowski E, Hudgins PA (2009) Failed endoscopic sinus surgery: spectrum of CT findings in the frontal recess. Radiographics 29: 177-195.

5. Levine HL (1995) Endoscopic Sinus Surgery: reasons for failure. Op Tech Otolaryngol. Head & Neck Surg 6:176-179.

6. Kennedy DW, Senior BA (1997) Endoscopic sinus surgery. A review. Otolaryngol Clin North Am 30: 313-330.

7. Stammberger H, Posawetz W (1990) Functional endoscopic sinus surgery. Concept, indications and results of the Messerklinger technique. Eur Arch Otorhinolaryngol 247: 63-76.

8. Kuhn FA (1996) Chronic Frontal Sinusitis: the endoscopic frontal recess approach. Operative techniques. Otlaryngolo Head Neck Surg 7:222-229.

9. Tschopp KP, Thomaser EG (2008) Outcome of functional endonasal sinus surgery with and without CT-navigation. Rhinology 46: 116-120.

10. Masterson L, Agalato E, Pearson C (2012) Image-guided sinus surgery: practical and financial experiences from a UK centre 2001-2009. J Laryngol Otol 126: 1224-1230.

11. Batra PS, Kanowitz SJ, Citardi MJ (2008) Clinical utility of intraoperative volume computed tomography scanner for endoscopic sinonasal and skull base procedures. Am J Rhinol 22: 511-515.

12. Acclarent, Inc. 1525-B O'Brien Drive, Menlo Park, CA 94025, USA.

13. Medtronic, Inc., 710 Medtronic Parkway, Minneapolis, MN 55432-5604, USA.

14. Bolger WE, Brown CL, Church CA, Goldberg AN, Karanfilov B, et al. (2007) Safety and outcomes of balloon catheter sinusotomy: a multicenter 24-week analysis in 115 patients. Otolaryngol Head Neck Surg 137: 10-20.

15. Levine HL, Sertich AP 2nd, Hoisington DR, Weiss RL, Pritikin J; PatiENT Registry Study Group (2008) Multicenter registry of balloon catheter sinusotomy outcomes for 1,036 patients. Ann Otol Rhinol Laryngol 117: 263-270.

16. Wormald PJ (2008) Surgical Approach to the Frontal Sinus and Frontal Recess. In: Endoscopic Sinus Surgery, Anatomy, Three-Dimensional Reconstruction, and Surgical Technique. (2nd Edn), Thieme Medical Publishers, New York.

17. Wormald PJ (2005) Surgery of the frontal recess and frontal sinus. Rhinology 43: 82-85.

18. Wormald PJ (2002) The axillary flap approach to the frontal recess. Laryngoscope 112: 494-499.

19. Plaza G, Eisenberg G, Montojo J, Onrubia T, Urbasos M, et al. (2011) Balloon dilation of the frontal recess: a randomized clinical trial. Ann Otol Rhinol Laryngol 120: 511-518.

20. Catalano PJ, Payne SC (2009) Balloon dilation of the frontal recess in patients with chronic frontal sinusitis and advanced sinus disease: an initial report. Ann Otol Rhinol Laryngol 118: 107-112.

21. Batra PS, Ryan MW, Sindwani R, Marple BF (2011) Balloon catheter technology in rhinology: Reviewing the evidence. Laryngoscope 121: 226-232.

22. Chan Y, Melroy CT, Kuhn CA, Kuhn FL, Daniel WT, et al. (2009) Long-term frontal sinus patency after endoscopic frontal sinusotomy. Laryngoscope 119: 1229-1232.

23. Schaefer SD, Close LG (1990) Endoscopic management of frontal sinus disease. Laryngoscope 100: 155-160.

24. Wormald PJ (2003) The agger nasi cell: the key to understanding the anatomy of the frontal recess. Otolaryngol Head Neck Surg 129: 497-507.

14

Harmonious Team Approach for Safe Airway Management - The Keio University Experience

Haruna Yabe[1], Koichiro Saito[1]*, Kosuke Uno[1], Takeyuki Kono[1], Hiroshi Morisaki[2] and Kaoru Ogawa[1]

[1]Department of Otolaryngology-Head and Neck Surgery, Keio University School of Medicine, Tokyo, Japan
[2]Department of Anesthesiology, Keio University School of Medicine, Tokyo, Japan

Abstract

Surgical Tracheostomy (ST) has been a standard procedure for surgical airway management for a long time. Recently, Percutaneous Dilatational Tracheostomy (PDT) is getting more and more popular in the US and Europe in this field. In Japan, PDT is becoming well-known following the trend in other countries mainly due to its relatively easy procedure even for non-surgeons to secure the airway. However, part of the multidisciplinary participants in preparing/performing tracheostomy and postoperative care do not have opportunities to understand the (contra) indications of PDT, or to precisely learn the technical difference between ST and PDT. Furthermore, instruction for use is hard to be strictly followed in diverse situations to potentially induce multiple accidents.

In our institution, PDT was adopted under the collaboration between anesthesiologists and otolaryngologists in January 2008. However, at that time, responsibilities and roles of every participant engaged in the tracheostomy were not clarified, while multiple responsible decisions were necessary for harmonious procedure, e.g. necessity of tracheostomy for the candidate, timing to perform the procedure, selection of proper surgical procedure, and the place where the tracheostomy should be performed. Considering such a muddled situation, we organized a committee consisted of surgeons, anesthesiologists, nurses and administrative organizers to comprehend the recent complicated situations surrounding tracheostomy. The final purpose of organizing the committee was to build a unique intramural rule to prepare and perform elective tracheostomy safely and harmoniously.

In this communication, multiple issues to produce the present confused situation for harmonious elective tracheostomy are summarized. We show our current intramural protocol for elective tracheostomy, delivered in July 2010, which clarifies the sequential role and responsibility of every multidisciplinary participant at each indispensable decision for safe procedure. Furthermore, current practice of tracheostomy in our institution, especially in the intensive care unit, was assessed.

Keywords: Tracheostomy; Percutaneous dilatational tracheostomy; Multidisciplinary teams' approach; Airway management; Protocol

Introduction

Tracheostomy is a common surgical procedure to secure the airway in critically ill patients. Surgical Tracheostomy (ST) has long been the gold standard tracheostomy procedure since Jackson first standardized the technique in 1909 [1]. Shelden et al. [2] described Percutaneous Dilatational Tracheostomy (PDT) concept in 1955 to simplify the tracheostomy procedure. In 1985, Ciaglia et al. [3] introduced an epoch-making PDT method using the relatively easy Seldinger technique to introduce the serial dilators and a tracheostomy tube into the trachea. The Griggs Guidewire Dilating Forceps (GWDF) technique, introduced in 1990, was based on an idea to enlarge a small tracheal aperture with a guidewire-dilating forceps especially manufactured for this technique [4]. In 1998, a modification of Ciaglia technique which utilizes a single sharply tapered dilator was introduced (Ciaglia Blue Rhino Percutaneous Tracheostomy Introducer Kit, Cook Critical Care Inc., Bloomington, IN). The Ciaglia Blue Rhino (CBR) technique allowed the complete dilation of the stoma in one step [5]. Recently, a meta-analysis study showed the superiority of the CBR technique in terms of safety and success rate among multiple PDT techniques [6]. Multiple studies have proved the advantages of PDT compared with ST [7-10], and PDT is gaining popularity as a procedure to secure the airway especially in the Intensive Care Units (ICUs) worldwide [11, 12]. In Japan, PDT is becoming a well-known procedure following the trend in other countries. In our institution, the CBR technique was adopted under the collaboration between anesthesiologists and otolaryngologists in 2008. Firstly, sequential multiple decisions are necessary for the successful tracheostomy by a team consisted of multidisciplinary participants. Additionally, PDT's entry into the airway management field allowed the non-surgeons to perform the tracheostomy using the Seldinger technique, as long as the indications and contraindications of the procedure were strictly followed. Thus, at this point, the role and responsibility of each participant engaged in the tracheostomy became complicated in order to accomplish safe and harmonious procedure [13]. Although, only anesthesiologists were the non-surgically trained members of the airway management team to perform PDT in our institution, it had not been clarified who was responsible for each step and who was to make specific decisions among sequential responsible decisions required for successful tracheostomy. We organized a committee to comprehend such recent complicated situations surrounding tracheostomy and to build a multidisciplinary collaborative system with unequivocal rules for safe and smooth elective tracheostomy. Our original intramural protocol for successful tracheostomy was delivered in 2010. Our protocol clarified

*Corresponding author: Koichiro Saito, Assistant Professor and Director, Division of Laryngology, Department of Otolaryngology-Head and Neck Surgery, Keio University School of Medicine, 35 Shinanomachi Shinjuku, Tokyo 160-8582, Japan; E-mail: koichiro@ja2.so-net.ne.jp

the respective roles and responsibilities of each multidisciplinary participant at each of the respective indispensable decisions. In this communication, our intramural protocol for tracheostomy is shown expecting to be one practical reference for the ideal system in the future. At present, PDT is routinely performed in our institution as the first choice tracheostomy procedure for adult patient receiving long-term mechanical ventilation in the ICU. Current practice of tracheostomy in our institution, especially in the ICU, was further assessed to speculate the validity of our current tracheostomy protocol in this report.

Our Multidisciplinary Protocol for Safe and Harmonious Tracheostomy

In our institution, anesthesiologists invited us to observe them from the airway surgeon's point of view on adopting the PDT procedure in the ICU. Anesthesiologists preferred and desired to adopt the CBR technique as they were familiar with the Seldinger technique, and our collaborative approach to the PDT started in January 2008. During the first 3 months period, otolaryngologists performed PDT as experienced airway surgeons, while anesthesiologists assisted the procedure by performing the bronchoscopy. During this training period, anesthesiologists learned the PDT technique as well as the internal anatomy of the subglottic-tracheal region as an important knowledge for safe PDT procedure [13]. Since April 2008, anesthesiologists started to perform PDT by themselves at the bedside in the ICU. At present, PDT is routinely performed by anesthesiologists in our institution and considered the first choice tracheostomy procedure for adult patient receiving long-term mechanical ventilation in the ICU. Our collaboration has been providing the on-site or on-call otolaryngologist available on each PDT case as needed.

While adopting the CBR technique under cooperation of two departments, we organized a committee consisted of airway surgeons, anesthesiologists, nurses and administrative organizers to build an original, multidisciplinary collaborative system with unequivocal rules for safe and smooth elective tracheostomy. As airway surgeons, a thoracic surgeon and an otolaryngologist (KS in this manuscript) were incorporated.

One GWDF PDT kit (Portex® Percutaneous Tracheostomy Kit, Smiths Medical Japan Ltd., Tokyo, Japan), and three CBR PDT kits (Ciaglia Blue Rhino® G2 Advanced Percutaneous Tracheostomy Introducer Set, Cook Japan Inc., Tokyo, Japan; Neo Perc™ Percutaneous Tracheostomy Kit, Covidien Japan Inc., Tokyo, Japan; Portex® ULTRAperc® Single Stage Dilator Technique Kit, Smiths Medical Japan Ltd.) are currently available in Japan. To comprehend the recent complicated situation surrounding tracheostomy and to understand the details of newly adopted PDT technique, we first read and compared the instructions for use (IFU) package inserts of these PDT kits thoroughly. It has been emphasized that PDT could be a safe method of choice for performing elective tracheostomy in the appropriately selected patients receiving mechanical ventilation [7-9]. However, several contraindications for PDT performance provided in the IFU package inserts of four PDT kits were not shared among all of these kits as absolute contraindications to possibly cause confusions and raise the related morbidity. In other words, several conditions were considered as absolute contraindications in some PDT kits, while IFU package inserts of other PDT kits not mentioned these conditions or rated these conditions as relative contraindications. While shared absolute contraindications included 1) emergency case, 2) inability to palpate the cricoid cartilage, 3) pediatric patients, 4) active cervical infection, and 5) presence of a midline neck mass, the following conditions were

not mentioned as absolute contraindications in all of the four PDT kits available in Japan. These confusing contraindications included 6) thyroid hypertrophy, 7) coagulopathy, 8) difficult airway (patients with difficult tracheal intubation), 9) unprotected airway (patients not intubated), 10) patients requiring high PEEP, 11) inability to extend the neck, 12) previous surgery in the neck/tracheal area, and 13) deformity of the neck/tracheal area. Additionally, detailed description of the proper environment for PDT to prefer the performance in the ICU or OR under control of critical care specialists was observed in the IFUs supplied by Smiths Medical Japan Ltd. (Portex® Percutaneous Tracheostomy Kit; Portex® ULTRAperc® Single Stage Dilator Technique Kit). Intraoperative visual support by bronchoscopy was recommended, but not mentioned, as mandatory in all of the available IFU package inserts. To perform the newly adopted PDT procedure with minimal risk, the committee decided to consider all the possible contraindications as absolute contraindications in our institution. Furthermore, the committee decided that PDT should be performed only in the ICU or OR under the bronchoscopic visual guidance. The committee preferred to perform ST in the OR rather than to perform in the ward in consideration of the quick access to the required resources and critical care specialists. Intramural unified Informed Consent (IC) form of the tracheostomy was revised to include PDT as a surgical option additional to ST. The IC form clearly mentioned that the procedure might be shifted from PDT to ST as needed during surgical procedure.

As we have mentioned before [13], sequential responsible decisions are necessary for the success of cooperative tracheostomy by multidisciplinary participants. When there is a candidate for tracheostomy, the necessity of the procedure is the first topic to be determined. Subsequently, the timing to perform the tracheostomy is determined, and in case of emergency, ST is performed immediately. In an elective case, subsequent decisions include the selection of the proper procedure (ST or PDT) and place (ICU, OR, or ward) to perform tracheostomy for the patient. It is necessary to clarify the respective roles and responsibilities of each multidisciplinary participant at each indispensable decision necessary for safe and harmonious tracheostomy. Our original intramural protocol for tracheostomy was established July 2010. This protocol is summarized in Figure 1. This protocol was established mainly for elective cases, and in emergency cases, this chart could be modified to meet the situations. In every case, multidisciplinary teams consist of attending physicians, airway surgeons (mainly otolaryngologists in our institution), anesthesiologists, and nurses. Sequential decisions and "respective roles" of *each participant* were clarified as follows (Figure 1).

1) When there arises a candidate for tracheostomy, *attending physicians* and *airway surgeons* are responsible to "determine the necessity of tracheostomy". *Anesthesiologists* "cooperate with them to make a better decision as needed".

2) Once the tracheostomy performance is decided, *attending physicians* take the responsibility to explain the necessity of tracheostomy to the patient and the persons concerned to "acquire the informed consent regarding the necessity of the procedure". At the same time, *anesthesiologists* receive the mandatory notification of the tracheostomy performance from the airway surgeons and "join the team as critical care specialists".

3) *Airway surgeons* and *anesthesiologists* take the subsequent responsibility to "decide the timing of the procedure (elective or immediate)". In emergency cases, ST is performed immediately

by airway surgeons with the modification of the following steps to secure the patient's life.

4) In elective cases, *airway surgeons* and *anesthesiologists* "determine the proper method of tracheostomy (ST or PDT)".

5) *Airway surgeons* and *anesthesiologists* further take the responsibility to "determine the place to perform the procedure (ICU, OR, or ward)".

6) *Nurses* are responsible to "prepare the resources and environments" to perform safe and smooth surgical procedure.

7) At this point, *either airway surgeons or anesthesiologists who are to perform the procedure* explain the surgical procedure and potential risks to the patient and the persons concerned to "acquire the informed consent regarding the surgical performance". As PDT is the first choice tracheostomy procedure for the patient receiving long-term mechanical ventilation in the ICU, "PDT is mostly performed in the ICU"

by *anesthesiologists* at the bedside. *Airway surgeons* "perform ST on most of the residual cases in the OR" with the potential PDT performance in the OR.

8) *Airway surgeons* and *anesthesiologists* "cooperate with each other during the procedure either in a PDT case or in a ST case". In all PDT cases, a surgical tracheostomy tray and on-site or on-call otolaryngologist are available in the event that conversion to open tracheostomy is necessary.

Our Current Practice of Tracheostomy

Based on the retrospective chart review, current practice of tracheostomy in our institution, especially in the ICU was assessed to speculate the validity of our current protocol. Fifty-seven consecutive patients who underwent elective tracheostomy from April 2012 to September 2013 were incorporated in this assessment. Of these, 7 patients (2 boys and 5 girls) were under 15 y.o. and these pediatric cases were excluded from this assessment to focus on the elective adult tracheostomies. Of the residual 50 adult patients (30 males and 20 females; mean age, 67.8 y.o.; range, 31-95 y.o.), 39 patients were ICU cases (23 males and 16 females; mean age, 67.7 y.o.; range, 31-88 y.o.). Choice of procedure was reviewed, and the delay from the decision to perform a tracheostomy to the procedure being performed (waiting period), and perioperative complications were compared between ST group and PDT group in all the cases. Subgroup analyses were further performed on the ICU cases. In our institution, currently, the first choice tracheostomy procedure for the intubated patient in the ICU is PDT, while most of the other patients underwent ST in our institution as a teaching hospital for airway surgeons. However, some of the patients in the ICU underwent ST and the conditions being contraindications for PDT in these patients were assessed. Furthermore, the waiting period, duration of intubation, and ICU stay after tracheostomy were compared between ST group and PDT group. The results are summarized in Tables 1 and 2. Statistical analyses were performed using Mann-Whitney U test, and the significant level was set at $p<0.05$. All PDT

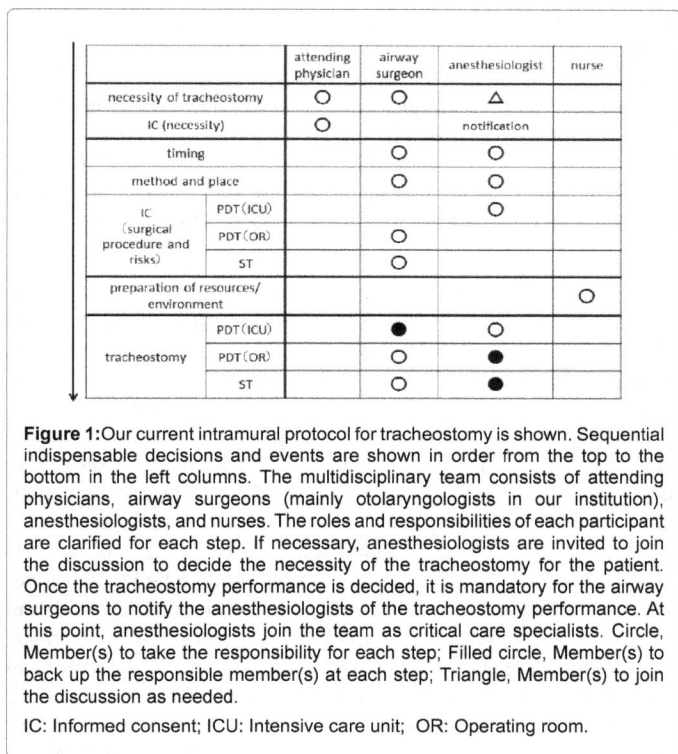

Figure 1: Our current intramural protocol for tracheostomy is shown. Sequential indispensable decisions and events are shown in order from the top to the bottom in the left columns. The multidisciplinary team consists of attending physicians, airway surgeons (mainly otolaryngologists in our institution), anesthesiologists, and nurses. The roles and responsibilities of each participant are clarified for each step. If necessary, anesthesiologists are invited to join the discussion to decide the necessity of the tracheostomy for the patient. Once the tracheostomy performance is decided, it is mandatory for the airway surgeons to notify the anesthesiologists of the tracheostomy performance. At this point, anesthesiologists join the team as critical care specialists. Circle, Member(s) to take the responsibility for each step; Filled circle, Member(s) to back up the responsible member(s) at each step; Triangle, Member(s) to join the discussion as needed.

IC: Informed consent; ICU: Intensive care unit; OR: Operating room.

Procedure	Cases Sex; Age	Waiting Period* Average ± SD; Range (Days)	Perioperative Complications
ST	M, 17; F, 11; 31-95 y.o. (mean, 68.4 y.o)	4.0 ± 4.1; 0-14	1**
PDT	M, 13; F, 9; 43-88 y.o. (Mean 67.2 y.o.)	2.6 ± 1.6; 1-7	0

M: Male; F: Female; *: Delay from the decision to perform a tracheostomy to the procedure being performed; **: Bleeding required local suture

Table 1: Fifty consecutive patients who underwent elective tracheostomy from April 2012 to September 2013.

Procedure	Cases Sex; Age	Waiting Period* Mean ± SD; Range (Days)	Endotracheal Intubation Before Tracheostomy Mean ± SD; Range (Days)	ICU Stay After Tracheostomy Mean ± SD; Range (Days)	Conditions Being Contraindications For PDT
ST	M, 10; F, 7; 31-87 y.o. (Mean 68.4 y.o.)	2.4 ± 2.8; 0-9	8.3 ± 4.6; 0-15; n=14**	5.3 ± 3.3; 2-13; n=15***	coagulopathy, 6; previous surgery in the neck, 4; no intubation, 3; inability to palpate the cricoid cartilage, 2; thyroid hypertrophy, 1; other****, 1
PDT	M, 13; F, 9; 43-88 y.o. (Mean 67.2 y.o.)	2.6 ± 1.6; 1-7	8.6 ± 3.3; 2-14	6.0 ± 4.6; 1-18	n.a

M: Male; F: Female; *: Delay from the decision to perform a tracheostomy to the procedure being performed; **:As shown in the right panel, 3 patients were not intubated at the tracheostomy, and 14 patients were incorporated in this group; ***: Two patients died during ICU stay after tracheostomy, and 15 patients were incorporated in this group; ****: Serious heart failure which required circulation control with OR resources during surgery

Table 2: ICU patients who underwent elective tracheostomy.

procedures were performed at the bedside in the ICU using the CBR kit (Neo Perc™ Percutaneous Tracheostomy Kit, Covidien Japan Inc.), while all ST procedures were performed in the OR. There was a trend that ST need shorter waiting period compared with PDT, however, the difference was not statistically significant (ST, 4.0 ± 4.1 days; PDT, 2.6 ± 1.6 days; p=0.70). One patient in the ST group required local suture to control the bleeding from the muscle in the anterior neck, however, no perioperative complication was observed in the PDT group (Table 1). Values of the waiting period (ST, 2.4 ± 2.8 days; PDT, 2.6 ± 1.6 days; p=0.27), endotracheal intubation before tracheostomy (ST, 8.3 ± 4.6 days; PDT, 8.6 ± 3.3 days; p=0.95), and ICU stay after tracheostomy (ST, 5.3 ± 3.3 days; PDT, 6.0 ± 4.6 days; p=0.89), were similar when ST group and PDT group were compared with each other in the ICU patients. Two patients died during ICU stay because of their original diseases (1 patient suffered upper mesentery arterial thrombosis and the other suffered end-stage lung cancer), and ICU stay after tracheostomy was assessed in the residual 15 patients. Conditions being contraindications for PDT consisted of coagulopathy (n=6), previous surgery in the neck (n=4), no intubation (n=3), inability to palpate the cricoid cartilage (n=2), thyroid hypertrophy (n=1), and serious heart failure to require careful circulation control with OR resources during surgery (n=1) (Table 2).

Discussion

Following multiple Randomized Clinical Trials (RCTs) comparing ST and PDT to define the superior procedure with respect to both resource use and morbidity, several meta-analyses of these RCTs have been performed [7-10]. These reports supported the idea to favor PDT in terms of perioperative bleeding, intraoperative drop of oxygen saturation level, operative time, wound infection, unfavorable scarring, waiting period, and costs [7-10]. As a result, combined with its relative technical ease, PDT is the favored tracheostomy technique for an adult intubated patient, especially in the ICUs worldwide [11,12].

On the other hand, advantages of performing PDT by collaborative multidisciplinary teams have been reported by Polderman et al. [14] and Blankenship et al. [15]. Their teams consisted of otolaryngologists, and either intensivists or pulmonary/critical care specialists. Their systems enabled the professional anesthesia support and airway management accompanied by an intensivist or anesthesiologist with a smooth conversion to ST as needed by a backup otolaryngologist. The main structure of their multidisciplinary team is similar to the members of our system, whereas our system incorporated attending physicians and nurses, as well as anesthesiologists and airway surgeons. Our protocol further clarified the respective roles and responsibilities of each multidisciplinary participant at each of the sequential indispensable decisions.

Although there was a trend that PDT patients have shorter waiting period compared with ST patients, the difference was not statistically significant in our current practice of tracheostomy. Furthermore, no perioperative complication was observed in the PDT group. Subgroup analysis of ICU patients showed no difference between ST and PDT in terms of waiting period, endotracheal intubation before tracheostomy, and ICU stay after tracheostomy. Partially due to the PDT performance at the bedside without OR scheduling, shorter waiting period prior to the performance, and shorter endotracheal intubation before procedure in the PDT group, have been reported when compared with the ST group [9,10]. Furthermore, early tracheostomy has been reported to reduce the duration of artificial ventilation and length of stay in the ICU [16]. Different from the previous RCTs comparing ST and PDT, most of the

STs were performed on the patients with serious complications being contraindications for PDT performance (n=14, 82 %) in our recent ICU practice. Residual ST patients were not intubated at the performance (n=3, 17 %). All PDT procedures were performed at the bedside and all ST procedures were performed in the OR. However, ST patients (2.4 ± 2.8 days) were not required the longer waiting period compared with PDT patients (2.6 ± 1.6 days). Thus, no difference was observed in terms of endotracheal intubation before tracheostomy and ICU stay after tracheostomy. These results suggest the potential of our protocol to assist the collaboration of multidisciplinary teams to complete the smooth tracheostomy without time-consuming OR scheduling even on the patients with serious complications. In our recent practice, perioperative complication was not observed in the PDT group, while one patient in the ST group suffered wound bleeding to require local suture. These results may support the idea that our choice of tracheostomy procedure strictly followed the (contra)indications of PDT to minimize perioperative morbidity. Although there may remain a potential for PDT to be an effective alternative procedure in challenging cases such as children [17] and trauma patients with difficult airways [18], it could never be overemphasized, at present, that PDT could be a safe method of choice for performing elective tracheostomy in the appropriately selected adult patients receiving mechanical ventilation [7-9]. In our recent ICU practice, there was one patient in the ST group who suffered serious heart failure which required circulation control with OR resources during surgery. PDT might not have been a contraindication procedure for this patient with a normal-size neck; however, the team preferred ST owing to the practical ST experiences of airway surgeons involved in the particular case.

It should be noted that false passage of a tracheostomy tube trends toward favoring ST [10]. To reduce the overall complication rate related to PDT [19], bronchoscopic visual guidance was determined as mandatory for PDT performance in our protocol. As we have reported before [13], intraoperative bronchoscopy enables the clear visualization of the subglottic-tracheal lesion including the subglottic bulge in the anterior wall as an anatomical landmark representing the lower edge of the cricoid to the first tracheal ring. Additionally, decannulation/obstruction of the tracheostomy tube were reported to be more likely to occur in the PDT group compared with the ST group, partially related to the less frequent use of a tracheostomy tube with an inner and outer cannula that facilitates nursing [10]. In the UK, more than half of the ICUs routinely use tracheostomy tubes with inner liners [12]. Considering these situations, revision of the current protocol is underway to define the proper tracheostomy tube either for ST or PDT in our institution. Although several revisions might be necessary after assessment of long-term outcomes [9, 10], our current system could be one of the practical references to build an ideal collaborative multidisciplinary team for successful airway management in the future.

Conclusions

PDT's entry into the airway management field allowed the non-surgeons to perform the tracheostomy in selected cases, and the cooperative multidisciplinary teams' approach is indispensable for successful tracheostomy at present. We have established an original tracheostomy protocol to clarify the respective role and responsibility of each participant at each of the sequential decisions required for smooth procedure with minimal risk. We believe our current protocol could be one practical reference as a system to enable the safe and harmonious multidisciplinary airway management. Future assessments and revisions of our current protocol are warranted.

Acknowledgement

We would like to thank Drs. Hideki Naganishi, Koji Inagaki, Yuko Takiuchi, and Hiromasa Nagata for their efforts to build our collaborative system successfully. We are also grateful to Dr. Reiko Watanabe for her helpful advice in making this work a success.

References

1. Jackson C (1909) Tracheostomy. Laryngoscope 19: 285-290.

2. Shelden CH, Pudenz RH, Freshwater DB, Crue BL (1955) A new method for tracheotomy. J Neurosurg 12: 428-431.

3. Ciaglia P, Firsching R, Syniec C (1985) Elective percutaneous dilatational tracheostomy. A new simple bedside procedure; preliminary report. Chest 87: 715-719.

4. Griggs WM, Worthley LI, Gilligan JE, Thomas PD, Myburg JA (1990) A simple percutaneous tracheostomy technique. SurgGynecolObstet 170: 543-545.

5. Byhahn C, Lischke V, Halbig S, Scheifler G, Westphal K (2000) [Ciaglia blue rhino: a modified technique for percutaneous dilatation tracheostomy. Technique and early clinical results]. Anaesthesist 49: 202-206.

6. Cabrini L, Monti G, Landoni G, Biondi-Zoccai G, Boroli F, et al. (2012) Percutaneous tracheostomy, a systematic review. ActaAnaesthesiolScand 56: 270-281.

7. Cheng E, Fee WE Jr (2000) Dilatational versus standard tracheostomy: a meta-analysis. Ann OtolRhinolLaryngol 109: 803-807.

8. Freeman BD, Isabella K, Lin N, Buchman TG (2000) A meta-analysis of prospective trials comparing percutaneous and surgical tracheostomy in critically ill patients. Chest 118: 1412-1418.

9. Delaney A, Bagshaw SM, Nalos M (2006) Percutaneous dilatational tracheostomy versus surgical tracheostomy in critically ill patients: a systematic review and meta-analysis. Crit Care 10: R55.

10. Higgins KM, Punthakee X (2007) Meta-analysis comparison of open versus percutaneous tracheostomy. Laryngoscope 117: 447-454.

11. Kluge S, Baumann HJ, Maier C, Klose H, Meyer A, et al. (2008) Tracheostomy in the intensive care unit: a nationwide survey. AnesthAnalg 107: 1639-1643.

12. Veenith T, Ganeshamoorthy S, Standley T, Carter J, Young P (2008) Intensive care unit tracheostomy: a snapshot of UK practice. Int Arch Med 1: 21.

13. Saito K, Morisaki H (2013) Percutaneous dilatational tracheostomy: collaborative team approach for safe airway management. J Anesth 27: 161-165.

14. Polderman KH, Spijkstra JJ, de Bree R, Wester JP, Christiaans HM, et al. (2001) Percutaneous tracheostomy in the intensive care unit: which safety precautions? Crit Care Med 29: 221-223.

15. Blankenship DR, Gourin CG, Davis WB, Blanchard AR, Seybt MW, et al. (2004) Percutaneous tracheostomy: don't beat them, join them. Laryngoscope 114: 1517-1521.

16. Griffiths J, Barber VS, Morgan L, Young JD (2005) Systematic review and meta-analysis of studies of the timing of tracheostomy in adult patients undergoing artificial ventilation. BMJ 330: 1243.

17. Toursarkissian B, Fowler CL, Zweng TN, Kearney PA (1994) Percutaneous dilational tracheostomy in children and teenagers. J PediatrSurg 29: 1421-1424.

18. Ben-Nun A, Altman E, Best LA (2004) Emergency percutaneous tracheostomy in trauma patients: an early experience. Ann ThoracSurg 77: 1045-1047.

19. Kost KM (2005) Endoscopic percutaneous dilatational tracheotomy: a prospective evaluation of 500 consecutive cases. Laryngoscope 115: 1-30.

15

Role of Neck Dissection in Locoregionally Advanced Head and Neck Cancer Treated with Primary Chemoradiotherapy

Martin M, García J*, Lopez M, Hinojar A, Manzanares R, Fernandez L, Prada J and Cerezo L

Hospital Universitario de La Princesa, Madrid, Spain

Abstract

Introduction: Planned neck dissection after chemoradiotherapy (CRT) in locoregionally advanced head and neck cancer is controversial. The objective of the present study was to evaluate the influence of neck dissection on the long-term locoregional control and survival of patients with stage III-IV head and neck squamous cell carcinoma (HNSCC) after primary CRT.

Methods/patients: We retrospectively analysed locoregional control, locoregional relapse-free survival (LRFS), and overall survival (OS) in 67 patients with locally-advanced HNSCC treated with exclusive CRT at our department between January 1998 and December 2013.

Results: Complete clinical response was achieved in 36 of 67 patients (53.7%), partial response $\geq$ 50% in 17 pts (25.4%), stable disease in 3 (4.5%); 9 patients (13.4%) developed disease progression during treatment. At a median follow-up of 35 months, LRFS and OS were 100% in patients with complete response and neck dissection versus 77.9% and 79.8%, respectively, in patients who did not undergo neck dissection (p = ns). The only independent prognostic factor for locoregional control was complete response to CRT.

Conclusions: Patients who achieve a complete clinical response to CRT have a very low risk of isolated neck recurrence and, therefore, planned neck dissection may not be justified in such cases. Clinical and radiographic identification of patients with residual disease following CRT who could benefit from neck dissection remains challenging.

Keywords: Carcinoma; Squamous cell of head and neck; Chemoradiotherapy; Neck dissection; Neoplasm recurrence local

Introduction

Concomitant chemoradiotherapy (CRT) is one of the pillars of organ preservation in the treatment of advanced tumours of the head and neck. However, the need to perform neck dissection (ND) in patients with complete clinical and radiological response remains controversial. While some authors support cervical dissection to improve control in patients with N2 - N3 disease, other authors and centres do not routinely perform ND after CRT in those patients.

The main argument for systematic ND is the premise that this procedure reduces the risk of recurrence in patients with large pre-treatment adenopathies and that any recurrence treated with salvage surgery in such patients will have a small likelihood of success. A review of the published literature reveals that the percentage of patients who achieve a complete clinical response in the neck after CRT varies widely, although the mean response rate is approximately 56%. In a phase II study carried out by Homma et al. in 41 patients with N2 disease, neck disease was successfully controlled by CRT in 44% of patients [1]. McHam et al. reviewed 109 patients with N2-N3 disease treated by CRT and found that neck disease was successfully controlled by CRT in 74% of patients [2]. Published reports indicate that patients who present complete clinical or radiographic response have a 20-30% incidence of pathologic disease at the time of dissection. Stenson et al. reported complete pathological response in 75% and 50%, respectively, of patients with N2 and N3 disease who underwent ND within 5-17 weeks after intensive concurrent CRT [3]. Although surgery can benefit some patients, it is worth noting that ND can contribute to morbidity

in terms of pain and shoulder disability, with significant complications reported in 26% of patients. In studies that have evaluated the clinical (but not radiological) response of lymph nodes to treatment, the percentage of salvage cervical dissections with pathologic positivity is higher. It is also important to note that pathologic positivity does not necessarily translate into a subsequent neck failure, particularly when ND is performed early (2-6 weeks) after completion of CRT when tumour cell viability in pathologic specimens is uncertain. In 27 patients with complete clinical/radiologic response, Brizel et al. found a 26% pathologic positivity rate but a neck failure rate of only 4% [4]. Argiris et al. reported that 39% of patients with complete response after CRT harboured residual tumours in elective ND specimens, even though only 7% of patients with complete response (CR) who did not undergo ND experienced a neck recurrence; these authors concluded that, in the majority of cases, microscopic residual disease indicates nonviable tumours [5]. In a 2008 study carried out by our group, we reported a 100% control rate in 28 node-positive patients who presented a CR after radical treatment and did not undergo ND [6]. Given the context described above particularly the risk of significant morbidity associated with neck dissection and the fact that only a small percentage of patients with residual disease will go on to develop a recurrence our team has long preferred to take a wait-and-see approach in patients with complete nodal response to CRT, irrespective of the initial extent of nodal disease. However, the optimal treatment approach to patients with stage III-IV head and neck squamous cell carcinoma (HNSCC) after primary CRT remains unclear. For this reason, we carried out the

---

*Corresponding author: García J, Otolaryngologist, Hospital Universitario de La Princesa, Madrid, Spain; E-mail: jesuscultivos@hotmail.com

present study to evaluate the influence of ND on long-term locoregional control and survival in this patient population.

Patients and Methods

We retrospectively reviewed the medical records of patients with squamous cell carcinoma of the oropharynx, hypopharynx, larynx, and oral cavity who received definitive radiotherapy at our institution (University Hospital La Princesa in Madrid, Spain) between January 1998 and December 2013. Patients who underwent ND or lymphadenectomy before radiation were excluded. Inclusion criteria were as follows: histologically-proven squamous cell carcinoma, tumour stage III/IV, ECOG 0-2 with normal renal and bone marrow function, absence of distant metastases, and treatment with curative intent. Variables evaluated included locoregional control, locoregional relapse-free survival (LRFS), and overall survival (OS).

Treatment modalities

Most of the patients in this study were treated with three-dimensional conformal radiotherapy (3D-CRT), although in recent years intensity-modulated radiotherapy (IMRT) with sliding dynamic multileaf collimators was used. Computed tomography (CT)-based treatment planning was used for all patients. The gross tumour volume (GTV) encompassed the primary tumour and involved lymph nodes, and the clinical target volume (CTV) consisted of the GTV with a standard margin of 1 cm that was adjusted to account for natural barriers to tumour spread and nodal areas at high risk of containing microscopic disease. CTV margins were expanded by 3 mm to form the planning target volumes (PTV). The high-dose PTV received a total dose of 66 Gy in 30 fractions using IMRT or 70 Gy in 35 fractions using 3D-CRT. Platinum based chemotherapy or Cetuximab was administered in various treatment schemes to all patients.

Response assessment and follow up

Staging procedures included clinical examination, endoscopy/laryngoscopy, contrast-enhanced neck CT or MRI and chest CT or X-ray. Eight weeks after completion of CRT, patients underwent a clinical examination/upper endoscopy and neck CT scan. Complete response was defined as no palpable tumour on physical examination, no evidence of local disease on radiographic examination, and no nodes > 1.5 cm and no nodes with irregular enhancement, round shape or a necrotic centre. In the event that any clinical or radiological abnormalities were found, patients were examined under anaesthesia and biopsies were performed. Our general policy was not to dissect the neck in patients with CR. However, the multidisciplinary team responsible for the patient made the final decision regarding whether to perform ND or not. Subsequently, patients were followed up with physical examination, and flexible endoscopy every 6-8 weeks in the first year after treatment, every 3 months for an additional 2 years, every six months for 5 years, and every year until final discharge at 10 years.

Statistical methods

All time-to-failure end points were calculated from the day of the final radiotherapy treatment. All-cause deaths are included in the overall survival estimates. Differences in locoregional control were tested by the Pearson chi-square test. Actuarial estimates for overall and disease-free survival were calculated by the Kaplan-Meier method and compared with the long-rank test. Cox's proportional hazard model was used for multivariate analysis to assess the effect of patient characteristics and other prognostic factors of significance on the end

points. Statistical significance was considered p<0.05. All statistical tests were performed using SPSS v.15 (Inc., Chicago, IL, USA).

Results

Treatment modalities

The study cohort comprised a total of 67 patients with a median follow up of 35 months. Patient and disease characteristics are detailed in Table 1. In 63 patients, 3D-CRT was administered to the primary tumour and involved nodes at a mean dose of 68 Gy (range 60-74 Gy) with 50 Gy to the elective nodal area. The remaining 4 patients received IMRT with concomitant boost technique in 30 fractions for a total of 66 Gy to the primary tumour and involved nodes and 54 Gy to the elective nodal area. The chemotherapy sequence was neoadjuvant taxol, platin, and 5-fluorouracil (TPF) followed by cetuximab in 1 patient and concurrent CRT in 66. Various chemotherapy regimens were administered, as follows: cisplatin, 75 mg/m^2 every 21 days (45 patients); the same cisplatin regimen plus tirapazamine (6 patients); cisplatin with 5-fluorouracil (2 patients); cetuximab 200 mg/m^2

Characteristics	N (%)
Gender	
Male	59 (88,1)
Female	8(11,9)
Smoker	
yes	64(95,5)
No	3 (4,5%)
ECOG	
0	41(61,2%)
1	25(37,3)
2	1(1,5%)
Primary site	
Oropharynx	41(62,7%)
Larynx	14 (20,9%)
Hipopharynx	11 (16,4%)
Oral cavity	1(1,5%)
T	
1	5 (7,5%)
2	11 (16,4%)
3	33 (49,3%)
4	18 (27%)
N	
1	13 (19,4%)
2a	8(11,9%)
2b	17 (25,4%)
2c	20 (29,9%)
3	9 (13,4%)
Estadio	
III	17 (25,4%)
IVa	41 (61,2%)
IVb	9 (13,4%)
Chemotherapy	
Cisplatin	45(67%)
Cetuximab	10(15%)
Cisplatin-Tirapazamine	6(9%)
Cisplatin-Panitumumab	2(3%)
Cisplatin-5FU	2(3%)
Cisplatin intra arterial	1(1,5%)
TPF-Cetuximab	1(1,5%)
Radiotherapy	69,3 Gy (64-74)

Table 1: Patients and treatment characteristics.

weekly (10 patients); cisplatin with panitumumab (2 patients); and intraarterial-cisplatin in 1 patient.

Treatment response

After completion of CRT, patients were evaluated by superior panendoscope and CT after a median of 65 days. Complete response was defined as no palpable tumour on physical examination, no evidence of local disease on radiographic examination, and no nodes >1.5 cm or with irregular enhancement, round shape or a necrotic centre, partial response as tumor reduction >50%, and stable disease as not tumor change. Complete clinical and radiological response was achieved in 36 of 67 patients (53.7%), partial response, in 17 cases (25.4%), and stable disease in 3 (4.5%). Nine patients (13.4%) experienced disease progression during treatment and were excluded from the univariate and multivariate analysis. The decision to perform ND or not was individualized and influenced by comorbidities, treatment toxicity, unresectable/progressive disease or personal patient preferences; nevertheless, radiological response to CRT highly influenced this decision. ND was performed in 5 of the 36 patients with complete response and in 11 of 20 with partial response or stable disease (p= 0.058). Most patients who underwent ND received modified radical treatment. The median time from completion of CRT to neck dissection was 107 days. None of the 5 patients with complete response had evidence of residual disease in the pathological specimens. In contrast, 6 of 11 patients with partial or no response harboured viable tumour cells in the resected specimens.

Nodal control

In the 36 patients with complete radiological response after CRT, 8 patients developed a recurrence, as follows: at the primary tumour site and lymph nodes (2 cases); the primary site alone (3 cases); bilateral nodal recurrence (1 case), and distant relapse (2 cases). No isolated homolateral regional recurrences were observed. No relapses were observed in the 5 patients with complete radiological response and ND. The actuarial 3-year LRFS rate was 100% for patients who underwent ND vs. 77.9% without ND (p = 0.22). OS was 100% for patients with ND vs. 79.8% for those who did not undergo ND, although this difference was not significant (p = 0.26) (Figures 1A and 1B). In the 20 patients with partial response or stable disease, 7 recurrences were recorded: 4 at the primary site and regionally; 2 at the primary site alone; and 1 case of distant recurrence. Of those 7 patients, 4 had undergone ND. The 3-year LRFS for patients with and without ND was 68.2% and 19.2%, respectively, while the corresponding OS rate was 54.5% vs 27.3% (p = 0.045) (Figures 2A and 2B). We evaluated the following to identify prognostic factors for locoregional control (Table 2): age, gender, primary tumour site, T/N classification, and CT response. On univariate analysis, only complete radiological response to chemotherapy was associated with better disease control (88.4% vs 55.9% p = 0.001). On multivariate analysis, complete response to chemotherapy was the only independent prognostic factor for locoregional control (Table 3).

Discussion

The present report is an update to our previous paper on the clinical outcomes of patients with node-positive HNSCC treated with definitive CRT [6]. Our present results confirm that high rates of nodal control can be achieved in selected patients (based on response to CRT) without the need to perform neck dissection. In patients with advanced N2-N3 disease, the benefits of elective post-radiotherapy ND regardless of the clinical response is still under debate. Authors who support neck dissection affirm that there are no definite criteria for complete nodal

response, and complete radiological response correlates poorly with pathological response. Some studies have defined complete response as "no evidence of disease". Nevertheless, assessing neck disease after CRT presents many difficulties and, moreover, the z criteria to determine what constitutes residual adenopathy have evolved over time [7-10]. According to the definition of response evaluation criteria in solid tumours (RECIST), nodes that shrink to <10mm on the short axis are considered normal [11]. However, some of the studies that have evaluated neck response after definitive CRT used criteria of <1 cm or ≤ 1.5 cm for maximum diameter without any focal abnormality [8,12]. In our study, we used the same criteria used by the University of Florida Health Science Center [12]. These criteria consider clinical and radiological response to be complete if there is no evidence of clinical

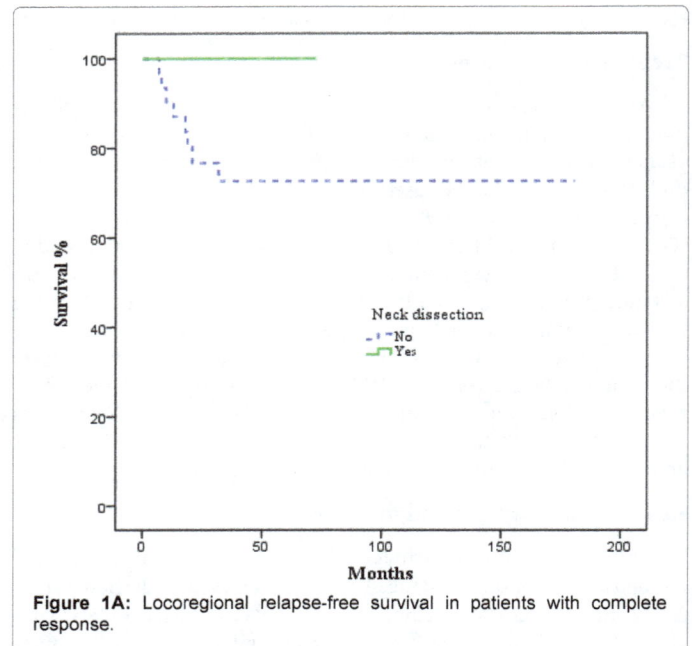

Figure 1A: Locoregional relapse-free survival in patients with complete response.

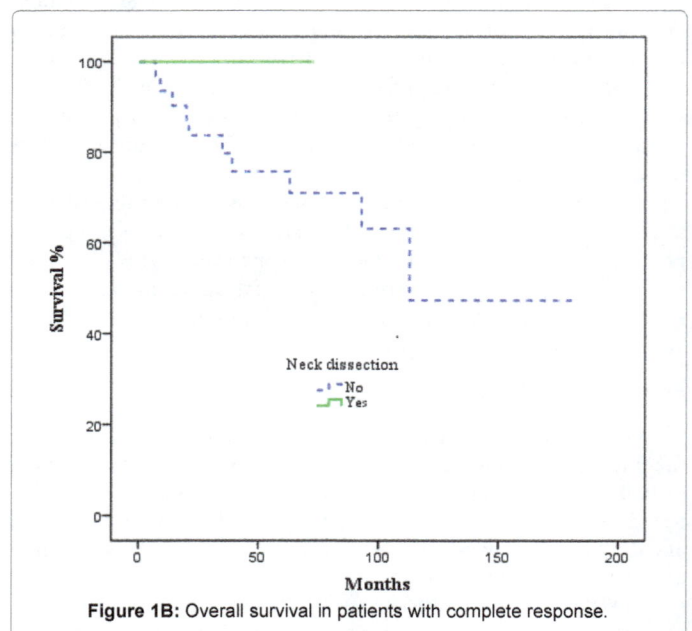

Figure 1B: Overall survival in patients with complete response.

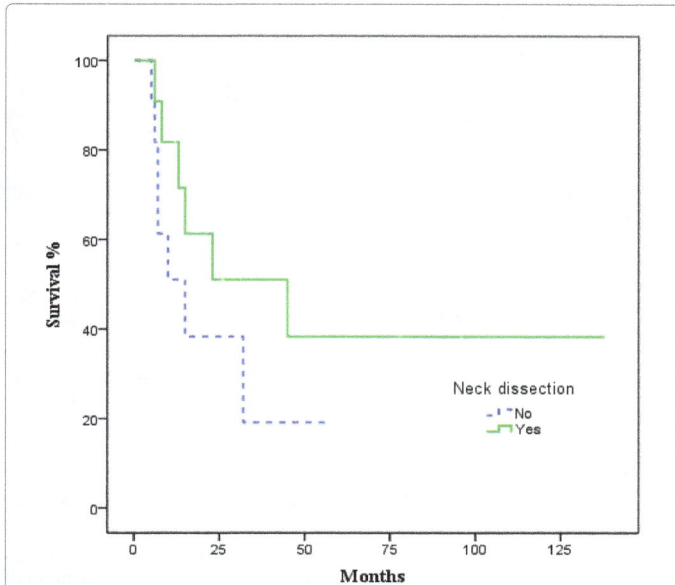

Figure 2A: Locoregional free survival in patients with partial response or stable disease.

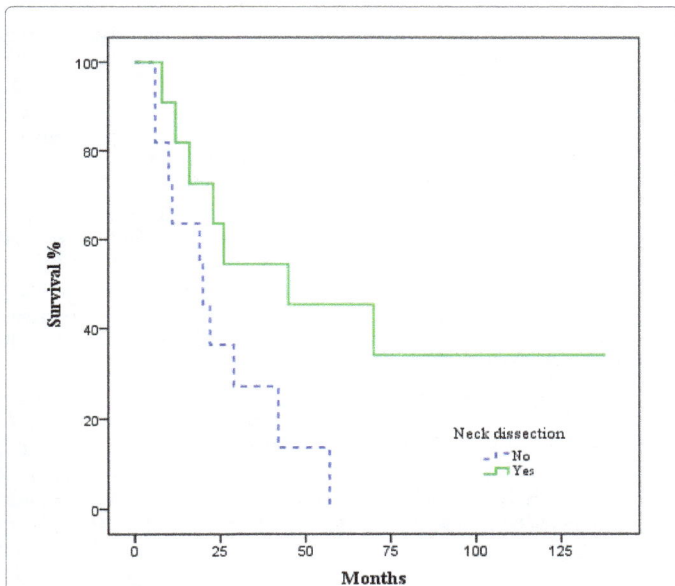

Figure 2B: Overall survival in patients with partial response or stable disease.

disease in the panendoscope and residual visualised nodes in CT are ≤ 1.5 cm in the short axis without irregular enhancement, round shape or necrotic centre.

The other point of controversy is that approximately 25% of patients with complete radiological response do not have complete pathological response [4,9]. According to some reports, the risk for residual tumour in ND specimens after CRT increases with initial cN-stage regardless of the clinical response. For example, in one series of 73 patients reported by Stenson et al. the risk for viable tumour cells in patients who had post-radiotherapy ND increased from 12% for initial N2b to 20% for N2c to 30% for N3[3]; rates up to 30-50%, have been reported for N3 [2,3]. Based on these pathological results, Stenson et al. concluded that,

in patients with ≥ N2 disease after CRT, ND is necessary to eradicate residual disease. In our case, we did not find any residual disease in the pathological specimens from five patients with radiological CR. A relatively new imaging technique-[18F]-fluorodeoxyglucose positron emission tomography (FDG-PET)-has proven to be highly accurate in the detection of persistent and recurrent disease in HNSCC patients, with a low false-negative rate after CRT. In patients with residual lymphadenopathy but negative FDG-PET [10,12,13] it appears reasonable to omit ND. FDG PET was only introduced during the last years of our study and, consequently, we did not assess the results of FDG-PET here. Several studies report beneficial effects of post-radiotherapy ND. Brizel et al. concluded that adjuvant modified ND confer a disease-free and overall survival advantage with acceptably low morbidity; in their study, overall survival was 77% in patients with N2/N3 disease with complete response plus ND compared to only 50% in patients with complete response but without ND [4]. Lavertu et al. found significantly better disease-specific survival in N2-N3 patients with complete response (p = 0.002). Disease-specific survival was not affected by ND (p = 0.40) but was significantly affected by viable tumour in the specimen (p = 0.03) [14]. Notwithstanding the evidence presented above, recent data provides support for the position that the strategy of planned ND is no longer justified in patients without clinically residual disease in the neck after CRT. More effective CRT regimens, together with improvements in response assessment, have

Variable	Locoregional control	p value
Age		
>60	68%	
<60	75,8	0,51
Gender		
Male	74%	
Female	62,5%	P:0,4
Primary site		
Hypopharynx	88,9%	
Larynx	76,9%	
Oropharynx	68,6%	
Oral cavity	0%	P:0,2
T		
T1-2	85,7%	
T3-4	68,2%	P:0,2
N		
N1-2a	70%	
N2b-3	73,6%	P:0,7
Response		
Complete	83,3%	
< 50% or stable	50%	P:0,008
Neck dissection		
Yes	81,2%	
No	69%	P:0,3

Table 2: Univariate analysis for locoregional control.

	HR	p value	95,0% IC	
			Inferior	Superior
CT response Others vs Complete	6,102	0,002	1,955	19,052
T stage T3-4 vs T1-2	1,144	0,872	0,224	5836
Primary site Oropharynx vs Others	1,752	0,352	0,537	5,709

Table 3: Multivariate Cox regression model with no locoregional relapse as end point.

further modified the paradigm of planned ND. In fact, both the University of Florida and the University of Chicago have changed their approach and now recommend ND only for patients with residual disease after CRT. The results of their studies showed no difference in outcomes regardless of whether patients underwent ND or not [3,15-17]. Ferlito et al. recently carried out a review of many recently-published studies on this topic. Those authors found that 24 studies indicate that regional control increased due to "planned" ND in patients with pre-treatment bulky neck disease. However, all of those 24 studies were retrospective and did not assess treatment response prior to surgery, although regional control rates were very good. In contrast, the same authors found that 26 other studies demonstrated no benefit from "planned" ND after complete clinical response. Based on their review, the authors concluded that there is now a large body of evidence based on long-term clinical outcomes that patients who have achieved a complete clinical (including radiologic) response to CRT have a low rate of isolated neck failure, and, therefore, the continued use of planned ND for these patients cannot be justified [18]. A retrospective study of 880 patients carried out by Thariat et al. confirmed these findings: those authors found no significant differences in regional control with or without neck dissection. Moreover, given the 92% 5-year neck control rate without ND after chemotherapy, there seems to be little justification for systematic neck dissection [19]. In our study, we found that the most important factor for locoregional control is radiological response rather than the pre-treatment nodal stage. None of our patients with complete response and without ND presented isolated homolateral nodal relapse during follow up. Consequently, we agree with the conclusions made by Thariat et al. and Ferlito et al. However, we found that-in line with Thariat et al. [19,20]. Our patients who did not exhibit complete response after CRT had significant better regional control and overall survival with ND. For this reason, in such patients, neck dissection remains a recommended treatment.

Conclusion

Patients who achieve a complete clinical response to CRT, regardless of initial nodal stage, have a very low risk of an isolated neck recurrence and such patients can be spared from planned ND. In order to better identify patients with residual anatomical abnormalities who do not harbour viable tumour cells, it will first be necessary to achieve a consensus regarding the definition of "complete response". This new definition will require the integration of newer, more sophisticated imaging techniques. In patients with residual viable tumour cells, neck dissection appears to significantly improve overall survival.

References

1. Homma A, Furuta Y, Oridate N, Suzuki F, Higuchi E, et al. (2006) "Watch-and-see" policy for the clinically positive neck in head and neck cancer treated with chemoradiotherapy. Int J Clin Oncol 11: 441-448.

2. McHam SA, Adelstein DJ, Rybicki LA, Lavertu P, Esclamado RM, et al. (2003) Who merits a neck dissection after definitive chemoradiotherapy for N2-N3 squamous cell head and neck cancer? Head Neck 25: 791-798.

3. Stenson KM, Haraf DJ, Pelzer H, Recant W, Kies MS, et al. (2000) The role of cervical lymphadenectomy after aggressive concomitant chemoradiotherapy: the feasibility of selective neck dissection. Arch Otolaryngol Head Neck Surg 126: 950-956.

4. Brizel DM, Prosnitz RG, Hunter S, Fisher SR, Clough RL, et al. (2004) Necessity for adjuvant neck dissection in setting of concurrent chemoradiation for advanced head-and-neck cancer. Int J Radiat Oncol Biol Phys 58: 1418-1423.

5. Argiris A, Stenson KM, Brockstein BE, Mittal BB, Pelzer H, et al. (2004) Neck dissection in the combined-modality therapy of patients with locoregionally advanced head and neck cancer. Head Neck 26: 447-455.

6. Lopez R M, Cerezo P L, Martin M M, Counago L F (2008) Neck dissection after radiochemotherapy in patients with locoregionally advanced head and neck cancer. Clin Transl Oncol 10: 812-816.

7. Chan AW, Ancukiewicz M, Carballo N, Montgomery W, Wang CC (2001) The role of postradiotherapy neck dissection in supraglottic carcinoma. Int J Radiat Oncol Biol Phys 50: 367-375.

8. Corry J, Peters L, Fisher R, Macann A, Jackson M, et al. (2008) N2-N3 neck nodal control without planned neck dissection for clinical/radiologic complete responders-results of Trans Tasman Radiation Oncology Group Study 98.02. Head Neck 30: 737-742.

9. Goguen LA, Posner MR, Tishler RB, Wirth LJ, Norris CM, et al. (2006) Examining the need for neck dissection in the era of chemoradiation therapy for advanced head and neck cancer. Arch Otolaryngol Head Neck Surg 132: 526-531.

10. Eisenhauer EA, Therasse P, Bogaerts J, Schwartz LH, Sargent D, et al. (2009) New response evaluation criteria in solid tumours: revised RECIST guideline (version 1.1). Eur J Cancer 45: 228-247.

11. Liauw SL, Mancuso AA, Amdur RJ, Morris CG, Villaret DB, et al. (2006) Postradiotherapy neck dissection for lymph node-positive head and neck cancer: the use of computed tomography to manage the neck. J Clin Oncol 24: 1421-1427.

12. Stenson KM, Huo D, Blair E, Cohen EE, Argiris A, et al. (2006) Planned post-chemoradiation neck dissection: significance of radiation dose. Laryngoscope 116: 33-36.

13. Chen AM, Khodayari B, Daly ME, Farwell G, Luu Q, et al. (2013) Observation Versus Neck Dissection for Residual, PET-Negative Lymphadenopathy After Chemoradiotherapy for Head-and-Neck Cancer. Pract Radiat Oncol 3: S5.

14. Khodayari B, Daly ME, Bobinski M, Farwell DG, Shelton DK, et al. (2014) Observation versus neck dissection for positron-emission tomography-negative lymphadenopathy after chemoradiotherapy. Laryngoscope 124: 902-906.

15. Yao M, Luo P, Hoffman HT, Chang K, Graham MM, et al. (2007) Pathology and FDG PET correlation of residual lymph nodes in head and neck cancer after radiation treatment. Am J Clin Oncol 30: 264-270.

16. Lavertu P, Adelstein DJ, Saxton JP, Secic M, Wanamaker JR, et al. (1997) Management of the neck in a randomized trial comparing concurrent chemotherapy and radiotherapy with radiotherapy alone in resectable stage III and IV squamous cell head and neck cancer. Head Neck19: 559-566.

17. Mendenhall WM, Million RR, Cassisi NJ (1986) Squamous cell carcinoma of the head and neck treated with radiation therapy: the role of neck dissection for clinically positive neck nodes. Int J Radiat Oncol Biol Phys 12: 733-740.

18. Langerman A, Plein C, Vokes EE, Salama JK, Haraf DJ, et al. (2009) Neck response to chemoradiotherapy: complete radiographic response correlates with pathologic complete response in locoregionally advanced head and neck cancer. Arch Otolaryngol Head Neck Surg 135: 1133-1136.

19. Ferlito A, Corry J, Silver CE, Shaha AR, Thomas Robbins K, et al. (2010) Planned neck dissection for patients with complete response to chemoradiotherapy: a concept approaching obsolescence. Head Neck 32: 253-261.

20. Thariat J, Ang KK, Allen PK, Ahamad A, Williams MD, et al. (2012) Prediction of neck dissection requirement after definitive radiotherapy for head-and-neck squamous cell carcinoma. Int J Radiat Oncol Biol Phys 82: e367-374.

16

High-Resolution ENT Video Endoscope with Superior Image Quality Equivalent to that of Gastric Video Endoscopes

Atsunobu Tsunoda*, Koichi Tsunoda, Takuro Sumi, Seiji Kishimoto and Ken Kitamura

Department of Otolaryngology and Head and Neck Surgery, Tokyo Medical and Dental University, Japan

Abstract

Background and study aims: To assess the usability of high resolution fiberscope which has equivalent image quality to that of the esophageal and gastric video endoscopes

Patients and methods: Image resolution of this endoscope was estimated by the United States Air Force (USAF) resolution test chart. Clinical application was done between January and December 2010 and transnasal observation of the larynx and hypopharynx were performed during this period. These examinations were done for screening and follow-up for patients with hypopharyngeal and laryngeal disorders.

Results: This endoscope could distinguish features on a scale of nearly 20 μm, and abnormal vascular patterns on the mucosal surface characteristic of carcinomas were clearly observed under a conventional light source. In addition, these changes on the mucosal surface became more apparent with use of the i-SCAN®. Nevertheless, the handling of this video endoscope was similar to that of popular ENT video endoscopes, and all patients tolerated its use well.

Conclusion: This new device may dramatically improve pharyngolaryngeal examination in ENT clinics.

Keywords: Early diagnosis; Intraepithelial papillary capillary loops; Narrow-band imaging; Video endoscope

Introduction

At present, esophageal cancer can be detected at an early stage by observing characteristic vascular abnormalities such as abnormal Intraepithelial Papillary Capillary Loops (IPCLs) [1-4]. Pharyngeal carcinoma has been detected in the same manner, and carcinomas of the head and neck can be detected early with the use of video endoscopes in the upper gastrointestinal tract [5-8]. However, anatomical restrictions limit the size of the Charge-Coupled Device (CCD) used in video endoscopes. ENT video endoscopes with Narrow Band Imaging (NBI) are also reported to be useful in the detection of such vascular abnormalities; however, their image quality is lower compared to that of gastric video endoscopes [5]. The transnasal gastric video endoscope is much smaller and is becoming popular with clinicians. However, this scope t is designed for gastric observation; its handling is not suitable for observations in the ENT field. In addition, the image quality is not comparable to that of commonly used oral gastric video endoscopes. In this article, we report our experience using a new video endoscope with image quality equivalent to that of the latest gastric video endoscopes.

Materials and Methods

An ENT (ear nose throat) video endoscope (Pentax® VNL-1590 STi; Hoya Co., Ltd.; Tokyo, Japan) was used for this study. Its diameter was relatively large; the tip and middle diameters are φ 5.6 and 5.1, respectively. However, its radius of curvature was nearly the same as that of a general ENT fiberscope (Figure 1a and b). Both the diameter and radius of curvature were much smaller than those of gastric video endoscopes. The size of the CCD was nearly equivalent to that of the latest gastric video endoscopes. The focal length was slightly closer to the lens—the minimum distance was 3 mm-thus allowing for precise examination of the mucosa. Image resolution was estimated by the

United States Air Force (USAF) resolution test chart.

The development of this endoscopic system began from 2007. We started using this video endoscope in our office clinic in August 2009 after minor modifications and adjustments were made to it. Final specifications were decided in late 2009. Between January and December 2010, we observed the larynx and hypopharynx using this

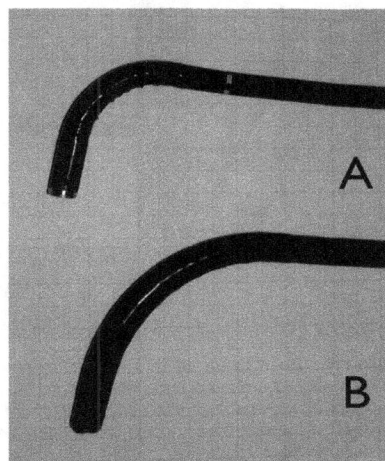

Figure 1: VNL-1590 STi (A diameter: 5.1 mm) and trans-nasal gastric endoscope (B: diameter: 5.9 mm). The VNL-1590 STi has smaller radius of curvature and is suitable for observation of pharynx and larynx.

*Corresponding author: Atsunobu Tsunoda, MD, Department of Otolaryngology and Head and Neck Surgery, Tokyo Medical and Dental University, Bunkyo-ku, Yushima 1-5-45, Tokyo 113-8519, Japan; E-mail: atsunoda@mac.com

scope. Prior to examination, all patients underwent application of nasal spray with adrenalin and lidocaine. All examinations were recorded as digital video throughout the procedure. The study protocol complied with the Declaration of Helsinki and the Institutional Review Board (Tokyo Medical and Dental University No 401). No financial supports were given to this study.

Results

This endoscope could distinguish at least 32 line pairs/mm on a USAF chart; hence, it could distinguish a line of at least 16 μm in width (Figure 2). Between January and December 2010, transnasal observation of the larynx and hypopharynx using this scope were performed 356 times during this period. Due to severe nasal deviation, one patient required the application of gauze soaked with adrenalin and lidocaine to the nasal cavity. Other patients safely underwent examination after nasal pretreatment, that is, no major side effects such as epistaxis were noted. Image quality was much better than that of general ENT video endoscopes (Figures 3 and 4). This video endoscope has an image modification function (i-Scan®), and all lesions, including vascular structures, were more clearly observed using this function (Figure 4). Abnormal IPCLs that appeared on the surface of carcinomas were directly and easily observed with the VNL-1590 STi.

Discussion

Several diagnostic techniques related to vascular abnormalities seen in cases of carcinoma have been reported. In particular, abnormal IPCLs have been reported as an early finding in esophageal and pharyngeal carcinomas [1-4]. Magnifying endoscopy coupled with NBI has been reported to be useful for detecting IPCLs [3,4]. With the use of these superior video endoscopes, hypopharyngeal as well as mesopharyngeal carcinomas were detected during diagnostic examinations for esophageal and gastric diseases by gastroenterologists

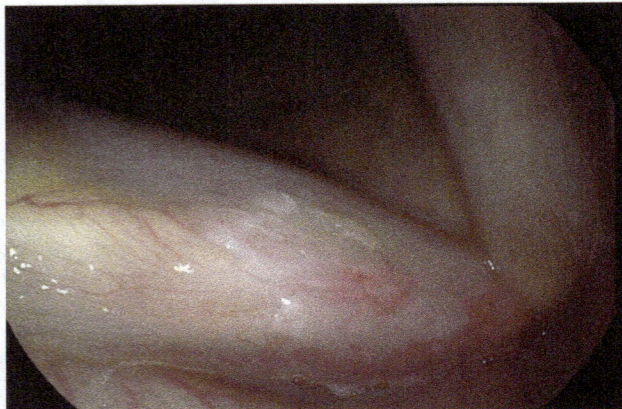

Figure 3: This image from a 76-year-old man shows a thin keratotic lesion involving a major portion of the right vocal cord. This lesion was pathologically diagnosed as parakeratosis. Fine blood vessels under the leukoplakic area are clearly depicted with the VNL-1590 STi.

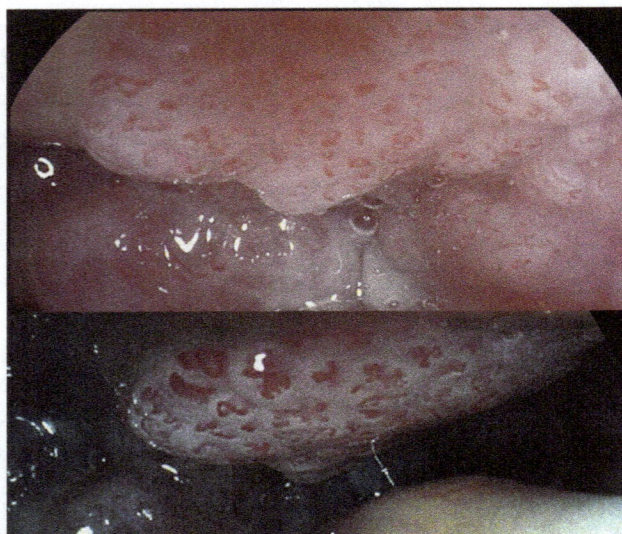

Figure 4: Images from a 66-year-old man with a hypopharyngeal carcinoma. Vascular changes such as abnormal IPCLs were observed in the left pyriform sinus on both the normal image (upper) and the i-SCAN® image (lower) obtained using the VNL-1590 STi.

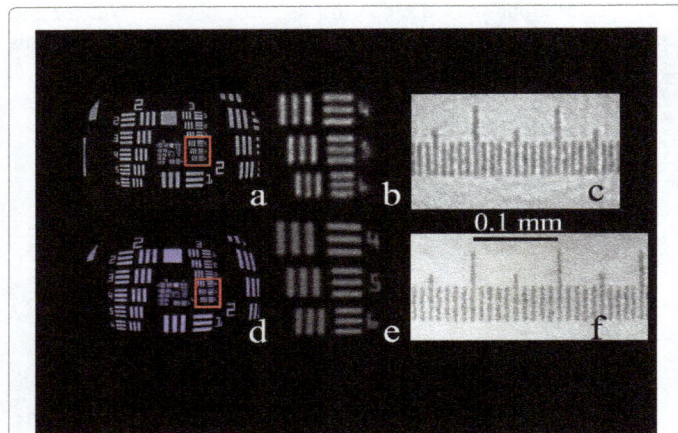

Figure 2: Estimation of resolution by USAF chart. Various sized white bars are spaced in a line at regular intervals equivalent to the width of a bar. The chart is consisted from 6 "Groups" and each group has 6 "Elements" which have thee vertical and horizontal bars. Size of bars gradually shrinks from Group 2, Element 2 to Group 5 Element 6 in this figure. Figure 2a shows an image obtained using a general ENT video endoscope, Figure 2c shows and image obtained using theVNL-1590 STi, Figure 2b and 2d show observation inside the frame: Group 3, Element 4 to 6. Compared to the conventional video endoscope, the VNL-1590 STi more clearly depicts these bars. Figure 2e (dotted frame) and 2f (dotted oval frame) are images of Group 4 and 5, respectively, on the USAF chart. The VNL-1590 STi can distinguish between 32 (line width = 16 μm) and 36 (line width = 14 μm) vertical line within 1 mm (Group 5, Element 1 and 2) and horizontal line pars of 22.62 (22 μm; Group 4, Element 4).

and surgeons [7]. ENT video endoscopes with NBI were also reported to be useful in the detection of such vascular abnormalities. These abnormalities were usually detected with NBI as demarcated brownish areas or scattered brown spots [5].

In the ENT clinic, transnasal examination of patients in a sitting position has several advantages compared to transoral examination with patients in the lateral position [8,9]. Examination in a sitting position is more natural and comfortable for patients. It also enables examination while the patient is performing various tasks or under certain conditions. For example, examinations during swallowing, the Valsalva maneuver, head torsion, and neck flexion enable clear visualization of the fossa of Rosenmuller, the pyriform sinus, and the posterior wall of the hypopharynx, subglottis, and glottic ventricle [10]. Therefore, these techniques are helpful for superior endoscopic examinations. The radius of curvature of the VNL-1590 STi is nearly the same as that of a general ENT video endoscope; therefore, the clinician can easily observe anatomical structures under various conditions that facilitate examination. Nevertheless, the VNL-1590 has higher resolution and can distinguish features on a scale of less than 20 μm. According to the reports of the size of abnormal vasculature in early esophageal carcinoma, the average caliber of an IPCL was 12.9 ± 3.9 μm in m1, 14.5 ± 3.9 μm in m2, and 18.1 ± 5.2 μm in m3 cancer [2]. For cancers that invade the submucosa, the average caliber of the tumor vessels was 26.1 ± 11.6 μm. The resolution of the VNL-1590 STi was nearly equivalent to these abnormal vessels themselves, and these vessels could be directly observed, rather than merely as brownish areas or scattered brown spots.

Some techniques and devices, including the use of dyes (such as iodine) and NBI, have facilitated detection of carcinoma at an early stage [3-7]. However, these procedures or devices require drug administration or a specialized light source. The VNL-1590 STi has an image modification function called i-Scan® that facilitates detection of not only the blood vessels but also other structures such as cartilage and ligaments [11-16]. Image modification is different from NBI and is done instantaneously, and modified images appear natural (Figure 4). However, the image resolution of the VNL-1590 STi is high enough to detect subtle changes on the mucosal surface and very tiny keratotic changes or abnormal IPCLs can be detected with this video endoscope with conventional examination procedures.

Conclusion

Despite its relatively large size, the VNL-1590 STi is easy to handle and can be used for daily clinical examinations. The image quality is excellent and nearly equivalent to that of the latest gastric video endoscopes. It is valuable for pharyngeal and laryngeal examinations in ENT clinics.

References

1. René Lambert (2013) Role of Endoscopy in Screening and Treatment of Gastrointestinal Cancer. J Gastrointest Dig Syst S2: 006.

2. Goda K, Dobashi A, Yoshimura N, Chiba M, Fukuda A, et al. (2013) Clinicopathological features of narrow-band imaging endoscopy and immunohistochemistry in ultraminute esophageal squamous neoplasms. Dis Esophagus.

3. Goda K, Tajiri H, Ikegami M, Yoshida Y, Yoshimura N, et al. (2009) Magnifying endoscopy with narrow band imaging for predicting the invasion depth of superficial esophageal squamous cell carcinoma. Dis Esophagus 22: 453-460.

4. Watanabe A, Tsujie H, Taniguchi M, Hosokawa M, Fujita M, et al. (2006) Laryngoscopic detection of pharyngeal carcinoma in situ with narrowband imaging. Laryngoscope 116: 650-654.

5. Katada C, Nakayama M, Tanabe S, Koizumi W, Masaki T, et al. (2008) Narrow band imaging for detecting metachronous superficial oropharyngeal and hypopharyngeal squamous cell carcinomas after chemoradiotherapy for head and neck cancers. Laryngoscope 118: 1787-1790.

6. Nonaka S, Saito Y (2008) Endoscopic diagnosis of pharyngeal carcinoma by NBI. Endoscopy 40: 347-351.

7. Katada C, Tanabe S, Koizumi W, Higuchi K, Sasaki T, et al. (2010) Narrow band imaging for detecting superficial squamous cell carcinoma of the head and neck in patients with esophageal squamous cell carcinoma. Endoscopy 42: 185-190.

8. Sato K, Nakashima T (2002) Office-based videoendoscopy for the hypopharynx and cervical esophagus. Am J Otolaryngol 23: 341-344.

9. Tsunoda A, Ishihara A, Kishimoto S, Tsunoda R, Tsunoda K (2007) Head torsion technique for detailed observation of larynx and hypopharynx. J Laryngol Otol 121: 489-490.

10. Hoffman A, Basting N, Goetz M, Tresch A, Mudter J, et al. (2009) High-definition endoscopy with i-Scan and Lugol's solution for more precise detection of mucosal breaks in patients with reflux symptoms. Endoscopy 41: 107-112.

11. Atkinson M, Chak A (2010) I-Scan: chromoendoscopy without the hassle? Dig Liver Dis 42: 18-19.

12. Hoffman A, Kagel C, Goetz M, Tresch A, Mudter J, et al. (2010) Recognition and characterization of small colonic neoplasia with high-definition colonoscopy using i-Scan is as precise as chromoendoscopy. Dig Liver Dis 42: 45-50.

13. Hoffman A, Kiesslich R, Goetz M, Tresch A, Mudter J, et al. (2010) High definition colonoscopy combined with i-Scan is superior in the detection of colorectal neoplasias compared with standard video colonoscopy: a prospective randomized controlled trial. Endoscopy 42: 827-833.

14. Dekker E, East JE (2010) Does advanced endoscopic imaging increase the efficacy of surveillance colonoscopy? Endoscopy 42: 866-869.

15. Kodashima S, Fujishiro M (2010) Novel image-enhanced endoscopy with i-scan technology. World J Gastroenterol 16: 1043-1049.

16. Lee CK, Lee SH, Hwangbo Y (2011) Narrow-band imaging versus I-Scan for the real-time histological prediction of diminutive colonic polyps: a prospective comparative study by using the simple unified endoscopic classification. Endoscopy 74-3: 603-609.

17

Locally Advanced Anaplastic Thyroid Carcinoma with Long-Term Survival of More Than 7 Years after Combined Surgery Including Tracheal Resection and Radiotherapy

Wei Zhong Ernest Fu[1]*, Ming Yann Lim[1], Khoon Leong Chuah[2], Khoon Leong Chuah[2] and Li-Chung Mark Khoo[1]

[1]Department of Otolaryngology, Tan Tock Seng Hospital, Singapore
[2]Department of Pathology, Tan Tock Seng Hospital, Singapore

Abstract

We present a case of locally advanced Anaplastic Thyroid Carcinoma (ATC) with tracheal invasion in a 67-year-old elderly Chinese man who was treated with radical surgery encompassing total thyroidectomy, neck dissection and tracheal resection followed by adjuvant radiotherapy. Long-term disease-free survival is more than 7 years to date. A 10-year literature review of locally advanced ATC with long-term survival (more than 2 years) is also presented.

Keywords: Anaplastic thyroid carcinoma; Long term survival; Tracheal invasion

Introduction

Anaplastic thyroid carcinoma (ATC) accounts for about 2% of all thyroid carcinomas and is one of the most aggressive human malignancies [1-4]. In most series, mean survival time from diagnosis is 6 months regardless of treatment [5-13]. Peak incidence is usually more than 60 years of age and it occurs more commonly in females than males. Patients usually present with symptoms of extensive local invasion such as pain, dysphagia, hoarseness, respiratory distress and a rapidly enlarging neck mass.

We present a case of locally advanced ATC with trachea invasion in an elderly male that was treated with radical surgery and adjuvant radiotherapy with long-term disease-free survival of more than 7 years.

Case Report

A 67-year-old Chinese man first presented to us with a left neck mass of 2 months' duration associated with hoarseness and compressive symptoms of 1 month.

He was a previous smoker and had a history of bilateral pulmonary silicosis, having previously worked in a granite quarry for more than 25 years. He has no family history of thyroid disease or previous exposure to irradiation.

On examination, there was a hard 4 cm left thyroid mass that was fixed to the larynx and trachea. There were no palpable cervical nodes. Nasoendoscopy examination revealed left vocal cord paresis in the adducted position. Computed tomography (CT) revealed a left thyroid lesion with possible tracheal invasion (Figure 1). The left vocal fold was abducted. There was no evidence of metastatic cervical lymphadenopathy and systemic review was negative for distant metastasis. Fine-needle aspiration cytology (FNAC) showed features of a high-grade malignant tumour with necrosis favouring an anaplastic carcinoma of the thyroid. Thyroid function tests were normal.

He underwent elective total thyroidectomy, bilateral level 6 neck dissection, and tracheal resection with primary end-to-end anastomosis. There was frank tracheal invasion with gross tumour seen intra-luminally. Frozen section analysis showed a malignant high-grade neoplasm. Surgery was otherwise uneventful and he recovered well post-operatively with no complications. He was discharged well 12 days after surgery.

Final histology showed anaplastic carcinoma of the isthmus and left hemithyroid measuring 5 × 3.7 × 2.5 cm. It was a high-grade neoplasm composed of epithelioid and spindle cells with marked anisonucleosis. Necrosis and mitotic activity including tripolar mitotic figures were present (Figure 2). The tumour had infiltrated posteriorly into the adjacent trachea reaching the connective tissue below the epithelial lining of the trachea and was 2 mm from the closest tracheal margin. No follicular or papillary component was noted despite extensive sampling. On immunohistochemistry, the tumour was positive for cytokeratin AE1/3 but not CD31. A total of 11 level 6 lymph nodes were negative for tumour.

He subsequently underwent adjuvant intensity-modulated

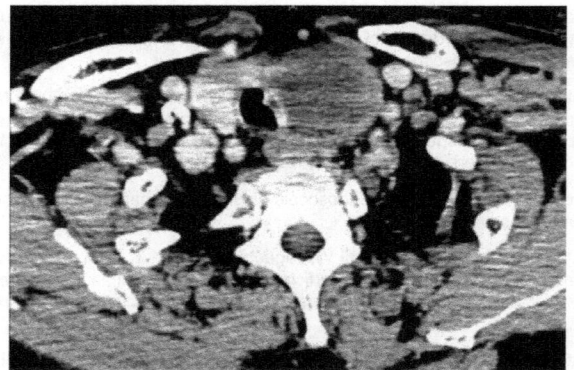

Figure 1: Hypodense left thyroid lesion 4.0 × 3.9 cm causing displacement of the trachea to the right with invasion of left lateral wall of the trachea with a polypoidal enhancing mass of tissue seen protruding into the tracheal lumen.

*Corresponding author: Ernest Fu, Department of Otolaryngology, Tan Tock Seng Hospital, 11 Jalan Tan Tock Seng, Singapore; E-mail: ernest.fu@gmail.com

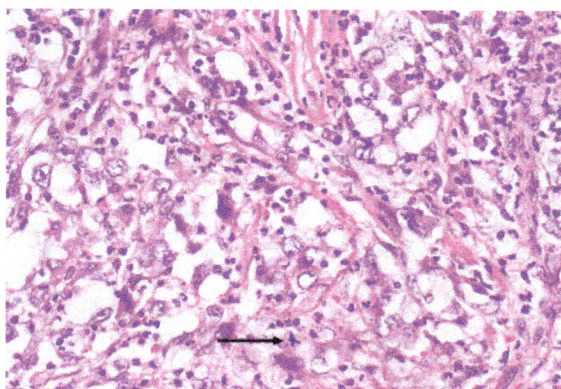

Figure 2: High-powered view of thyroid neoplasm disclosing a proliferation of epithelioid and spindle cells with nuclear pleomorphism amidst a fibrotic background. Note the presence of a tripolar mitotic figure (arrow). (Haematoxylin and eosin stain).

radiation therapy (IMRT) of 66Gy over 33 fractions. He has since been on regular follow-up and to date has been disease-free for more than 7 years. Post-treatment CT scans has showed no evidence of local recurrence or distant metastasis. He is on thyroxine replacement.

Discussion

ATC is one of the most lethal human cancers and to date, the management remains challenging and controversial. Based on the American Thyroid Guidelines on ATC published in 2012 [14], in patients with extra-thyroidal invasion, an en bloc resection should be considered if grossly negative margins (R1 resection) could be achieved.

There have been many studies looking at various prognostic factors affecting survival. Kebebew et al. [5] studied a cohort of 516 patients with ATC wherein multivariate analysis showed that although most patients with ATC had an extremely poor prognosis, patients less than 60 years old with intra-thyroidal tumours survived longer. Surgical resection with external beam radiotherapy was associated with lower cause-specific mortality.

Other studies have variably shown that younger age, tumour size less than 6 cm, localized disease, female gender, and tumour resectability are independent predictors of lower cause-specific mortality [8,15-17]. In particular, complete surgical resection appears to be an important determinant of survival. Haigh et al. [18] reported that the primary factor associated with survival was potential curative surgery. In their study, neither tumour size nor age influenced survival. Kobayashi et al. [19] also observed that complete tumour resection achieved better prognosis and that age did not significantly impact survival.

In contrast to the above findings, Sugitani et al. [9] performed a retrospective analysis of 44 patients with ATC and devised a novel prognostic index (PI) based on four prognostic factors to select patients for aggressive multimodal treatment. The features were the presence of acute symptoms, large tumour size (>5 cm), distant metastasis, and leukocytosis (white blood cell count >10,000/mm³), but notably did not include complete surgical resection. The presence of acute symptoms and large tumour size probably reflect rapid disease progression. Smaller tumour size may correlate with resectability. Patients with distant metastasis inevitably do poorly and the presence of leukocytosis likely represent the late stage of specific subtypes of ATC secreting granulocyte colony-stimulating factor (G-CSF) or related cytokines.

The PI is calculated by totaling the number of unfavourable prognostic factors a given patient possessed: 0 to 4. The study showed that patients whose PI was ≤ 1 had a 62% survival rate at 6 months. No patients whose PI was ≥ 3 survived more than 6 months and all patients whose PI was 4 died within 3 months. The authors also noted that the mean PI of the patients treated by multimodal therapy was 0.6 (either 0 or 1), whereas the PI of those who were not was 2.3, and hence proposed that multimodal treatment be advocated for PI of ≤1 while aggressive treatment is avoided when PI is ≥ 3.

Orita et al. [20] recently published the prospective application of this PI in the treatment strategy of 74 patients with ATC. 6-month survival rates for PI ≤ 1 and PI ≥ 3 were 72% and 12%, respectively. Both groups (P1 ≤ 1 and ≥ 3) demonstrated significantly better disease-specific survival as compared to the previous study above. Within each group, the survival rates did not differ between stages. The authors thus concluded that the PI is valid for anticipating prognosis and aiding timely decisions on treatment policy for ATC.

For our patient, long-term survival with no evidence of disease after 7 years is unusual, especially considering the presence of tracheal invasion. However, based on the above PI, he has a PI of 1 for tumour size, which indicated that he would have benefitted from the multimodal treatment he received.

In the past, there has been anecdotal evidence of cases of ATC with long-term survival. Since the mid-1980s, a group of poorly differentiated thyroid cancers (PDTC) has been recognized and considered to be tumours of biological aggressiveness intermediate between the more indolent well-differentiated thyroid carcinomas and ATC [21]. Historically, the distinction between poorly differentiated thyroid cancer (PDTC) and ATC has always been difficult. In our patient, there was no question that the tumour was an ATC.

We carried out a literature review of all ATC cases with survival greater than 2 years. Prior to review, we identified several features thought to influence survival as discussed above, namely age, tumour size, extent of tumour spread, adequacy of surgical resection, histopathology and neoadjuvant/adjuvant therapy. We restricted our review to papers published after January 1990. Exclusion criteria included papers not published in peer-reviewed journals as well as any case series in which the prognostic factors for the longest surviving cases were not specified. Medical subject headings and main keywords used were: 'undifferentiated', 'anaplastic' and 'thyroid', with variants of the main keywords also applied.

The initial review yielded a total of 37 articles, 10 case reports and 21 case series. 13 case series were further excluded due to insufficient data. We further excluded 3 case reports and 1 case series with only intra-thyroidal ATC tumours (T4a) for ease of comparison. A total of 7 case reports and 7 case series remained for our review.

A total of 22 cases of locally advanced ATC (T4b) with long-term survival of more than 2 years were compiled from the remaining 14 articles (Table 1). The length of survival varied from more than 2 to 12 years. The age at diagnosis ranged from 26 to 85 years. 4 cases [22-24] were diagnosed with ATC incidentally after surgery for presumed benign thyroid disease. Of cases that were known, most did not present with acute symptoms, usually that of a rapidly enlarging neck mass. Only 3 cases [22,25,26] had evidence of tracheal invasion while 1 case [27] had tumour extending to the cervical esophagus.

All cases received multi-modality treatment with most cases being treated with radical surgery followed by either concurrent

SN	Journal	Age/Gender	Presentation	Extent of surgery	Positive margins	Neoadjuvant / Adjuvant Therapy	Tumour size (cm)	Formal Histopathology	Presence of extrathyroidal spread & location	TMN Stage	Length of survival
1	Kanaseki et al. [25]	52/F	Enlarging anterior neck mass with vocal cord palsy	TT with tracheal wall resection Interval upper mediastinal LN dissection	No	Adjuvant CTX followed by CRT	9.0 × 6.5 × 3.0	ATC with tracheal invasion Positive superior mediastinal LN	Yes Tracheal wall and mediastinal LN	Stage IVB T4bN1bM0	>2 years
2	Shinohara et al. [27]	53/F	Anterior neck pain with left thyroid nodule	Total pharyngo–laryngo–esophagectomy with bilateral neck and upper mediastinum LN dissection	No	Neoadjuvant CTX followed by RT Tumour regrowth on MRI after RT, proceeded with surgery	4.1	Tumour replaced by granulation tissue and necrosis, no cancer cells (ATC on initial fine-needle aspiration cytology)	Yes Cervical esophagus	Stage IVB T4bN0MO	>2 years
3	Kurukahvecioglu et al. [22]	35/F	Rapidly growing right thyroid nodule initially Tracheal mass 9 months later Suspicious right neck nodes on PET-CT 5 months later	Right lobectomy Interval radical excision of tracheal mass and left lobectomy Interval right radical ND	No	Adjuvant CTX and RT after 2nd surgery	2.1 × 1.5	Right thyroid nodule: benign Tracheal mass: ATC, 3 LN positive Right ND: negative	Yes Trachea and strap muscles	Stage IVB T4bN1aM0	>3 years after second surgery
4	Noguchi et al. [28]	51/M	Rapidly growing right thyroid nodule with mild tenderness	Right lobectomy with right levels 2-4 and level 6 ND with intraoperative RT	No	Oral valproic acid daily Neoadjuvant CRT Adjuvant CTX	3 × 4.1 × 3.5	Tumour surrounded by fibrous tissue divided by thin ring of PTC; encapsulating fibrous tissue contained remnants of ATC LN: 4 out of 26 positive	Yes Strap muscles	Stage IVB T4bN1M0	>2 years
5	Olthof et al. [31]	76/F	Enlarging anterior neck mass	TT with left modified radical neck dissection (levels 2-6)	Yes	Adjuvant radioactive iodine therapy I131 Adjuvant RT	7 × 6 × 4	Hürthle cell carcinoma dedifferentiated to ATC with differentiation along rhabdomyoblastic cell lines Level 2 LN positive	Yes Regional cervical LN	Stage IVB T4aN1aM0	>3 years
6	Liu et al. [23]	68/M	Anterior neck mass with compressive symptoms and dyspnoea	TT with removal of enlarged LNs	No	Adjuvant RT	5 × 3 × 4	ATC LN negative	Yes Strap muscles	Stage IVB T4bN0M0	>10 years
7	Pichardo-Lowden et al. [26]	26/F	Rapidly growing anterior neck mass with odynophagia and voice change	TT and left modified radical ND	No	Adjuvant CRT	5 × 4	Undifferentiated carcinoma LN negative	Yes Tracheal wall, strap and sternocleidomastoid muscles, encasing left internal jugular vein and adhering to common carotid artery	Stage IVB T4bN0M0	>2 years
8	Akaishi et al. [24]	48/F	Not known	Now known but completely resected	No	No	<5	Incidental small focus of ATC	Yes Not known	Stage IVB	>12 years 7 months
9	Akaishi et al. [24]	68/F	Not kwown	Not known but debulking done	Not known	Adjuvant RT and CTX	<5	Incidental small focus of ATC	Yes Not known	Stage IVB	9 years
10	Akaishi et al. [24]	66/F	Not known	Not known but completely resected	No	Adjuvant RT and CTX	>5	ATC	Yes Not known	Stage IVB	>3 years

11	Kihara et al. [32]	82	Immobile thyroid mass	Subtotal thyroidectomy	Not known	Adjuvant CRT	4.9	ATC	Yes / Surrounding muscle	Stage IVB T4bN0M0	6 years 4 months
12	Kim et al. [33]	57/F	Not known	TT	Not known	Adjuvant RT and CTX	5	ATC	Yes / Not known	Stage IVB	4 years 4 months
13	Kim et al. [33]	55/F	Not known	TT	Not known	Adjuvant RT	4	ATC	Yes / Not known	Stage IVB	>3 years 5 months
14	Siironen et al. [34]	85/F	Not known	Thyroid lobectomy	Not known	Adjuvant RT	Not known	ATC	Yes / Recurrent laryngeal nerve	Stage IVB T4bN0M0	>6 years 6 months
15	Siironen et al. [34]	62/M	Not known	Radical surgery including TT	Not known	Adjuvant CRT	Not known	ATC	Yes / Not known	Stage IVB T4bN0M0	5 years 4 months
16	De Crevoisier et al. [29]	75/M	Not known	Macroscopically complete resection	Not known	Adjuvant CRT	Not known	ATC concomitant with PTC or FTC	Yes / Not known	Stage IVB T4bN1M0	6 years 6 months
17	De Crevoisier et al. [29]	72/F	Not known	Incomplete resection	No	Adjuvant CRT	Not known	ATC concomitant with PTC or FTC	Yes / Not known	Stage IVB T4bN0M0	>4 years
18	De Crevoisier et al. [29]	52/F	Not known	Macroscopically complete resection	Not known	Neoadjuvant CRT	Not known	ATC	Yes / Regional cervical LN	Stage IVB T4bN1M0	2 years 3 months
19	De Crevoisier et al. [29]	75/F	Not known	Macroscopically complete resection	Not known	Adjuvant CRT	Not known	ATC	Yes / Regional cervical LN	Stage IVB T4bN1M0	2 years 1 month
20	De Crevoisier et al. [29]	58/M	Not known	Incomplete resection	No	Adjuvant CRT	Not known	ATC concomitant with PTC or FTC	Yes / Regional cervical LN	Stage IVB T4bN1M0	2 years 1 month
21	Ito et al. [35]	77/F	Not known	TT and ND	Yes	Adjuvant CRT	Not known	ATC	Yes / Local spread and regional cervical LN	Stage IVB T4bN1M0	>4 years 6 months
22	Rodriguez et al. [36]	58/M	Not known	Total thyroidectomy and multiple LN dissections (5)	Not known	Adjuvant CTX	Not known	ATC with associated PTC	Yes / Local spread and regional cervical LN	Stage IVB T4bN1M0	>5 years 10 months

Table 1: Cases of locally advanced (T4b) ATC with long-term survival of >2 years.

chemoradiation or radiotherapy or radioactive iodine ablation. Only 3 cases [27-29] received neoadjuvant chemoradiation followed by surgery. The extent of thyroidectomy performed also differed and ranged from lobectomy to total thyroidectomy. All patients with clinically or radiologically positive cervical lymph nodes underwent neck dissections. Surgical resection included debulking surgery, macroscopically complete resections and microscopically complete resections. In general, most studies concluded that although the prognosis of most patients with ATC continues to be poor, complete resection combined with adjuvant chemotherapy and radiotherapy resulted in better survival.

There have been 3 cases with comparable survival in the literature with survival of more than 9, 10 and 12 years [23,24]. All cases were characterized by having just an incidental focus of ATC within an otherwise well-differentiated thyroid carcinoma with limited extra-thyroidal spread. Our case however, was different as our patient presented with a gross ATC tumour with tracheal invasion and we were fortunate that the disease was still surgically resectable.

A widely cited staging system by Shin et al. [30] for papillary thyroid cancer is based on the depth of tracheal invasion. Stage I disease abuts the external perichondrium of the trachea but without cartilaginous erosion. Stage II disease invades into the cartilage or causes cartilage destruction. Stage III disease extends into the lamina propria of the tracheal mucosa. Stage IV disease is full-thickness invasion through the tracheal mucosa. There is no similar staging system for ATC but based on the above, the degree of tracheal invasion for our case would be classified as Stage 3. Based on the histological examination, the tumour was about 2 mm from the closest tracheal resection margin with tumour seen beneath the epithelium of the trachea. The involved tracheal segment was completely resected and primary anastomosis was performed.

Our case represents an anecdotal case wherein it is possible to achieve cure with clear surgical margins. Although there is general reluctance to attempt surgical resection in anaplastic carcinoma due to uniformly poor prognosis, our case concurs with the American Thyroid Guidelines on ATC [14] in which patients with ATC and extra-thyroidal invasion should have en bloc resection if grossly negative margins can be achieved. In our opinion, being able to achieve clear negative margins is the single most important prognostic factor for patients with ATC.

Conclusion

The prognosis of ATC remains poor as it is characterized by aggressive and extensive disease at presentation, the inability in most patients to perform radical enough surgery in order to achieve clear margins, high morbidity of complete extirpation and limited response to radiotherapy or chemotherapy. However, if complete surgical resection is possible, patients should be treated aggressively with a combination of surgery and adjuvant radiotherapy.

References

1. Pasieka JL (2003) Anaplastic thyroid cancer. Curr Opin Oncol 15: 78-83.

2. Ain KB (1998) Anaplastic thyroid carcinoma: behavior, biology, and therapeutic approaches. Thyroid 8: 715-726.

3. Giuffrida D, Gharib H (2000) Anaplastic thyroid carcinoma: current diagnosis and treatment. Ann Oncol 11: 1083-1089.

4. O'Neill JP, O'Neill B, Condron C, Walsh M, Bouchier-Hayes D (2005) Anaplastic (undifferentiated) thyroid cancer: improved insight and therapeutic strategy into a highly aggressive disease. J Laryngol Otol 119: 585-591.

5. Kebebew E, Greenspan FS, Clark OH, Woeber KA, McMillan A (2005) Anaplastic thyroid carcinoma. Treatment outcome and prognostic factors. Cancer 103: 1330-1335.

6. Goutsouliak V, Hay JH (2005) Anaplastic thyroid cancer in British Columbia 1985-1999: a population-based study. Clin Oncol (R Coll Radiol) 17: 75-78.

7. Besic N, Auersperg M, Us-Krasovec M, Golouh R, Frkovic-Grazio S, et al. (2001) Effect of primary treatment on survival in anaplastic thyroid carcinoma. Eur J Surg Oncol 27: 260-264.

8. McIver B, Hay ID, Giuffrida DF, Dvorak CE, Grant CS, et al. (2001) Anaplastic thyroid carcinoma: a 50-year experience at a single institution. Surgery 130: 1028-1034.

9. Sugitani I, Kasai N, Fujimoto Y, Yanagisawa A (2001) Prognostic factors and therapeutic strategy for anaplastic carcinoma of the thyroid. World J Surg 25: 617-622.

10. Passler C, Scheuba C, Prager G, Kaserer K, Flores JA, et al. (1999) Anaplastic (undifferentiated) thyroid carcinoma (ATC). A retrospective analysis. Langenbecks Arch Surg 384: 284-293.

11. Nilsson O, Lindeberg J, Zedenius J, Ekman E, Tennvall J, et al. (1998) Anaplastic giant cell carcinoma of the thyroid gland: treatment and survival over a 25-year period. World J Surg 22: 725-730.

12. Junor EJ, Paul J, Reed NS (1992) Anaplastic thyroid carcinoma: 91 patients treated by surgery and radiotherapy. Eur J Surg Oncol 18: 83-88.

13. Demeter JG, De Jong SA, Lawrence AM, Paloyan E (1991) Anaplastic thyroid carcinoma: risk factors and outcome. Surgery 110: 956-961.

14. Smallridge RC, Ain KB, Asa SL, Bible KC, Brierley JD, et al. (2012) American Thyroid Association guidelines for management of patients with anaplastic thyroid cancer. Thyroid 22: 1104-1139.

15. Venkatesh YS, Ordonez NG, Schultz PN, Hickey RC, Goepfert H, et al. (1990) Anaplastic carcinoma of the thyroid. A clinicopathologic study of 121 cases. Cancer 66: 321-330.

16. Are C, Shaha AR (2006) Anaplastic thyroid carcinoma: biology, pathogenesis, prognostic factors, and treatment approaches. Ann Surg Oncol 13: 453-464.

17. Tan RK, Finley RK 3rd, Driscoll D, Bakamjian V, Hicks WL Jr, et al. (1995) Anaplastic carcinoma of the thyroid: a 24-year experience. Head Neck 17: 41-47.

18. Haigh PI, Ituarte PH, Wu HS, Treseler PA, Posner MD, et al. (2001) Completely resected anaplastic thyroid carcinoma combined with adjuvant chemotherapy and irradiation is associated with prolonged survival. Cancer 91: 2335-2342.

19. Kobayashi T, Asakawa H, Umeshita K, Takeda T, Maruyama H, et al. (1996) Treatment of 37 patients with anaplastic carcinoma of the thyroid. Head Neck 18: 36-41.

20. Orita Y, Sugitani I, Amemiya T, Fujimoto Y (2011) Prospective application of our novel prognostic index in the treatment of anaplastic thyroid carcinoma. Surgery 150: 1212-1219.

21. Patel KN, Shaha AR (2006) Poorly differentiated and anaplastic thyroid cancer. Cancer Control 13: 119-128.

22. Kurukahvecioglu O, Ege B, Poyraz A, Tezel E, Taneri F (2007) Anaplastic thyroid carcinoma with long term survival after combined treatment: case report. Endocr Regul 41: 41-44.

23. Liu AH, Juan LY, Yang AH, Chen HS, Lin HD (2006) Anaplastic thyroid cancer with uncommon long-term survival. J Chin Med Assoc 69: 489-491.

24. Akaishi J, Sugino K, Kitagawa W, Nagahama M, Kameyama K, et al. (2011) Prognostic factors and treatment outcomes of 100 cases of anaplastic thyroid carcinoma. Thyroid 21: 1183-1189.

25. Kanaseki T, Harabuchi Y, Wakashima J, Asakura K, Kataura A, et al. (1999) A case of anaplastic thyroid carcinoma surviving disease free for over 2 years. Auris Nasus Larynx 26: 217-220.

26. Pichardo-Lowden A, Durvesh S, Douglas S, Todd W, Bruno M, et al. (2009) Anaplastic thyroid carcinoma in a young woman: a rare case of survival. Thyroid 19: 775-779.

27. Shinohara S, Kikuchi M, Naito Y, Fujiwara K, Hori S, et al. (2009) Successful treatment of locally advanced anaplastic thyroid carcinoma by chemotherapy and hyperfractionated radiotherapy. Auris Nasus Larynx 36: 729-732.

28. Noguchi H, Yamashita H, Murakami T, Hirai K, Noguchi Y, et al. (2009) Successful treatment of anaplastic thyroid carcinoma with a combination of oral valproic acid, chemotherapy, radiation and surgery. Endocr J 56: 245-249.

29. De Crevoisier R, Baudin E, Bachelot A, Leboulleux S, Travagli JP, et al. (2004) Combined treatment of anaplastic thyroid carcinoma with surgery, chemotherapy, and hyperfractionated accelerated external radiotherapy. Int J Radiat Oncol Biol Phys 60: 1137-1143.

30. Shin DH, Mark EJ, Suen HC, Grillo HC (1993) Pathologic staging of papillary carcinoma of the thyroid with airway invasion based on the anatomic manner of extension to the trachea: a clinicopathologic study based on 22 patients who underwent thyroidectomy and airway resection. Hum Pathol 24: 866-870.

31. Olthof M, Persoon AC, Plukker JT, van der Wal JE, Links TP (2008) Anaplastic thyroid carcinoma with rhabdomyoblastic differentiation: a case report with a good clinical outcome. Endocr Pathol 19: 62-65.

32. Kihara M, Miyauchi A, Yamauchi A, Yokomise H (2004) Prognostic factors of anaplastic thyroid carcinoma. Surg Today 34: 394-398.

33. Kim TY, Kim KW, Jung TS, Kim JM, Kim SW, et al. (2007) Prognostic factors for Korean patients with anaplastic thyroid carcinoma. Head Neck 29: 765-772.

34. Siironen P, Hagstrom J, Maenpaa HO, Louhimo J, Heikkila A, et al. (2010) Anaplastic and poorly differentiated thyroid carcinoma: therapeutic strategies and treatment outcome of 52 consecutive patients. Oncology 79: 400-408.

35. Ito K, Hanamura T, Murayama K, Okada T, Watanabe T, et al. (2012) Multimodality therapeutic outcomes in anaplastic thyroid carcinoma: improved survival in subgroups of patients with localized primary tumors. Head Neck 34: 230-237.

36. Rodriguez JM, Pinero A, Ortiz S, Moreno A, Sola J, et al. (2000) Clinical and histological differences in anaplastic thyroid carcinoma. Eur J Surg 166: 34-38.

18

Microbial Prevalence and Antimicrobial Resistance in Children and Adolescents with Chronic Rhinosinusitis in South Indian Population

Madhavi Jangala[1,2], Raja Meganadh Koralla[1], Santoshi Kumari Manche[1,2] and Jyothy Akka[2*]

[1]MAA Research Foundation, Somajiguda, Hyderabad, Telangana, India

[2]Institute of Genetics and Hospital for Genetic Diseases, Osmania University, Hyderabad, Telangana, India

*Corresponding author: Jyothi Akka, Emeritus Professor, Institute of Genetics and Hospital for Genetic Diseases, Osmania University, Begumpet, Hyderabad, Telangana, India; E-mail: jyothycell@rediffmail.com

Abstract

Objective: Chronic rhinosinusitis (CRS) is a common multifactorial upper respiratory disease with a key role of microbes in worsening of disease and its associated co-morbidities. Further, significant region specific variation in patient demographics and antibiotic resistance of causative bacteria are reported to pose difficulty in diagnosis and treatment. In India, studies on the etiology and antibiotic resistance in chronic rhinosinusitis are very meager, especially in children. The present study aimed to determine the prevalence of common causative microbes and their antibiotic resistance in children and adolescents with chronic rhinosinusitis in South Indian population.

Subjects and methods: The present study was conducted on 89 children and 99 adolescents with chronic rhinosinusitis who visited MAA ENT Institute, Hyderabad, South India. The study samples were collected under the nasal endoscopic guidance from the middle meatus at first visit and sinuses at surgery. Conventional and VITEK-2 methods were used for identification and antibiotic sensitivity of the microbes. Chi-square test and multinomial logistic regression was applied to determine statistical differences between the variable using PASW v. 18.0 software (SPSS Inc., Chicago, IL).

Results: The male-female ratio was 2:1 with an average children age of 8.9 ± 3.65 years and 16.1 ± 1.23 years in adolescents. The risk for adenoids was seen in 49.2 % of children (OR; 2.6: 95% CI: 1.63-4.06) while allergic fungal sinusitis (18.1%, OR: 2.7; 95% CI: 1.12-6.57) and nasal polyps (26.6%, OR: 2.3; 95% CI: 1.07-4.86) was commonly seen in adolescents. About 26.6% of adolescents with fungal positivity also showed bacterial infection. Aspergillus flavus (68%) was the most common fungi identified. Bacterial culture rate was positive in 46.8% of the total subjects of which Streptococcus aureus was the most common bacteria (59.1%) followed by *Streptococcus pnuemoniae* (21.2%), *Klebsiella* sp. (11.4%), *Pseudomonas aeruginosa* (11.4%) and β hemolytic streptococci (1.1%). No Methicillin-resistant *Staphylococcus aureus* strains could be identified. *Streptococcus pneumonia* (63.2%) was commonly identified in younger children and *Pseudomonas aeruginosa* (80%) was mostly seen in adolescents. The frequency of bacterial positivity in adolescents with CRS when compared to CRS children was high and varied between different associated co-morbidities. High antibiotic resistance in *Staphylococcus aureus* was seen towards gentamicin (73%) and co-trimoxazole (64%), *Streptococcus pnuemoniae* to gentamicin (58%), co-trimoxazole (68%) and meropenem (32%), *Pseudomonas aeruginosa* to co-trimoxazole (100%), cefatoximine (60%) and cefatazidime (50%) while *Klebsiella* sp. to gentamicin (80%) and co-trimoxazole (60%). *Streptococcus aureus* showed high sensitivity to cefatoximine (95.8%) and *Streptococcus pneumoniae* for ofloxacin (100%), ciprofloxacin (89.5%) and cefazolin (89.5%). *Pseudomonas aeruginosa* showed high sensitivity for amikacin (100%) and ciprofloxacin (80%) and *Klebsiella* sp. for amikacin (100%)

Conclusion: Significant regional specific variation in bacterial etiology that differed with age, severity and co-morbidities was observed in children and adolescents with chronic rhinosinusitis. High antimicrobial resistance in the cultures of chronic rhinosinusitis patients at their first visit and also at sinus surgery warrants urgent need for early initiation of personalized interventions for better management of the infectious disease.

Keywords: Chronic rhinosinusitis; Allergic fungal sinusitis; Nasal polyps; Adenoids; Antibiotic sensitivity; Functional endoscopic sinus surgery; Chronic suppurative otitis media

Introduction

Chronic rhinosinusitis (CRS) is a common multifactorial inflammatory disorder of the upper airway system that drastically affects the patient's quality of life across all ages and socioeconomic conditions of millions of people worldwide [1]. About 5-15% of the worldwide population is affected with chronic rhinosinusitis yet paucity of data exists in relation to etiopathogenesis, especially in children [2]. Various demographic and socioeconomic factors are reported to cause differences in CRS manifestation which affects management and recurrence rate of the disease [3,4]. Clinico-pathophysiological mechanisms such as immaturity of the immune system, smaller ostia of the sinuses, increased respiratory tract infections and adenoidal hypertrophy in children while tissue remodeling and greater irreversible scarring due to inflammation in adults contribute to the disease worsening in chronic rhinosinusitis [5]. Further, presence of nasal pathogens leads to longer mean duration of symptoms and greater severity of the inflammation [6]. The role of bacteria differed with respect to different chronic rhinosinusitis comorbidities which further increase variation in disease management in children as well as in adults [7,8].

Sinusitis and its associated complications are more frequently treated with antibiotics to prevent the onset of complications and the need for surgical interventions [9]. Antibiotic treatment can promote subsequent growth of various bacteria, often to new multidrug resistant strains, on the mucosal epithelium with frequencies and changes that may vary with the use of different antibiotics, between age groups and clinical entities [10,11]. Misdiagnosis of the symptoms in many cases with upper respiratory tract infections, indiscriminate prescribing of antibiotics by general practitioners including broad-spectrum antibiotics, and ease of obtaining antibiotics has promoted the microbial resistance for many antibiotics [12,13]. The susceptibility trends among common pathogens appear to have stabilized over the past years as measures have been taken up in many countries but high prevalence of multidrug resistance remains as a major concern [13,14]. Also, the Center for Disease Control and Prevention (CDC) recently estimated that antimicrobials usually prescribed often to treat acute respiratory tract infections in children and adults are still at inappropriately high rates. Continuing research is therefore needed to refine physician awareness and to evaluate regional differences in antibiotic resistance that may result in variations with significant effects upon disease progression and management.

In India, very meager studies are been reported on etiology of chronic rhinosinusitis, especially in children. The choice of antibiotics is discretionary and usually not made based on microbial culture and sensitivity results which promotes the high risk for bacterial resistance. Misconceptions exist about the use and indications of antibiotics and lack of knowledge regarding antibiotic resistance is prevalent in India [15]. The purpose of this study was to determine the etiology, and the prevalence of major bacterial and fungal pathogens and antibiotic resistance of the identified bacteria in children and adolescents of South Indian population.

Study, Subjects and Methods

188 CRS subjects including 89 children and 99 adolescents who underwent treatment at MAA ENT Hospitals, Hyderabad were considered for the study. Clinical diagnosis was based upon presence of two or more symptoms of nasal obstruction, nasal congestion, anterior nasal discharge, posterior nasal drip, facial pain, cough; atleast one of the endoscopic signs of nasal polyps, mucosal obstruction and/or mucopurulent discharge mainly from middle meatus, oedema and mucosal changes within the ostiomeatal complex and/or sinuses as seen through computed tomography. The criteria for the diagnosis of

nasal allergy were mainly by the symptoms such as nasal discharge, nasal itching and sneezing for more than 5 times a day. Diagnosis of adenoids was made when greater than 50% of nasopharyngeal space occupied by soft tissue in the X-ray neck lateral view. The confirmation of diagnosis was by X-ray in subjects less than 13 yrs and computed tomography scan in subjects more than 13 yrs. Subjects who have not been on antibiotic therapy during the first visit and who have stopped their antibiotic use for atleast 3 weeks before surgery were included in the study. CRS subjects with immune compromised conditions, cystic fibrosis and nasocominal infections were excluded. The study samples were collected in the first visit if purulent discharge was present in the middle meatus and in patients when discharge was not seen in the middle meatus due to blockage of sinus opening the samples were collected at the surgery under the nasal endoscopic guidance. Surgical interventions were done when the condition could not be managed by the therapeutic interventions. Identification and antibiotic sensitivity of the microbes were performed by the conventional and VITEK-2 method. Data related to detailed medical history, clinical findings and the findings of endoscopic examination, computed tomography scanning and microbiological assessments were recorded and the data obtained was analyzed using PASW ver. 18.0 (SPSS Inc. Chicago, US). Continuous data was presented as means and standard deviations. Chi-square test and multinomial logistic regression was used to determine statistical differences between the age, sex, co-morbidities, type of microbial pathogen and their antibiotic sensitivity and resistance. The study was performed after approval of the institutional research ethics committee for biomedical research.

Results

The mean age of children was 8.9 ± 3.65 years and 16.1 ± 1.23 years in adolescents. Male preponderance of 2:1 was noticed in both children and adolescents. 51.6% of the CRS children with adenoids were affected with allergic rhinitis, 32.2 % cases with CSOM and 16.6% cases with asthma. Allergic fungal sinusitis (AFS) was commonly found in adolescents (18.1%) of which 57.1% of cases had nasal polyposis while 19.9% had asthma. Allergic Rhinitis was the most common co-morbidity in both the age groups. Allergic rhinitis with nasal polyps was present in 21.2% of CRS subjects and 4.2% of CRS subjects had allergic rhinitis with nasal polyps and asthma. Of the total subjects, 36.7% of cases underwent primary and 10.1% of cases had revised functional endoscopic sinus surgery (FESS). The distribution of risk factors and co-morbidities of CRS in children and adolescents is given in Table 1.

Characteristic	Total	Children	Adolescents	p-value	Odds Ratio (95% CI)
Sex	188	89 (47.3)	99 (52.7)		
Male	130 (69.1)	61 (68.5)	69 (69.7)	0.876	1.056 (0.568-1.962)
Female	58 (30.9)	28 (31.5)	30 (30.3)		
Risk Factors/Co-morbidities					
Adenoids	63 (33.5)	44 (49.4)	19 (19.2)	<0.001	2.6 (1.63-4.06)

Allergic rhinitis	102 (54.2)	43 (48.3)	59 (59.6)	0.143	0.81 (0.62-1.06)
Fungal Sinusitis	26 (13.8)	8 (9)	18 (18.1)	0.035	2.7 (1.12-6.57)
Nasal Polyps	38 (20.2)	12 (13.5)	26 (26.3)	0.045	2.3 (1.07-4.86)
Tonsillitis	78 (41.5)	38 (42.7)	40 (40.4)	0.769	1.06 (0.75-1.48)
Otitis Media	79 (42.0)	32 (36)	47 (47)	0.139	0.75 (0.54-1.07)
Asthma	23 (12.2)	14 (15.7)	9 (9.1)	0.186	1.73 (0.79-3.80)
History of sinus surgery					
No Surgery required	100 (53.2)	48 (53.9)	52 (52.5)	0.615	ref a
Sinus Surgery	69 (36.7)	34 (38.2)	35 (35.4)	0.87	0.950 (0.514 - 1.755)
Sinus Surgery Revision	19 (10.1)	7 (7.9)	12 (12.1)	0.374	1.582 (0.576 - 4.351)

Table 1: Demographic and clinical characteristics of children and adolescents with chronic rhinosinusitis (N=188), a p-value significance is based on multinomial logistic regression (2-sided), p-value significance is based on Fisher's Exact Test (2-sided), Odds ratio computed based on chi-square test.

A total of 88 bacterial isolates were recovered of which 94.3% were positive for single culture and 5.7% had multiple cultures. 80.6% of the cultures were Gram-positive cocci, 22.7% gram-negative rods and 5.6% were mixed cultures of gram positive cocci and gram negative rods. Co-infection of bacteria and fungus was noted in 4.4% of adolescents. S.aureus was the most frequently cultured organism (59.9%), followed by *S. pneumonia* (21.5%), *P. aeruginosa* (11.4%), *Klebsiella* sp. (11.4%) while no methicillin resistant *Staphylococcus aureus* strains could be identified. *Klebsellia* sp. was identified more frequently (60%) in polymicrobial infections. *Aspergillus flavus* was the most common fungi identified. *Staphylococcus aureus* was the most common pathogen in both the age groups, *Streptococcus pneumonia* was commonly identified in younger children and *Pseudomonas aeruginosa* was mostly seen in adolescents at their first visit. The distribution of microbes with respect to age in CRS subjects is given in Figure 1. The prevalence of bacteria with respect age and severity is given in Figure 2.

Bacterial culture rate was positive in 46% of the total subjects and varied with comorbidities, 44.7% of cases presented with allergy, 47.1% with nasal polyps, 54.5% asthma, 30.4% otitis media, 36.7% adenoids, 42.9% tonsillitis subjects. 57% of allergic fungal sinusitis subjects had nasal polyps. The bacterial prevalence in CRS subjects with regard to comorbidities and age is given in Figure 3. In CRS children with adenoids the microbial culture rate was 35.5% of which *S. aureus* was present in 72.7% of cases and *S. pneumonia* was seen in 18.1% of cases. In subjects with CSOM, bacterial positivity was found in 29.7% of the cultures of which *S. aureus* was 45.4% and *Streptococcus pneumonia* was identified in 36.3% cases. *Staphylococcus aureus* was seen in 59%

of bacterial positive cases in CRS subjects with allergic rhinitis. About 77% of isolates from adolescents with nasal polyps showed bacterial positivity. The prevalence of gram positive bacteria also differed with co morbidities, *S. aureus* was seen in 72.7% and *S. pneumonia* was seen 18.1% in CRS subjects with adenoids while in case of CRS subjects with CSOM, *S. aureus* was identified in 45.4% and *Streptococcus pneumonia* in 36.3% cases.

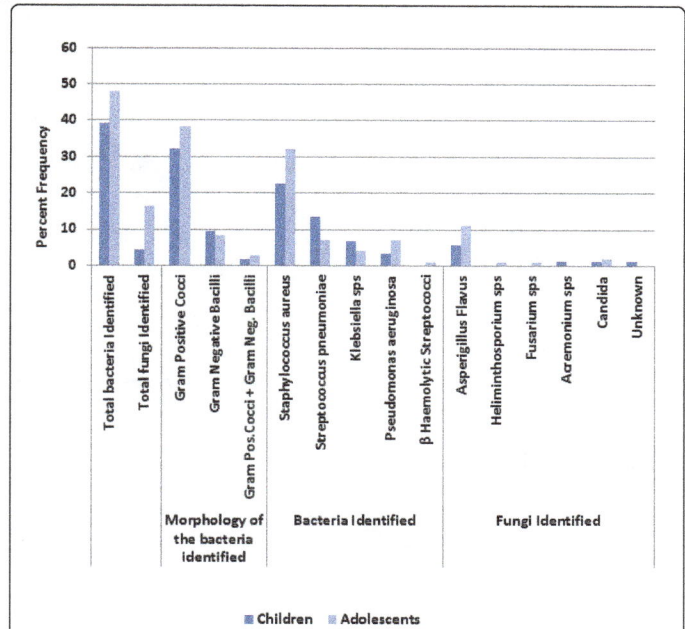

Figure 1: Distribution of microbes identified in CRS subjects with respect to age.

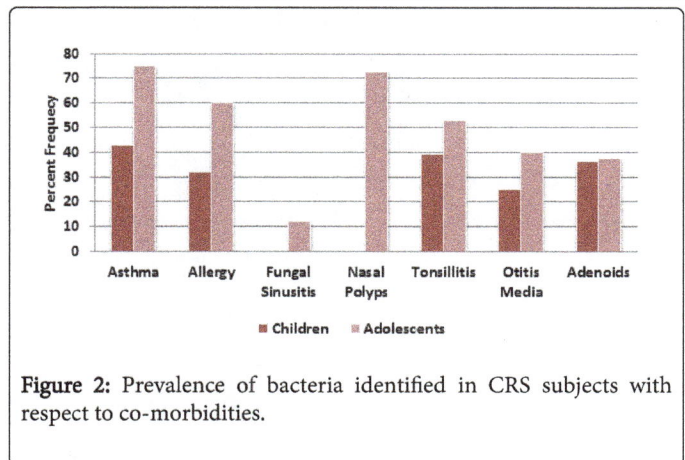

Figure 2: Prevalence of bacteria identified in CRS subjects with respect to co-morbidities.

Antibiotic resistance was observed in all the gram positive and gram negative bacterial isolates which differed with comorbidities and severity of the disease (Figure 4). High antibiotic sensitivity of *Staphylococcus aureus* was seen against cefatoximine (95.8%), *Streptococcus pnuemoniae* for ofloxacin (100%), cefazolin (89.5%), and cefatoximine (89.5%), *Pseudomonas aeruginosa* for amikacin (100%) and ciprofloxacin (80%) and *Klebsiella pnuemoniae* for amikacin (80%). All the *Staphylococcus aureus* isolates obtained at revision surgery were resistant to cotrimoxazole, 75% to amoxicillin clavunate and 50% to gentamicin. However, no difference in the antibiotic sensitivity was observed between the children and adolescents.

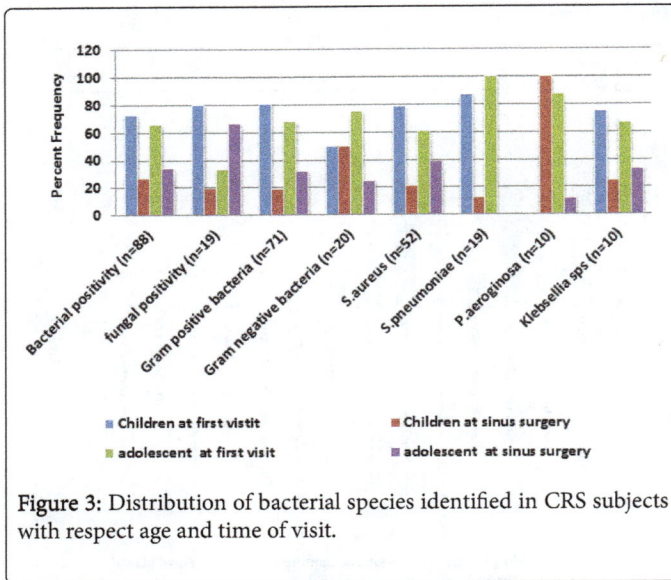

Figure 3: Distribution of bacterial species identified in CRS subjects with respect age and time of visit.

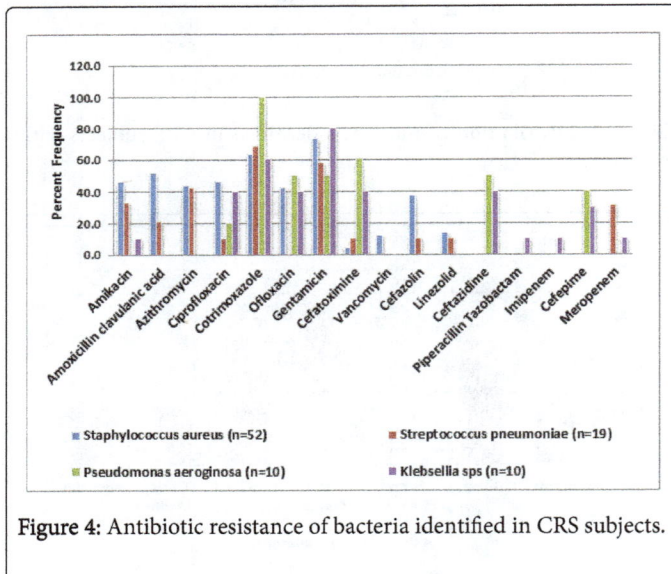

Figure 4: Antibiotic resistance of bacteria identified in CRS subjects.

Discussion

Chronic Rhinosinusitis (CRS) is the common upper respiratory disorder but continues to remain as a neglected disorder, especially in developing countries [16]. Bacterial infection plays a key role in worsening of CRS that can lead to asthma exacerbation, otitis media, recurrent polyps and refractory symptoms during post-sinus surgery [17]. The predominance of aerobic and anaerobic organisms cultured in children was reported to be different from adults and also with reference to site of isolation [18]. In the present study, identical potential pathogens were noticed in middle meatus *and sinus aspirates* which is in agreement with the earlier reports [19-21].

In a recent metanalysis study by Thanasumpun et al. [22] conducted on endoscopically derived bacterial cultures of adults with chronic rhinosinusitis reported Coagulase Negative Staphylococcus followed by *Staphylococcus aureus, Haemophilus influenza* and *Pseudomonas aeruginosa* to be the most common aerobes and Peptostreptococcus species and bacteroides species as the common anaerobes [22]. In pediatric chronic rhinosinusitis, polymicrobial infections and positive cultures of three major bacteria: *Haemophilus influenzae* (37.3%), *Streptococcus pneumoniae* (28.4%) and *Moraxella catarrhalis* (11.8%) were in Taiwan population whereas in chronic rhinosinusitis children of German population *Streptococcus pneumoniae* (33%) was the predominant followed by *Haemophilus influenzae* (27%), *Staphylococcus aureus* (13%), *Moraxella catarrhalis* (11%) and Streptococci (7%) [23,24]. In children of Chinese population both alpha-hemolytic Streptococcus (20.8%) and *Haemophilus influenzae* (19.5%) predominated followed by *Streptococcus pneumoniae* (14.0%), Coagulase-Negative Staphylococcus (13.0%), *Staphylococcus aureus* (9.3%) and anaerobes (8.0%) [25]. Unlike the above reported studies, the present study identifies *Staphylococcus aureus* (35%) to be the most common pathogen in both the age groups while other bacteria identified were *S. pneumonia* (22.3%) and *P. aeruginosa* (9%) showing variation with respect to severity and age of the chronic rhinosinusitis subjects. 64.7% subjects undergoing sinus surgery were positive for *S. aureus*. Polymicrobial infection was seen in only in 2.7% of study subjects. Also, no anaerobes were identified in children and adolescents with CRS which is not in agreement with the study conducted by Slack et al. [26].

Methicillin-resistance *Staphylococcus aureus* (MRSA) is known to be a common causative pathogen for chronic rhinosinusitis with greater recurrence rate and high prevalence and rising incidence in almost all countries [27]. According to a meta analysis study conducted by Macoul et al. the prevalence of MRSA was 1.8%-20.7% for CRS subjects [28]. The present study could not identify any MRSA strains and other predominant bacteria as reported in other studies in chronic rhinosinusitis children and adolescents. Also, a study from Karnataka, South India, reported only 3% of MRSA strains in CRS which indicates lesser burden of MRSA in community acquired infectious diseases in South Indian population [29].

Nasopharyngeal carriage of the *S. pneumoniae* was associated with younger age and considered to protect against colonisation by major pathogens such as *Staphylococcus aureus* and *Haemophilus influenzae* and thereby reducing their likelihood of causing invasive disease [30]. Reduction of pneumococcal carriage in children and increase in the incidence of *S. aureus* related infections was also attributed due to immunization with pneumococcal conjugate vaccine [31]. The present study finds *Streptococcus aureus* in 42.6% of bacterial isolates identified from younger children and 55.7% of subjects, who underwent sinus surgery, thereby supports the study conducted by Shaikh et al. [32].

Multiple co-morbidities like adenoids, otitis media, allergic rhinitis, asthma and nasal polyps are associated with chronic rhinosinusitis [1]. Significant correlation was seen between bacterial isolation rate of adenoid cultures to sinusitis grade and chronic suppurative otitis media [33,34]. Pathogens isolated from adenoids were also resistant to antibiotics that allowed infection to persist with an increased incidence of acute and unresolved otitis media [35]. Recent evidence suggests that the degree of atopy, is not associated with progression to chronic rhinosinusitis in pediatric age group but asthma is significantly associated which suggests a link between upper and lower airways and independent of allergic etiology [36]. In the present study, the prevalence of adenoids was more common in CRS children while nasal polyps were more commonly seen in CRS adolescents. Allergic rhinitis was the predominant comorbidity seen in children as well as in adolescents. Further, an association higher rate of *Staphylococcus aureus* was seen with allergic rhinitis as reported by Refaat et al. [37]. A significant correlation between allergy, asthma, rhinosinusitis and high positive rate of bacteria was also observed which is in accordance with earlier reports [38-40]. Increase in bacterial positivity in allergic rhinitis subjects with nasal polyps and asthma was found which is similar to the observation made by Ramakrishna et al. [41]. A very high frequency of bacterial positivity was noticed in CRS adolescents with nasal polyps. However, the study could not identify any microbes in the isolates from CRS children with nasal polyps.

With regard to allergic fungal sinusitis (AFS), Ferguson et al, noted a geographical variability in the incidence of AFS and fungal species associated with the disease process. In the Southern United States, dermatiaceous fungi are the most common when compared with the Northern United States, while Aspergillus species was the cause in most cases reported in the Middle East [42]. However, none of the allergic fungal sinusitis case was noticed in the northwest of Turkey [43]. In the present study, prevalence of 13.8% of allergic fungal sinusitis was noted in the study subjects and was more commonly seen in adolescents (68%). *Asperigillus flavus* being the most common fungi noted in both the age groups. Incidence of fungal sinusitis with nasal polyposis was reported to be 7% by Braun et al. [44]. Telmesani [45] reported allergic fungal sinusitis with nasal polyposis as 12.1% and with asthma as 30% to 40% [45]. In the present study, a very high prevalence of 57.1% of allergic fungal sinusitis with nasal polyposis was observed. Asthma was observed in 19.9% of allergic fungal sinusitis subjects.

Different survival strategies and mechanisms are adopted by the pathogens causing difficulty in management of severe infections [11]. Increase in evolution of antibiotic resistance usually to multiple drugs in almost all bacterial pathogens has enhanced the chances of survival and extension into the community [11,46]. Since the present study has observed ethnic variation in the prevalence of microbes and antibiotic resistance in isolates of both the age groups it signifies the importance of microbial evaluation before initiations of any therapeutic interventions.

Conclusion

To our knowledge this is the first study to report etiology and antibacterial resistance in chronic rhinosinusitis children and adolescents in Indian population. The bacterial and fungal prevalence varied with respect to age, severity and co-morbiditites. High rate of antibiotic resistance in all the microbial isolates, *Staphylococcus aureus*, *Streptococcus pnuemoniae*, *Pseudomonas aeruginosa* and *Klebsiella pneumoniae* warrants utmost need for early initiation of personalized interventions and management measures in chronic rhinosinusitis children and adolescents.

Acknowledgement

I thank ICMR for supporting me in the form of SRF grant. I would also like to thank Ms. B. Sunita G Kumar, CMD, MAA ENT Hospitals for her support and cooperation in carrying out the work. I thank all my labmates, JV Ramakrishna, D Dinesh and P Padmavathi for helping me to carry out this work.

References

1. Bachert C, Pawankar R, Zhang L, Bunnag C, Fokkens WJ, et al. (2014) ICON: Chronic rhinosinusitis. World Allergy Organ J 7: 25.

2. Jarvis D, Newson R, Lotvall J, Hastan D, Tomassen P, et al. (2012) Asthma in adults and its association with chronic rhinosinusitis: The GA2LEN survey in Europe. Allergy 67: 91-98.

3. Soler ZM, Mace JC, Litvack JR, Smith TL (2012) Chronic rhinosinusitis, race and ethnicity. Am J Rhinol Allergy 26: 110-116.

4. Smith WM, Davidson TM, Murphy C (2009) Regional variations in chronic rhinosinusitis, 2003-2006. Otolaryngol Head Neck Surg 141: 347-352.

5. Sacre-Hazouri JA (2012) [Chronic rhinosinusitis in children]. Rev Alerg Mex 59: 16-24.

6. Kristo A, Uhari M, Kontiokari T, Glumoff V, Kaijalainen T, et al. (2006) Nasal middle meatal specimen bacteriology as a predictor of the course of acute respiratory infection in children. Pediatr Infect Dis J 25: 108-112.

7. Scheid DC, Hamm RM (2004) Acute bacterial rhinosinusitis in adults: part I. Evaluation. Am Fam Physician 70: 1685-1692.

8. Beule A (2015) Epidemiology of chronic rhinosinusitis, selected risk factors, comorbidities and economic burden. GMS Curr Top Otorhinolaryngol Head Neck Surg 14: Doc11.

9. Kenealy T, Arroll B (2013) Antibiotics for the common cold and acute purulent rhinitis. Cochrane Database Syst Rev 6: CD000247.

10. Slack CL, Dahn KA, Abzug MJ, Chan KH (2001) Antibiotic-resistant bacteria in pediatric chronic sinusitis. Pediatric Infectious Disease Journal 20:247–

11. Davies J, Davies D (2010) Origins and evolution of antibiotic resistance. Microbiol Mol Biol Rev 74: 417-433.

12. Llor C, Bjerrum L (2014) Antimicrobial resistance: Risk associated with antibiotic overuse and initiatives to reduce the problem. Ther Adv Drug Saf 5: 229-241.

13. Sahm DF, Brown NP, Thornsberry C, Jones ME (2008) Antimicrobial susceptibility profiles among common respiratory tract pathogens: A Global perspective. Postgrad Med 120:16-24.

14. Harris AM, Hicks LA, Qaseem A (2016) Appropriate antibiotic use for acute respiratory tract infection in adults: Advice for high-value care from the American College of Physicians and the Centers for Disease Control and Prevention. Ann Intern Med 164: 425-434.

15. Agarwal S, Yewale VN. Dharmapalan D (2015) Antibiotics use and misuse in children: A knowledge, attitude and practice survey of parents in India. J Clin Diagn Res 9: SC21-24.

16. Wu AW, Shapiro NL, Bhattacharyya N (2009) Chronic rhinosinusitis in children: What are the treatment options? Immunol Allergy Clin North Am 29: 705-717.

17. Leiberman A, Dagan R, Leibovitz E, Yagupsky P, Fliss DM (1999) The bacteriology of the nasopharynx in childhood. Int J Pediatr Otorhinolaryngol 49 Suppl 1: S151-153.

18. Bernstein JM, Dryja D, Murphy TF (2001) Molecular typing of paired bacterial isolates from the adenoid and lateral wall of the nose in children undergoing adenoidectomy: Implications in acute rhinosinusitis. Otolaryngol Head Neck Surg 125: 593-7.

19. Uhliarova B, Karnisova R, Svec M, Calkovska A (2014) Correlation between culture-identified bacteria in the middle nasal meatus and CT score in patients with chronic rhinosinusitis. J Med Microbiol 63 :28-33.

20. Ramakrishnan VR, Feazel LM, Abrass LJ, Frank DN (2013) Prevalence and abundance of *Staphylococcus aureus* in the middle meatus of patients with chronic rhinosinusitis, nasal polyps and asthma. Int Forum Allergy Rhinol 4: 267-271.

21. Corriveau MN, Zhang N, Holtappels G, Van Roy N, Bachert C (2009) Detection of *Staphylococcus aureus* in nasal tissue with peptide nucleic acid-fluorescence *in situ* hybridization. Am J Rhinol Allergy 23: 461-465.

22. Thanasumpun T, Batra PS (2015) Endoscopically-derived bacterial cultures in chronic rhinosinusitis: A systematic review. Am J Otolaryngol 36: 686-691.

23. Huang WH, Fang SY (2004) High prevalence of antibiotic resistance in isolates from the middle meatus of children and adults with acute rhinosinusitis. Am J Rhinol 18: 387-391.

24. Fickweiler U, Fickweiler K (2005) [The pathogen spectrum of acute bacterial rhinitis/sinusitis and antibiotic resistance]. HNO 53: 735-740.

25. Hsin CH, Su MC, Tsao CH, Chuang CY, Liu CM (2008) Bacteriology and antimicrobial susceptibility of pediatric chronic rhinosinusitis: A 6 year result of maxillary sinus punctures. Am J Otolaryngol 31:145-9.

26. Slack CL, Dahn KA, Abzug MJ, Chan KH (2001) Antibiotic-resistant bacteria in pediatric chronic sinusitis. Pediatr Infect Dis J 20: 247-250.

27. Penttilä M, Savolainen S, Kiukaanniemi H, Forsblom B, Jousimies-Somer H (1997) Bacterial findings in acute maxillary sinusitis--European study. Acta Otolaryngol Suppl 529: 165-168.

28. Rujanavej V, Soudry E, Banaei N, Baron EJ, Hwang PH, et al. (2013) Trends in incidence and susceptibility among methicillin-resistant *Staphylococcus aureus* isolated from intranasal cultures associated with rhinosinusitis. American Journal of Rhinology & Allergy 27: 134–137.

29. Panduranga KM, Vijendra SS , Nithin M, Nitish S (2013) Microbiological analysis of paranasal sinuses in chronic sinusitis - A South Indian coastal study Egyptian Journal of Ear, Nose, Throat and Allied Sciences 14: 185-189.

30. Charalambous BM (2007) *Streptococcus pneumoniae*: Pathogen or protector? Reviews in Medical Microbiology 18: 73-78.

31. Olarte L, Hulten KG, Lamberth L, Mason EO, Kaplan SL (2014) Impact of the 13-valent pneumococcal conjugate vaccine on chronic sinusitis associated with *Streptococcus pneumoniae* in children. Pediatr Infect Dis J 33:1033-6.

32. Shaikh N, Wald ER, Jeong JH, Kurs-Lasky M, Bowen A, et al. (2014) Predicting response to antimicrobial therapy in children with acute sinusitis. J Pediatr 164: 536-541.

33. Shin KS, Cho SH, Kim KR, Tae K, Lee SH, et al. (2008) The role of adenoids in pediatric rhinosinusitis. Int J Pediatr Otorhinolaryngol 72: 1643-1650.

34. Rajeshwary A, Rai S, Somayaji G, Pai V (2013) Bacteriology of symptomatic adenoids in children. N Am J Med Sci 5: 113-118.

35. Wald ER (2011) Acute otitis media and acute bacterial sinusitis. Clin Infect Dis 52 Suppl 4: S277-283.

36. Compalati E, Ridolo E, Passalacqua G, Braido F, Villa E, et al. (2010) The link between allergic rhinitis and asthma: The united airways disease Expert Review of Clinical Immunology 6: 413-442.

37. Refaat MM, Ahmed TM, Ashour ZA, Atia MY (2008). Immunological role of nasal *Staphylococcus aureus* carriage in patients with persistent allergic rhinitis. The Pan African Medical Journal 1: 3.

38. Chalermwatanachai T, Velásquez LC, Bachert C (2015) The microbiome of the upper airways: Focus on chronic rhinosinusitis. World Allergy Organ J 8: 3.

39. Gelardi M, Iannuzzi L, Tafuri S, Passalacqua G, Quaranta N (2014) Allergic and non-allergic rhinitis: relationship with nasal polyposis, asthma and family history. Acta Otorhinolaryngol Ital 34: 36-41.

40. Staikuniene J, Vaitkus S, Japertiene LM, Ryskiene S (2008) Association of chronic rhinosinusitis with nasal polyps and asthma: Clinical and radiological features, allergy and inflammation markers. Medicina (Kaunas) 44: 257-265.

41. Ramakrishnan VR, Hauser LJ, Feazel LM, Ir D, Robertson CE, Frank DN. (2015) Sinus microbiota varies among chronic rhinosinusitis phenotypes and predicts surgical outcome. J Allergy Clin Immunol 136: 334-342.

42. Ferguson BJ, Barnes L, Bernstein JM, Brown D, Clark CE 3rd, et al. (2000) Geographic variation in allergic fungal rhinosinusitis. Otolaryngol Clin North Am 33: 441-449.

43. Hidir Y, Tosun F, Saracli MA, Gunal A, Gulec M, et al. (2008) Rate of allergic fungal etiology of chronic rhinosinusitis in Turkish population. Eur Arch Otorhinolaryngol 265: 415-419.

44. Braun H, Buzina W, Freudenschuss K, Beham A, Stammberger H (2003) 'Eosinophilic fungal rhinosinusitis': A common disorder in Europe? Laryngoscope 113: 264-269.

45. Telmesani LM (2009) Prevalence of allergic fungal sinusitis among patients with nasal polyps. Ann Saudi Med 29: 212-214.

46. Fair RJ, Tor Y (2014) Antibiotics and bacterial resistance in the 21st century. Perspect Medicin Chem 6: 25-64.

19

Multi-nodular Goiter with Intra-tracheal Thyroid Tissue: Ectopic or Implanted? and Ectopic Nasopharyngeal Thyroid Tissue

Muhammad Sami Jabbr*, Jamal Kassouma, Hussain Talib Salman and Gamal Youssef

Dubai Health Authority, Dubai Hospital, Albaraha, Alkhalij Street, Dubai, UAE

Abstract

We present a case of intra-tracheal thyroid tissue in a 44 year old woman who had been treated for multi-nodular goiter with left thyroidectomy 26 years earlier, the thyroid tissue was found in the trachea lumen which may appears to have been implanted at the time of this operation or it is a case of ectopic thyroid tissue. The patient presented with progressive right thyroid lobe swelling. Clinical examination and investigations were carried out. Right thyroidectomy was performed first, then after discovering in laryngostroboscopy, CT scan and MRI, the presence of intra-tracheal lesion narrowing the airways, patient had another procedure to remove the residual left thyroid lobe and the intra-tracheal tissue which was thyroid tissue as confirmed by histology examination. Post-operative I131 whole body-scan showed ectopic thyroid tissue in nasopharynx and residual tissue in thyroid bed. Currently the patient is free of complaint, but further investigation: SPECT-CT Scan was requested for better localization.

Keywords: Thyroid gland; Ectopic thyroid; Implanted thyroid tissue; Trachea

Background

The ectopic thyroid is uncommon with the prevalence rate of approximately 1 per 100,000 – 300,000 persons. More than 440 cases have been reported in Europe, America, and Asia to date [1-5]. Anatomically, the most common sites of ectopic thyroid tissue are lingual, sublingual, thyroglossal and laryngotracheal. In rare cases, esophageal, mediastinal, cardiac, aortic, adrenal, pancreatic, duodenal, gallbladder, mesentery of the small intestine, cutaneous and intra-tracheal sites have been found [6-15]. There is also unique cases of ectopic thyroid tissue include pituitary fossa, sphenoid sinus and uterus [16-18]. To our knowledge, this is the first case of ectopic nasopharyngeal thyroid tissue have been reported or published to date. Additionally there have been rare reports of Implantation of thyroid tissue following blunt trauma, fine needle aspiration biopsy and endoscopic thyroid surgery [19-23].

Case Presentation

A 44- year- old woman, nonsmoker, presented with progressive painless right sided neck swelling since more than 2 years, on examination she has right thyroid lobe enlargement, freely movable, not fixed to the skin, nodular, diffuse and about 4*4 cm in size, with other complaints of increasing dyspnea and swallowing difficulty since few months, she had been treated for asthma by her general practitioner. 26 years earlier, the patient had been treated for multi-nodular goiter with left hemi-thyroidectomy with subsequent thyroxin replacement therapy. There is family history of thyroid goiter in her sisters and she is allergic to penicillin. During the current presentation, clinical examination showed painless nodular right thyroid lobe swelling adherent and displacing the trachea, together with tremor, tachycardia and some stridor in deep inspiration, thyroid function tests were normal. Indirect laryngoscopy showed restricted mobility of left vocal cord only. The patient underwent completion thyroidectomy by right hemi-thyroidectomy, during the surgery, there was infiltration of thyroid tissue in between the tracheal rings, and small air leak was detected from trachea after shaving off the thyroid tissue which repaired

by using prolene 4-0 suture. Histologically: nodular hyperplasia (multi-nodular goitre), no evidence of malignancy.

On post-operative first day, patient developed biphasic stridor without any sign of neck swelling or hematoma, laryngostroboscopy showed restricted mobility of left vocal cord and submucosal rounded smooth intraluminal lesion on the right side causing marked narrowing in subglottic area, and this low mobility of left vocal cord can be attributed to the previous surgery on left side (Figure 1). Computed Tomography Scanning of the neck showed submucosal intraluminal mass extending from subglottic area to about the level of third tracheal ring, causing narrowing more than 50% of the airways (Figures 2-5). Magnetic Resonance Imaging (MRI) of the neck showed enhancing nodule mainly in the left side of the tracheal lumen in close relation to the left thyroid lobe, suggestive of either an ectopic thyroid nodule or abnormally implanted thyroid tissue post prior surgeries (Figure 6).

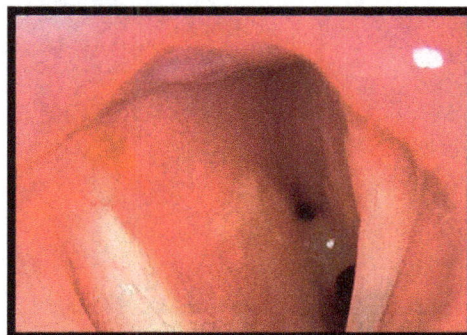

Figure 1: Laryngostroboscopy showed right sided intraluminal submucosal lesion narrowing the airways.

*Corresponding author: Muhammad Sami Jabbr, Dubai Health Authority, Dubai Hospital, Albaraha, Alkhalij Street, Dubai, UAE; Fax: 0097142195613; E-mail: msamijabbr@dha.gov.ae

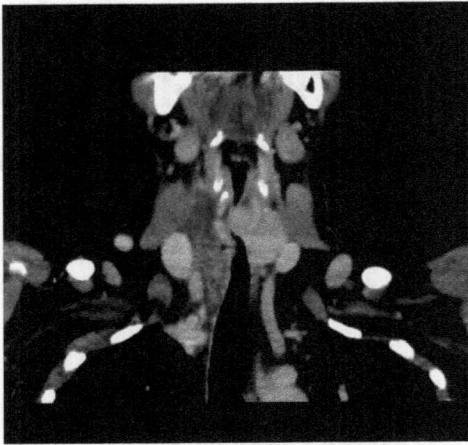

Figure 2: Neck CT Scan- coronal view showed submucosal subglottic mass narrowing the airways.

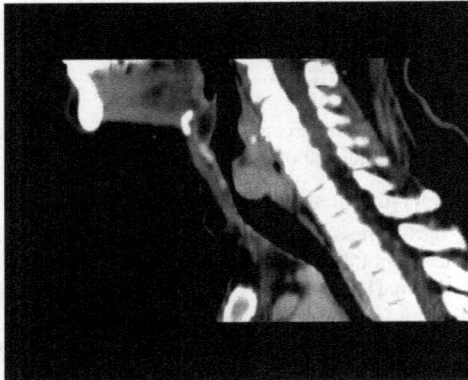

Figure 3: Neck CT Scan- sagittal view showed submucosal subglottic mass narrowing the airways.

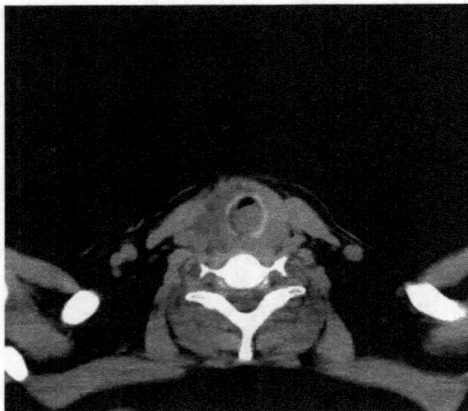

Figure 4: Neck CT Scan- axial view showed submucosal subglottic mass narrowing the airways.

Drain was removed next day, patient still complains of stridor, so patient was planned for excision of the tracheal lesion with or without surgical tracheostomy and tracheal stenting. Surgery was done two days later, starting with surgical tracheostomy and then we were unable to remove the intra-tracheal lesion sub-mucosally using debrider and bronchoscope, so we did an external approach (Laryngofissure) by median cricoidotomy extending through first three tracheal rings, exposing the endo-sublglottis area and endo upper trachea, sub-mucosal removal of lesion, re-approximating and suturing mucosal edges, suturing of cricoid and trachea bu absorbable sutures, following by completion thyroidectomy in left side and finishing by closure of tracheostomy, frozen section of this intra-tracheal lesion confirmed thyroid tissue.

Following surgery, the patient was kept intubated in ICU for 6 days to keep endotracheal tube in place as a stent, and then Micro-laryngotracheoscopy under general anesthesia was done and revealed patent airways so patient was extubated with uneventful postoperative course without any stridor or respiration difficulty, patient was discharged few days later. Endoscopic control after two weeks showed fixed left vocal cord, mobile right vocal cords and clear subglottic area (Figure 7).

I131 whole body Scan was performed after 1 month and showed

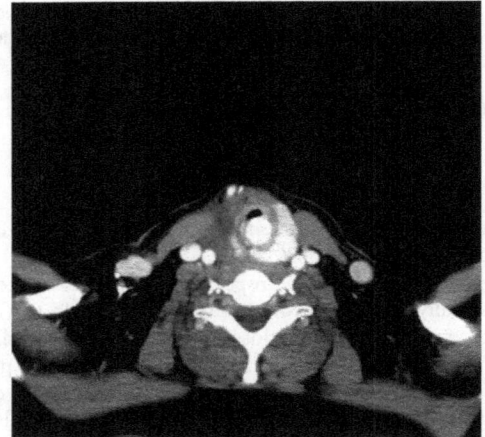

Figure 5: Neck CT Scan- axial view with contrast showed submucosal subglottic mass narrowing the airways.

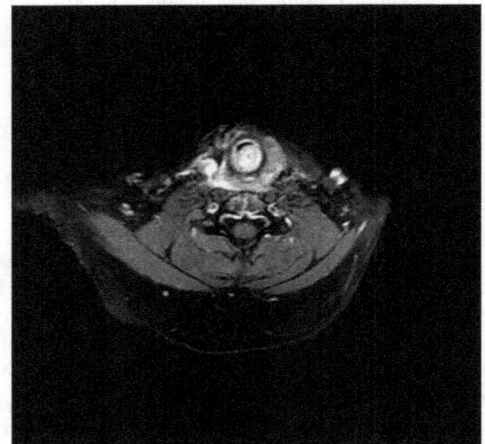

Figure 6: Magnetic Resonance Imaging (MRI) of the neck showed enhancing nodule mainly in the left side of the tracheal lumen in close relation to the left thyroid lobe narrowing the airways.

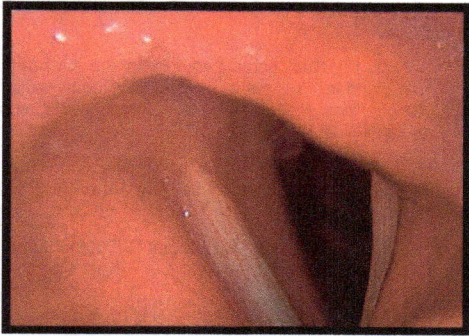

Figure 7: Post-operative Laryngostoboscopy showed clear airways.

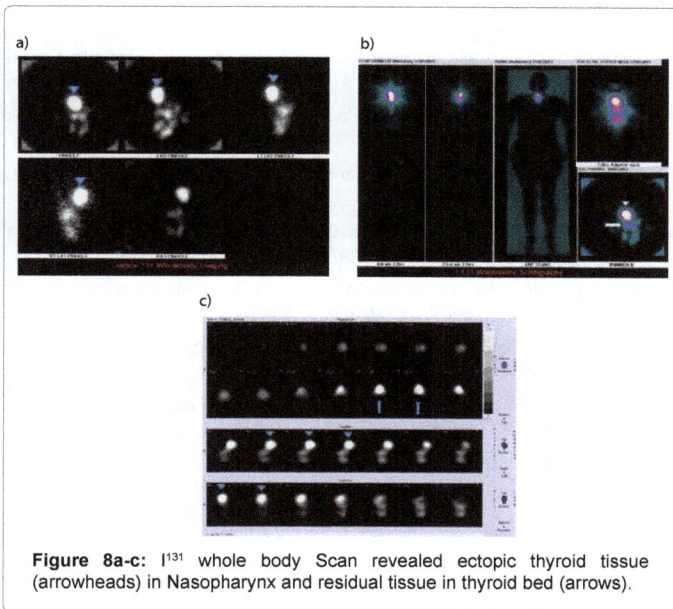

Figure 8a-c: I[131] whole body Scan revealed ectopic thyroid tissue (arrowheads) in Nasopharynx and residual tissue in thyroid bed (arrows).

ectopic thyroid tissue in nasopharynx and residual tissue in thyroid bed (Figures 8).

Endocrinologist advised to do SPECT-CT Scan for better localization and Radio ablation of this residual thyroidal tissue but patient refused. At present, patient attends the voice clinic for voice therapy without any symptoms of airway obstruction and endocrinology clinic for follow up her thyroid function.

Discussion

First ectopic thyroid case was reported as a lingual thyroid by Hickman in the year of 1869 [24]. Ectopic thyroid is a developmental defect of thyroid gland that leads to presence of thyroid tissue at sites other than its normal cervical location. Presence of two ectopic foci of thyroid tissue is rare, only a very few cases of dual ectopia have been reported in the world literature and it is extremely rarer to have dual ectopic thyroid with a normally located pre-tracheal thyroid gland as our presented case [25-27]. Scintigraphy, using Technetium-99m, I-131, or I-123, is the most important diagnostic tool for ectopic thyroid but CT scan and MRI may help in defining the extension and location of the ectopic thyroid gland and fiberoptic laryngoscopy is recommended in order to visualize directly the intra-tracheal mass and biopsy is required for a histologic diagnosis

[28-30]. Intra-tracheal ectopic thyroid tissue can cause progressive dyspnea, airway obstruction, stridor, cough, swallowing difficulty, and hemoptysis. The symptoms of ectopic intra-tracheal thyroid can easily be mistaken for those of asthma as in our case [31]. Treatment choices of ectopic thyroid tissue are: surgery, radioiodine ablation, and thyroid-suppression therapy [18]. Asymptomatic and euthyroid patients with ectopic thyroid tissue do not require any treatment, but when medical treatment fails in dysfunction thyroid patients or there are obstructive symptoms, haemorrhage or suspicion of malignancy, then surgery should be considered. Some surgeons consider excision in all cases [32]. The mainstay of treatment for ectopic intra-tracheal thyroid tissue is surgical excision and the endocrinologist advised the radioiodine ablation for the ectopic nasopharyngeal thyroid tissue in our present case. A variety of surgical techniques have been applied in the management of ectopic intra-tracheal thyroid tissue. Patients have two options: removal of the lesion via an open cricoid procedure, as we did in this case, or removal via an endoscopic laser-assisted approach [31,32].

In this case report, the intra-tracheal thyroid tissue was most probably dual ectopic foci with the other foci in the nasopharynx, but there is another weak probability that it was directly implanted into the tracheal lumen during the patient's initial treatment for multi-nodular goitre in right lobe of the thyroid gland, while details of that surgical procedure were not available, implantation might occurred during surgery and the resultant remnant remained quiescent for 26 years before enlarging and ecoming symptomatic. There are rare reported cases of thyroid tissue implantation following blunt trauma, fine needle aspiration biopsy and endoscopic thyroid surgery, and there are only five documented cases of intra-tracheal thyroid tissue associated with previous thyroidectomy [33-36]. These patients presented 4 to 21 years after their original thyroid surgery, with dyspnea or stridor, the tissue was resected or iopsied in all cases, and found to contain benign thyroid tissue.

In this case a pre-op indirect laryngoscopy to assess vocal cord movement and airway patency was not enough to put a pre-op diagnosis and therefore a better surgical strategy and plan, also there was no any preoperative radiologic investigations such as ultrasound or CT Scan that would be helpful in planning surgery and would know the presence of thyroid remnants in the bed of the previous surgery so it may prevent severe subsequent morbidity.

Conclusions

Even ectopic intra-tracheal thyroid tissue is rare, it should be considered as a possible cause of airway obstruction, particularly in those who have goiters. The current case highlights the possibility of Intra-operative thyroid tissue implantation in the trachea and shows the need for careful tissue handling during thyroid surgery, so ectopic thyroid tissue should be considered in the differential diagnosis even in the presence of a normal thyroid gland.

Standard thyroid workup before any surgical intervention should include imaging such as thyroid ultrasound or CT Scan and an assessment of the vocal cords by fiberoptic nasolaryngoscopy or laryngostroboscopy to ensure the status following previous surgery and prior to any further surgical treatment.

Authors' Contributions

MSJ: conception and design, writer, revision and approval of the final version. JK, HT: conception and design, revision and approval of the final version. GY: conceived of the study, and participated in its design and coordination and helped to draft the manuscript. AA: revision and approval of the final version.

References

1. Di Benedetto V (1997) Ectopic thyroid gland in the submandibular region simulating a thyroglossal duct cyst: a case report. J Pediatr Surg 32: 1745-1746.

2. Babazade F, Mortazavi H, Jalalian H, Shahvali E (2009) Thyroid tissue as a submandibular mass: a case report. J Oral Sci 51: 655-657.

3. Ulug T, Ulubil SA, Alagol F (2003) Dual ectopic thyroid: report of a case. J Laryngol Otol 117: 574-576.

4. Kalan A, Tariq M (1999) Lingual thyroid gland: clinical evaluation and comprehensive management. Ear Nose Throat J 78: 340-34, 345-9.

5. Yoon JS, Won KC, Cho IH, Lee JT, Lee HW (2007) Clinical characteristics of ectopic thyroid in Korea. Thyroid 17: 1117-1121.

6. Salam MA1 (1992) Ectopic thyroid mass adherent to the oesophagus. J Laryngol Otol 106: 746-747.

7. Gamblin TC, Jennings GR, Christie DB 3rd, Thompson WM Jr, Dalton ML (2003) Ectopic thyroid. Ann Thorac Surg 75: 1952-1953.

8. Rieser GD, Ober KP, Cowan RJ, Cordell AR (1988) Radioiodide imaging of struma cordis. Clin Nucl Med 13: 421-422.

9. Williams RJ, Lindop G, Butler J (2002) Ectopic thyroid tissue on the ascending aorta: an operative finding. Ann Thorac Surg 73: 1642-1643.

10. Shiraishi T, Imai H, Fukutome K, Watanabe M, Yatani R (1999) Ectopic thyroid in the adrenal gland. Hum Pathol 30: 105-108.

11. EyÃ¼boÄŸlu E, Kapan M, Ipek T, Ersan Y, Oz F (1999) Ectopic thyroid in the abdomen: report of a case. Surg Today 29: 472-474.

12. Maino K, Skelton H, Yeager J, Smith KJ (2004) Benign ectopic thyroid tissue in a cutaneous location: a case report and review. J Cutan Pathol 31: 195-198.

13. Takahashi T, Ishikura H, Kato H, Tanabe T, Yoshiki T (1991) Ectopic thyroid follicles in the submucosa of the duodenum. Virchows Arch A Pathol Anat Histopathol 418: 547-550.

14. Ihtiyar E, Isiksoy S, Algin C, Sahin A, Erkasap S, et al. (2003) Ectopic thyroid in the gallbladder: report of a case. Surg Today 33: 777-780.

15. Güngör B, Kebat T, Ozaslan C, Akilli S (2002) Intra-abdominal ectopic thyroid presenting with hyperthyroidism: report of a case. Surg Today 32: 148-150.

16. Malone Q, Conn J, Gonzales M, Kaye A, Coleman P (1997) Ectopic pituitary fossa thyroid tissue. J Clin Neurosci 4: 360-363.

17. Yilmaz F, Uzunlar AK, Sögütçü N (2005) Ectopic thyroid tissue in the uterus. Acta Obstet Gynecol Scand 84: 201-202.

18. Noussios G, Anagnostis P, Goulis DG, Lappas D, Natsis K (2011) Ectopic thyroid tissue: anatomical, clinical, and surgical implications of a rare entity. Eur J Endocrinol 165: 375-382.

19. Harach HR, Cabrera JA, Williams ED (2004) Thyroid implants after surgery and blunt trauma. Ann Diagn Pathol 8: 61-68.

20. Ito Y, Tomoda C, Uruno T, Takamura Y, Miya A, et al. (2005) Needle tract implantation of papillary thyroid carcinoma after fine-needle aspiration biopsy. World J Surg 29: 1544-1549.

21. Tamiolakis D, Antoniou C, Venizelos J, Lambropoulou M, Alexiadis G, et al. (2006) Papillary thyroid carcinoma metastasis most probably due to fine needle aspiration biopsy. A case report. Acta Dermatovenerol Alp Pannonica Adriat 15: 169-172.

22. Lee YS, Yun JS, Jeong JJ, Nam KH, Chung WY, et al. (2008) Soft tissue implantation of thyroid adenomatous hyperplasia after endoscopic thyroid surgery. Thyroid 18: 483-484.

23. Love RL, Ahsan F, Allison R, Keast A, Lambie N (2012) Multinodular goitre arising in the tracheal lumen: implantation or ectopic? J Laryngol Otol 126: 100-102.

24. Hickman W (1869) Congenital tumor of the base of the tongue, pressing down on the epiglottis and causing death by suffocation sixteen hours after birth. Trans Pathol Soc Lond 20:160–161.

25. Harisankar CNB (2013) Dual ectopic thyroid in the presence of atrophic orthotopic thyroid gland in a patient with acquired hypothyroidism: Evaluation with hybrid Single-Photon Emission Computed Tomography/Computed Tomography. Indian J Nucl Med. 28: 26–27.

26. Choudhury BK, Saikia UK, Sarma D, Saikia M, Choudhury SD, et al. (2011) Dual Ectopic Thyroid with Normally Located Thyroid: A Case Report. Journal of Thyroid Research.

27. Sood A, Sood V, Sharma DR, Seam RK, Kumar R (2008) Thyroid scintigraphy in detecting dual ectopic thyroid: a review. Eur J Nucl Med Mol Imaging 35: 843-846.

28. Bersaneti JA, Silva RD, Ramos RR, Matsushita Mde M, Souto LR (2011) Ectopic thyroid presenting as a submandibular mass. Head Neck Pathol 5: 63-66.

29. Sauk JJ Jr (1970) Ectopic lingual thyroid. J Pathol 102: 239-243.

30. Peters P, Stark P, Essig G Jr, Lorincz B, Bowman J, et al. (2010) Lingual thyroid: an unusual and surgically curable cause of sleep apnoea in a male. Sleep Breath 14: 377-380.

31. Yinlong Y, Quan L, JinMiao Q, Youqun X, Yifei P, et al. (2010) Ectopic Intratracheal Thyroid: case report. Southern Medical Journal.

32. Ramaniraj M, Jousal CP (2012) Dual ectopic thyroid – A case report of a very rare disease. JORL 2 Issue: 201.

33. Soylu L, KiroÄŸlu F, ErsÃ¶z C, Ozcan C, Aydogan B (1993) Intralaryngotracheal thyroid. Am J Otolaryngol 14: 145-147.

34. Byrd MC, Thompson LD, Wieneke JA (2003) Intratracheal ectopic thyroid tissue: a case report and literature review. Ear Nose Throat J 82: 514-518.

35. Dowling EA, Johnson IM, Collier FC, Dillard RA (1962) Intratracheal goiter: a clinico-pathologic review. Ann Surg 156: 258-267.

36. Osammor JY, Bulman CH, Blewitt RW (1990) Intralaryngotracheal thyroid. J Laryngol Otol 104: 733-736.

20

Oral Carcinoma, HPV Infection, Arsenic Exposure-their Correlation in West Bengal, India

Pritha Pal[1*], Ranjan Raychowdhury[2] and Ajanta Halder[1]

[1]Department of Genetics, Vivekananda Institute of Medical Sciences, Ramakrishna Mission Seva Pratishthan, 99 Sarat Bose Road, Kolkata, West Bengal, India

[2]Department of Otolaryngology, Vivekananda Institute of Medical Sciences, Ramakrishna Mission Seva Pratishthan, 99 Sarat Bose Road, Kolkata

*Corresponding author: Pritha Pal, Research Scholar, Department of Genetics, Vivekananda Institute of Medical Sciences, Ramakrishna Mission Seva Pratishthan, 99 Sarat Bose Road, Kolkata- 700026, West Bengal, India; E-mail: pritha.mcbt@gmail.com

Abstract

Objective: The aim is to find out any possible correlation between HPV infection and oral carcinoma along with this metal toxicity.

Methods: Ethical clearance for this study was obtained from the Ethics Committee of Vivekananda Institute of Medical Sciences, Ramakrishna Mission Seva Pratishthan. Patients attending our hospital were screened for the presence of oral premalignant and malignant lesions. The subjects were administered a standard questionnaire. The buccal swab and hair samples (107 cases and 50 controls) were collected after obtaining informed consent from all the corresponding subjects, and were analysed for detection of HPV 16 DNA and arsenic level analysis, respectively.

Results: 22.5% of malignant samples showed the presence of HPV 16 DNA. 80% of cases showed their arsenic count above the safe limit (0.8 µg/g).

Conclusion: A considerable percentage of malignant samples showed the presence of HPV16 DNA, indicating that there may be a correlation between HPV infection and oral malignancy in this population. A higher percentage of cases showing an elevated arsenic count states a possible link between arsenic toxicity and the development of this disease. However, a higher population size and statistical analysis are required for a proper conclusion.

Keywords: Human papilloma virus; Koilocytes; Arsenic toxicity; Buccal swab; Hair; Oral cancer; West Bengal

Abbreviations HPV: Human Papilloma Virus; OSCC: Oral Squamous Cell Carcinoma; OM: Oral Malignant; OPM: Oral Premalignant; PBS: Phosphate Buffer Saline; SD: Standard Deviation; As: Arsenic

Introduction

Oral squamous cell carcinoma (OSCC) accounts for the second most common cancer in adult males and third most common cancer in adult females worldwide. Incidence rates for oral cancer vary in men from 1 to 10 cases per 100,000 populations in many countries. In India, the age standardized incidence rate of oral cancer is reported as 12.6 per 100,000 populations. It is estimated that around 43% of cancer deaths are due to tobacco use, unhealthy diets, alcohol consumption and various infections. The prevalence of oral cancer is reportedly particularly high among men than in women but also contradicted to be opposite in some western countries [1]. The widespread use of various forms of tobacco, betel quid chewing, smoking habits and alcohol intake are considered as the main risk factors behind oral cancer. But, in recent years, many research studies suggest that there have been many cases developing this cancer without any history of habits related to these risk factors, which brings out the rise of another potent factor, namely the viral infection [2]. This has been attributed to

the human papilloma virus in various Western countries [1]. The reports of HPV prevalence in oral cancer from southern India seem to be highly variable [3]. High association rate of HPV-16 in OSCC cases, between 62% and 95%, have been well documented by various studies. Another factor namely, heavy metal toxicity has very shortly come into play for the development of cancer. These metals include lead, nickel, arsenic etc. whose presence in soils may exert their effects on human health through the food grown on them, which may put people under a higher risk of cancer development, if the metal is proved to be a carcinogen [4]. Arsenic (As) exposure leading to skin, lung and bladder cancer has already been established [5]. Moreover, many countries like Taiwan (mainly Central and Eastern parts) have alarming levels of oral cancer incidence [6], many cases accounting to the arsenic exposure. Since West Bengal has been known to be an arsenic prone state [7], we have chosen this zone in our study to find out a possible correlation between the arsenic toxicity and the development of oral malignancy.

Materials and Methods

Study population

In this case-control prospective study, a stratified sampling method was used to select 157 participants (54 oral malignant (OM), 53 oral premalignant (OPM), 50 control) to be interviewed after being informed about the research. Ethical clearance for this study was obtained from the Ethics committee of Ramakrishna Mission Seva Pratishthan and VIMS, Kolkata. 30785 patients were screened in the Department of ENT, Head and Neck Surgery and Oral and Maxillo Facial Surgery of our hospital. Among these, 54 patients with histopathologically confirmed cases of oral carcinoma, 53 with premalignant oral lesions and conditions were recruited for this study between November 2012 and July 2015. All cases were newly diagnosed and previously untreated. Clinical characteristics including basic medical data were obtained from medical records. All were resident of different districts of West Bengal. 50 controls (cancer free) were recruited simultaneously from the relative of the patients residing in similar geographic area. Controls were selected among the relatives of the cases who accompanied them and staying in the same localities. Age distribution for the controls was comparable to that of the cases. Cases and controls were matched primarily by frequency of geographic and social origin and secondly by age distribution. They mostly belong to medium to low economic classes having similar lifestyle and level of education.

Questionnaire administration

After signing the informed consent, subjects were interviewed to collect their demographic data (age, gender and residential history), their daily life style and occupation. Data relating to arsenic contamination in 129 blocks of 8 districts of the state of West Bengal and 100 wards of the city of Kolkata were obtained from literature [8].

Collection and analysis of samples

Buccal smear and swab samples, hair samples were collected after obtaining informed consent from all the subjects. 54 malignant, 53 premalignant and 50 control hair samples were analyzed by the method of flow injection-hydride generation-atomic absorption spectrometry for arsenic count and their buccal smears were taken on slides, Pap stained and examined under microscope for detecting the presence of koilocytes. The corresponding buccal swab samples were dissolved in Phosphate Buffer Saline (PBS) solution and DNA was extracted from all the sample solutions following the standard Qiagen

protocol, using the Qiagen DNA Mini Kit. Further PCR was performed with all the DNA samples, positive control (HPV 16 plasmid DNA) using the HPV 16 L1 consensus primers [MY11/MY09].

Primers	Sequence	Amplimer size (approx. bp)
MY11	5'GCCCAAGGACATAACAATGG	
MY09	5'CGTCCAAGGGGAAACTGATC	450

Analysis

Descriptive analysis was conducted comparing cases with malignant and premalignant oral lesions to the control group in terms of demographic factors, arsenic level in hair samples and the presence of micronuclei and apoptosis in buccal smear. To compare the case and control groups a student t-test was used for continuous variables (arsenic level in hair). The Arsenic (As) level mean, standard deviation (SD), quartiles and medians for all these groups were calculated. Statistical analysis was done using Graph-pad prism software. All tests were two-sided with a significant level of p value < 0.001.

Results

Figure 1 shows the overall association of various risk factors with the patients and controls. The age-sex distribution, source of drinking water and the various risk factor associations is depicted in Table 1. In the literature, the state of West Bengal has been divided into three groups of arsenic affected areas, based on the maximum permissible limit of arsenic concentration in groundwater being 50µg/L (recommended by World Health Organization). These are: highly affected (Out of 149 blocks in 8 districts and 100 wards of Kolkata, 107 blocks and 30 wards are affected), mildly affected (Out of 29 blocks in 5 districts, 4 blocks are affected) and unaffected (Out of 63 blocks in 5 districts, none is affected). In our study, patients and control individuals came from different districts of West Bengal. 123 (75%) patients came from the highly arsenic affected areas and 41 came from the unaffected areas, none came from the mildly affected areas.

Type	Sex M	Sex F	N	Age 15-35	Age 36-55	Age 56-75	Municipality Corporation – Mineral water	Municipality Corporation – Direct	Municipality Corporation – Treated	Tube well Deep – Direct	Tube well Deep – Treated	Tube well Shallow – Direct	Tube well Shallow – Treated	Pond water – Direct	Pond water – Treated	Betel quid	Oral tobacco	Smoking tobacco	Alcohol	Non-user
Control	37	13	50	12	32	6	1	20	12	10	0	6	0	0	1	4	1	0	0	46
Premalignant	39	14	53	13	33	7	1	21	13	11	0	6	0	0	1	12	17	22	9	4
Malignant	38	16	54	11	35	8	1	20	15	10	0	7	0	0	1	20	14	20	9	3

Table 1: The age and sex distribution, sources of drinking water and various addictions of malignant, premalignant and control individuals are presented here, *please note: Some of the malignant and premalignant cases and control individuals have more than one addiction.

The data relating to the highly arsenic affected and unaffected districts of West Bengal is compared to the data of the geographic distribution of the patients coming from those districts in the maps of West Bengal in Figure 2 and the tabular comparison is shown through Table 2.

Arsenic Exposure in West Bengal	Districts	% of blocks affected	% of patients came
Highly affected	Nadia	100	~2
	North 24 Parganas	95.4	~17
	Murshidabad	92.3	~2
	South 24 Parganas	64.7	~14
	Howrah	58.3	~12
	Kolkata	30	~45
Unaffected	Purulia	0	~2
	Midnapur (East)	0	~4
	Midnapur (West)	0	~2

Table 2: Tabular representation of the percentage of affected blocks in different highly arsenic affected and unaffected districts of West Bengal with the percentage of patients coming from those areas.

The statistics of distribution of As level in hair samples of our study population is shown in Table 3. The medians and ranges are presented in addition to the mean, SD and the quartiles. Out of 164 cases, 80% showed their arsenic count above the safe limit (0.8 μg/g; recommended by WHO), whereas, 96% of the controls' arsenic count were within the safe limit. This is shown in Figure 3.

Cases	Statistical Data					
	n	Mean	25-75th percentile	Range	Median	95% of CI of mean
Malignant	54	2.071 (1.102)	1.17- 2.615	0.72-4.78	1.88	1.616, 2.526
Premalignant	53	1.746 (1.067)	0.935- 2.52	0.39-4.23	1.45	1.306, 2.187
Control	50	0.544 (0.11)	0.44- 0.63	0.40-0.76	0.52	0.513, 0.576
p value	< 0.001*					

* denotes that the difference of mean values between control group and case (premalignant and malignant) group w.r.t. arsenic count is highly significant

Table 3: Statistical representation of arsenic levels of malignant, premalignant and control groups.

Out of 54 malignant cases, 27.78% (15/54) showed the presence of koilocytes, where out of these 15 cases, 80% (12/15) showed the presence of HPV 16 after PCR analysis. On the contrary, none of the premalignant and control cases showed the presence of HPV 16 DNA (Figure 4), both of which are related to each other. 9.25% (5/54) of the malignant cases showed the presence of both high arsenic count and HPV 16 DNA as well.

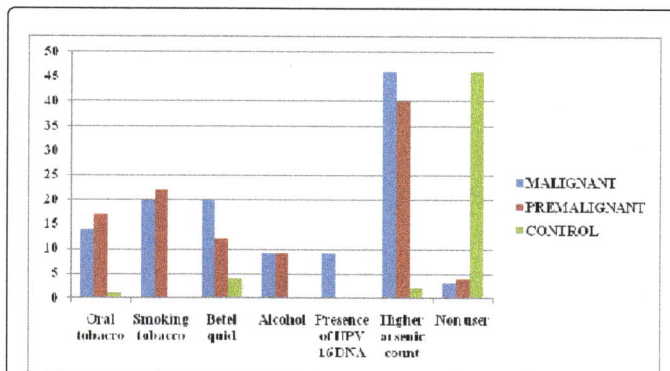

Figure 1: The histogram shows the association of various risk factors (including non user) with patients in malignant, premalignant groups and control individuals.

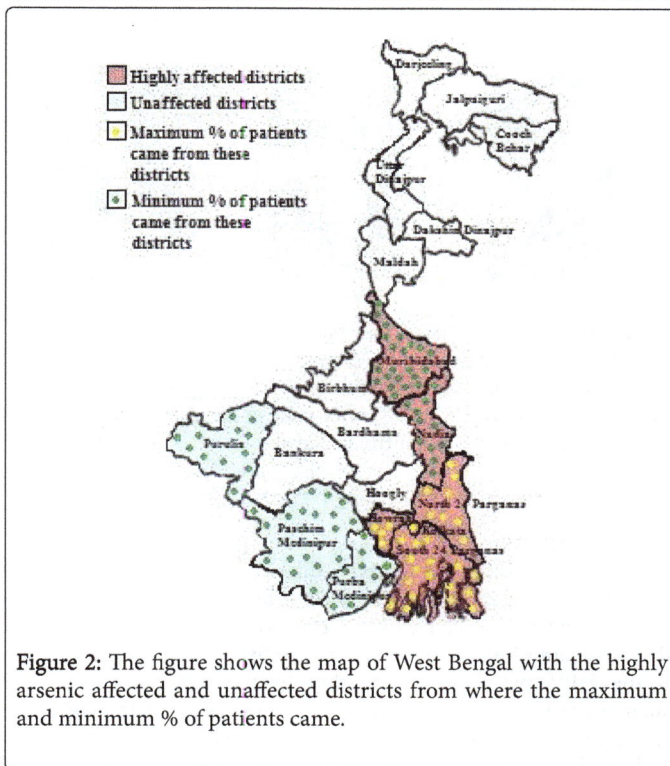

Figure 2: The figure shows the map of West Bengal with the highly arsenic affected and unaffected districts from where the maximum and minimum % of patients came.

Discussion

Increased incidence of oral cancer in younger adults with non-smoking habits and decline in the number of tobacco and alcohol related OSCC has been recorded over the past 30 years. Recently, women are reportedly at risk of this infection apart from much susceptible male in places like Vietnam [9]. Some estimates suggest that 70-90% of new oropharyngeal cancers have evidence of HPV [10]. Viral regulation of miRNA expression in oral cancer diagnosis including that of Epstein-Barr virus apart from HPV has also been stated in India [11].

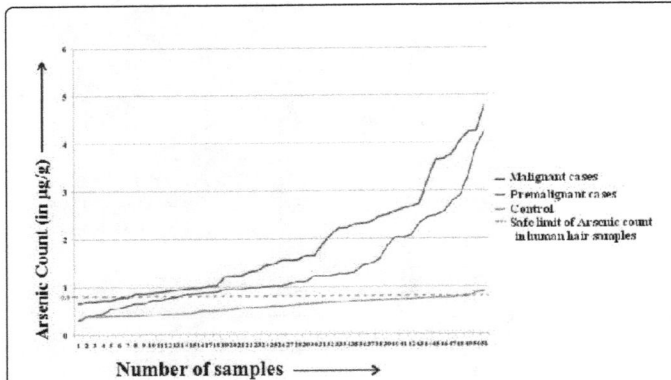

Figure 3: The graph shows the arsenic count (in μg/g) analyzed from human hair samples of premalignant and malignant cases and control groups.

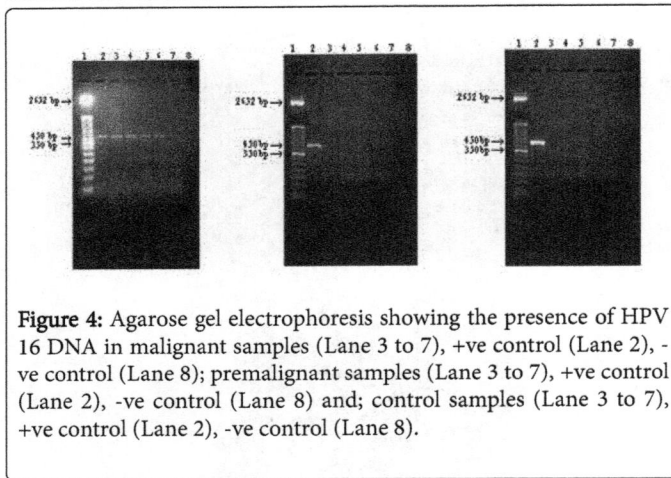

Figure 4: Agarose gel electrophoresis showing the presence of HPV 16 DNA in malignant samples (Lane 3 to 7), +ve control (Lane 2), -ve control (Lane 8); premalignant samples (Lane 3 to 7), +ve control (Lane 2), -ve control (Lane 8) and; control samples (Lane 3 to 7), +ve control (Lane 2), -ve control (Lane 8).

cytogenetic damage like micronuclei (MN), chromosomal aberrations (CA), sister chromatid exchanges (SCE) and aneuploidy have also been reported from the human populations exposed to arsenic through drinking water in various countries like Mexico, Finland, Argentina, etc. [17]. So, arsenic has become an alarming risk factor for the development of oral malignancy. Potential involvement of the mutated genes of Glutathione S-transferases (GSTs) enzymes leads to carcinoma caused by arsenic toxicity, which can be easily analyzed by CA and MN assays [17]. The two worst affected areas in the world are Bangladesh and West Bengal, India. In nine districts in West Bengal approx. 42.7 million people are exposed to ground water arsenic concentrations that are above the WHO maximum permissible limit of 50 μg/L. In both these areas the source of arsenic is mainly geological in origin contaminating aquifers which provide water for over one million tube-wells. The mechanism of arsenic accumulation in the Bengal Delta Plain is thought to have occurred during the late Quaternary age (Holocene age) with arsenic–containing alluvial sediments deposited by the Ganges, Brahmaputra, Meghna and other smaller rivers that flow across the Bengal Delta Plain in to the Bay of Bengal. The total As content in the farm soil of contaminated areas has profoundly negative impacts on nearby residents. Several studies have addressed the association between heavy metals in the environment and heavy metals inside the human body. The high concentrations of specific metals in the environment may be responsible for the high concentrations of these metals in the blood, urine and hair. Since arsenic toxicity is a proven factor of skin cancer, lung cancer and bladder cancer [18] and this metal is highly prevalent in the groundwater of West Bengal [19] at a concentration above 50 μg/L (recommended by World Health Organization; Erstwhile), we are trying to focus on its effect over the occurrence of oral malignancy, the latter being on an increasing level in this zone.

Conclusion

In this study, a considerable percentage of malignant cases showing the presence of HPV 16 DNA may suggest that this viral infection is acting as a potent factor of the development of this disease in this population of West Bengal, taking the other common risk factors into consideration. Some of the previous studies [3] also suggest this association playing an important role in the development of oral and oropharyngeal malignancy. Moreover a high percentage of cases bearing elevated arsenic count may also focus on its effect in contributing to this malignancy. Contrary to our findings a recent case-control study in central Taiwan revealed the absence of significant association between As blood levels and oral malignant and premalignant lesions [20]. However previous studies, it was found positive associations between this metal and risk of various type of cancers [21-24].

Moreover, a small yet considerable percentage of cases showing both the parameters simultaneously may state that these two factors (HPV infection and arsenic toxicity) when acting at a time, may contribute to this carcinoma to a larger extent. For such conclusion, much higher population size and proper statistical analysis is definitely required. This work also opens up into a new phase of research where further studies can be carried out to find out any possible correlation between these two factors, may be suggesting their additive role or whether this viral infection gets promoted in such in vivo environment of metal toxicity, contributing to the development of carcinoma on a larger scale.

Genetic polymorphisms and HPV infection has also been correlated [12]. HPV 16 antibodies are said to contribute to the increased risk of HPV associated oral cancer [13]. However, malignant potential of HPV is hypothesised but not definitely confirmed [14]. Various studies on the HPV prevalence accounting to the development of oral squamous cell carcinoma have also been done in countries like- Chile [15], China, California etc. In developing countries like India, not much study on this correlation has been yet focussed except some of the southern places of this country. So, we have chosen the population of West Bengal in our study to find out any possible link between this viral factor and the causation of this malignancy. In our study, a small yet considerable percentage of malignant cases showing the presence of this viral may contribute to the hypothesis of this viral infection playing as a factor in the development of oral carcinoma. However, since other risk factors are also taken into consideration in this study, we cannot bring out the independent role of HPV in this field. Further studies with higher sample size and appropriate statistical analysis are required to ascertain this phase of causation. On the other hand, the level of heavy metal exposure to the human body is reflected through the elevated concentrations of heavy metals in the soil [16]. Such findings of heavy metal toxicity have proven out to be a carcinogen in many places of Taiwan [6], Greece, etc. Higher incidences of

Acknowledgement

We are grateful to Swami Satyadevananda, Secretary of Ramakrishna Mission Seva Pratishthan to kindly allow us to conduct the study in this institution. We are also indebted to DST Inspire Fellowship, New Delhi for giving the financial assistance used in buying all the necessary chemicals, reagents and instruments required for DNA extraction, PCR apparatus and arsenic estimation procedure. There is no conflict of interest related to this study.

References

1. Chaturvedi AK, Anderson WF, Lortet-Tieulent J, Curado MP, Ferlay J, et al. (2013) Worldwide trends in incidence rates for oral cavity and oropharyngeal cancers. J Clin Oncol 31: 4550-4559.

2. Rakesh S, Janardhanan M, Vinodkumar RB, Vidya M (2010) Association of human papilloma virus with oral squamous cell carcinoma-A brief review. Oral & Maxillofacial Pathology Journal 1: 1-9.

3. Jamaly S, Khanehkenari MR, Rao R, Patil G, Thakur S, et al. (2012) Relationship between p53 overexpression, human papillomavirus infection, and lifestyle in Indian patients with head and neck cancers. Tumour Biol 33: 543-550.

4. Navarro Silvera SA, Rohan TE (2007) Trace elements and cancer risk: A review of the epidemiologic evidence. Cancer Causes Control 18: 7-27.

5. Guha Mazumder DN (2008) Chronic arsenic toxicity and human health. Indian J Med Res 128: 436-447.

6. Su C, Lin Y, Chang T, Chiang C, Chung J, et al. (2010) Incidence of oral cancer in relation to nickel and arsenic concentrations in farm soils of patients' residential areas in Taiwan. Bio Med Central Public Health 10: 67.

7. Patra M, Halder A, Bhowmick N, De M (2005) Use of black tea in modulating clastogenic effects of arsenic in mice in vivo, West Bengal, India. Journal of Environmental Pathology, Toxicology and Oncology 24: 201-210.

8. Chakraborti D, Das B, Rahman MM, Chowdhury UK, Biswas B, et al. (2009) Status of groundwater arsenic contamination in the state of West Bengal, India: A 20 year study report. Mol Nutr Food Res 53: 542-551.

9. Bui TC, Tran LT, Markham CM, Huynh TT, Tran LT, et al. (2015) Self-reported oral health, oral hygiene and oral HPV infection in at-risk women in Ho Chi Minh City, Vietnam. Oral Surg Oral Med Oral Pathol Oral Radiol 120: 34-42.

10. Young D, Xiao CC, Murphy B, Moore M, Fakhry C, et al. (2015) Increase in head and neck cancer in younger patients due to human papillomavirus (HPV). Oral Oncol 51: 727-730.

11. Chawla JP, Iyer N, Soodan KS, Sharma A, Khurana SK, et al. (2015) Role of miRNA in cancer diagnosis, prognosis, therapy and regulation of its expression by Epstein-Barr virus and human papillomaviruses: With special reference to oral cancer. Oral Oncol 51: 731-737.

12. Sun Y, Zhang Y, Liu L, Song X, Li G (2015) Genetic polymorphisms and HPV infection in oral squamous cell carcinomas. Curr Opin Virol 14: 1-6.

13. Anderson KS, Dahlstrom KR, Cheng JN, Alam R, Li G, et al. (2015) HPV16 antibodies as risk factors for oropharyngeal cancer and their association with tumor HPV and smoking status. Oral Oncol 51: 662-667.

14. Gupta S, Gupta S (2015) Role of human papillomavirus in oral squamous cell carcinoma and oral potentially malignant disorders: A review of the literature. Indian J Dent 6: 91-98.

15. Reyes M, Rojas-Alcayaga G, Pennacchiotti G, Carrillo D, Muñoz JP, et al. (2015) Human papillomavirus infection in oral squamous cell carcinomas from Chilean patients. Exp Mol Pathol 99: 95-99.

16. Li Y, Wang YB, Gou X, Su YB, Wang G (2006) Risk assessment of heavy metals in soils and vegetables around non-ferrous metals mining and smelting sites, Baiyin, China. J Environ Sci 18: 1124-1134.

17. Ghosh P, Basu A, Mahata J, Basu S, Sengupta M, et al. (2006) Cytogenetic damage and genetic variants in the individuals susceptible to arsenic-induced cancer through drinking water. Int J Cancer 118: 2470-2478.

18. Saha JC, Dikshit AK, Bandyopadhyay M, Saha KC (1999) A review of arsenic poisoning and its effects on human health. Critical Reviews in Environmental Science and Technology 29: 281-313.

19. Das D, Samanta G, Mandal BK, Roy Chowdhury T, Chanda CR, et al. (1996) Arsenic in groundwater in six districts of West Bengal, India. Environ Geochem Health 18: 5-15.

20. Yuan TH, Lian IB, Tsai KY, Chang TK, Chiang CT, et al. (2011) Possible association between nickel and chromium and oral cancer: A case-control study in central Taiwan. Sci Total Environment 409: 1046–1052.

21. Kazi TG, Wadhwa SK, Afridi HI, KaziN, Kandhro GA, et al. (2010) Interaction of cadmium and zinc in biological samples of smokers and chewing tobacco female mouth cancer patients. J Hazard Mater 176: 985–991.

22. Su CC, Lin YY, Chang TK, Chiang CT, Chung JA, et al. (2010) Incidence of oral cancer in relation to nickel and arsenic concentrations in farm soils of patients' residential areas in Taiwan. BMC Public Health.

23. Kazi TG, Wadhwa SK, Afridi HI, Kazi N, Kandhro GA, et al. (2010) Evaluation of cadmium and zinc in biological samples of tobacco and alcohol user male mouth cancer patients. Hum Exp Toxicol 29: 221-230.

24. Feki-Tounsi M, Olmedo P, Gil F, Khlifi R, Mhiri MN, et al. (2013) Cadmium in blood of Tunisian men and risk of bladder cancer: Interactions with arsenic exposure and smoking. Environ Sci Pollut Res Int 20: 7204-7213.

21

Ossicular Chain Erosion in Chronic Suppurative Otitis Media

Hassan Haidar, Rashid Sheikh, Aisha Larem, Ali Elsaadi, Hassanin Abdulkarim, Sara Ashkanani and Abdulsalm Alqahtani

Otolaryngology Department, Hamad Medical Corporation, Doha, Qatar

Corresponding author: Hassan Haidar, Otolaryngology Department, Hamad Medical Corporation, Doha, Qatar; E-mail: hassanhaidarmd@gmail.com

Abstract

Objectives: Hearing restoration surgery in chronic otitis media consists of myringoplasty for drum repair and ossiculoplasty for ossicular defect if present which carries a lower success rate and higher probability of revision surgery. Our objective is to evaluate the frequency of ossicular erosion in chronic suppurative otitis media which could be utilized to predict the probability of need for ossiculoplasty preoperatively then patients could be properly consented about these potential issues.

Materials and Methods: A prospective study was conducted in Otolaryngology unit of Hamad Medical Corporation. 279 ears that underwent surgery for chronic otitis media were studied and their ossicular status was reported.

Results: Ossicular chain was eroded in 66 (23.66%) out of the 279 ears. Erosion was more frequent in cholesteatoma ears (69.3%) than in safe ears (13.9%). The most frequently impaired ossicle was the incus and was found eroded in 62 (22.2%) ears. Malleus was found to be the most resilient ossicle and was eroded only in 13 (4.7%) ears. The stapes was eroded in 31 (11.1%) ears.

Conclusion: Our study shows that in chronic otitis media, approximately one-third patients have ossicular chain discontinuity. More than two thirds of patients with cholesteatoma have ossicular chain discontinuity. Otolaryngologists should be competent enough to do ossiculoplasty during ear surgery to give the best hearing results to their patients.

Keywords: Ossicles; CSOM; Erosion; Cholesteatoma

Introduction

Chronic Suppurative Otitis Media (CSOM) is a prevalent middle ear pathology that constitutes of tympanic membrane perforation together with a chronically inflamed middle ear mucosa.

CSOM can occur with or without cholesteatoma which is an in-growth of eardrum skin into the middle ear cavity.

CSOM is the leading cause of conductive hearing impairment in adults which is secondary to damage of the ear drum and middle ear ossicles induced by chronic inflammation present in the tympanic cavity. Ossicular erosion, a frequent complication of CSOM, may lead to total failure of middle ear mechanics and resulting in substantial hearing loss [1].

Hearing restoration surgery comprises ear drum repair and ossicular chain reconstruction in ears housing defective ossicles. The later scenario is associated with higher rate of long term acoustic failure that may reach 50% [2,3]. Myringoplasty in the absence of ossicular damage is bracketed with a much higher long-term success rate more than 90% even in wet ears [4].

Ossicular integrity or erosion can only be confirmed intra-operatively. The preoperative information given to the patient must be comprehensive, and should include details of the probabilities of having OCD and the associated risks of acoustic failure and need for revision surgery.

This study was conducted to assess middle ear ossicles state of in 279 ears that required surgery for CSOM. The findings of this study could be exploited to predict preoperatively the probability of having OCD in CSOM ears and thus patients could be therefore properly consented about these potential issues before surgery.

Materials and Methods

Ethical approval for this study was received from the JIRB (Joint Institutional review board) of our institution (IRB Number 14-00133).

We conducted a prospective study in our institution in the period running from January 2014 to June 2015.

Patients older than 18 who underwent tympanoplasty for CSOM during this period were recruited to our study. Patients younger than 18 or posted for revision tympanoplasty were excluded. Written informed research consent was obtained from recruited subjects.

Recruited subjects were interviewed preoperatively by the senior author for history taking and proper ear examination.

Intraoperatively, all patients had proper exploration of middle ear using microscope and endoscope looking and the status of each ossicle were checked. The presence of cholesteatoma was also checked.

Statistical analysis was done using Statistical Package for Social Sciences v.13.0 (SPSS inc., Chicago, USA). P values less than 0.05 were considered to be statistically significant.

Results

211 patients with CSOM were recruited for this study and a total of 279 ears were included. 34 patients had both ears included which were operated sequentially. The average age was (33.4 ± 8.9). 179 (84.8%) out of the 211 patients were younger than 40. There was 141 male (66.8%) and 70 female (33.1%). The most common complaint was recurrent otorrhea present the majority of the ears (89.2%), the next most common complaint was hypoacusia and was present in 213 ears (76.3%). Examination findings showed that most of the ears had safe CSOM (230 ears; 82.5%). While only 49 ears (17.5%) had cholesteaomatous or unsafe ear.

Intra-operative findings

Intra-operative middle ear exploration matched completely our pre-operative diagnosis; none of the patient who presumed to have safe ear turned to have cholesteatoma and vice versa. Overall, the ossicular chain was eroded in 66 ears out of the 279 (23.66%). In non-cholesteatomous ears, the ossicular status was intact in 198 ears (83.8%), eroded in 32 ears (13.9%). In cholesteatoma ears, the ossicular status was intact in 15 cases (30.8%), eroded in 34 ears (69.3%).

Ossicular erosion

Malleus (Table 1): It was found intact in 266 (95.34%), eroded in 13 (4.66%) ears. Malleus erosion was associated with incus erosion in all of the cases except one ear. In safe CSOM (total of 230), 228 (99.13%) of the ears had intact malleus. Only two ears (0.87%) had erosion of the malleal handle; one of the two ears had isolated erosion of the handle, the second one was associated with incus long process erosion. In cholesteatomous ears (total of 49), the malleus was found intact in 38 (77.5%), eroded in 11 (22.4%). Erosion involved the head of malleus in 7 ears, the handle of the malleus in 3 ears and the whole malleus (head and handle) in 1 ear.

Malleus	CSOM (%) n=279	Non-cholesteatomous ears (%) n= 230	Cholesteatomous ears (%) n=49	P value
Intact	266 (95.3%)	228 (99.1%)	38 (77.5%)	0.028*
Handle necrosed	5 (1.8%)	2 (0.9%)	3 (6.1%)	0.000*
Head necrosed	7 (2.5%)	-	7 (14.1%)	0.016*
Handle+ Head	1 (0.4%)	-	1 (2%)	0.223
* Statistically significant				

Table 1: Malleus status in chronic suppurative otitis media (CSOM).

Incus (Table 2): We found the incus intact in 216 (77.4%) and eroded in 63 (22.6%) ears. Incus erosion was most frequently localized to the lenticular process (34 ears) and to the long process (29 ears). In non-cholesteatomous ears, it was intact in 199 ears (86.5%) and eroded in 31 ones (13.5%) in which erosion were most frequently localized to the lenticular process 19 ears. In cholesteatoma ears, it was found intact in 17 (34.7%) and eroded in 32 (65.3%). Lenticular process was anew the most frequently involved portion in 16 ears (32.6%), next most common was the long process in 15 (30.6%) ears. The incus was completely absent in 1 case.

Incus	CSOM (%) n=279	Non-cholesteatomous ears (%) n= 230	Cholesteatomous ears (%) n=49	P value
Intact	216 (77.4%)	199 (86.5%)	17 (34.7%)	0.000*
Lenticular process	35 (12.5%)	19(8.3%)	16 (32.6%)	0.54
Long process	27 (9.6%)	12 (5.2 %)	15 (30.6%)	0.016*
Absent	1 (0.4)	-	1 (2%)	0.000*
* Statistically significant				

Table 2: Incus status in chronic suppurative otitis media (CSOM).

Stapes (Table 3): It was respected in 248 (88.9%) ears and eroded in 31 (11.1%) ones. The disease respected the footplate in all the cases and erosion was localized solely to stapes superstructure and was associated with incus erosion in all of the cases. Stapes erosion was infrequent in safe ears; it was present in 5.6% of the cases only. Conversely, the presence of cholesteatoma was associated with stapes superstructure erosion in most of the ears (63.3%).

Stapes	CSOM (%) n=279	Non-cholesteatomous ears (%) n= 230	Cholesteatomous ears (%) n=49	P value
Intact	248 (88.9%)	217 (94.3%)	18 (36.7%)	0.008*
Superstructure erosion	31 (11.1%)	13(5.6%)	31 (63.3%)	0.000*
* Statistically significant				

Table 3: Stapes status in chronic suppurative otitis media (CSOM).

Discussion

We analyzed data collected from a sample size of 279 ears with CSOM to ascertain their ossicular chain status. 49 out of the 279 operated CSOM ears (17.6%) had associated cholesteatoma.

Most of our patients were young which likely reflect increased health awareness among the population of Qatar with easy access to government sponsored medical care, especially, when hearing impairment affects work efficiency. The male to female ratio in our study was almost 2:1 in contrast to previously reported literature which showed almost equal gender distribution [1-4]. The possible explanation for males predominance could be that in the rapidly developing State of Qatar, the majority of the population is male expatriate workers and laborers.

OCD was evident in 66 (23.6%) ears. The most frequently impaired ossicle in both types of CSOM was the incus. It was found unscathed in 216 (77.4%) cases, eroded in 62 (22.2%) cases and absent in 1 (0.4%) case. The majority of the observed erosions were localized to the lenticular process in 35 (12.5%) ears and the long process in 27 (9.6%) ears. Hence, incudal erosion was observed to be the most prevailing ossicular pathology in cases of CSOM correlating with preceding studies in which the prevalence ranged from 20 to 30% [5,6].

Malleus was the most defiant and resilient middle ear ossicle. It was respected in more than 95% of studied ears. In cases of rare malleal involvement, erosion affects mostly the head of the malleus and spares the handle. This could be is attributed to the firm attachment of the handle to the tympanic membrane which acts as a mechanical barricade and allows adequate blood flow to the handle . The combined effect diminishes the risk of malleus handle necrosis.

The stapes was unviolated in 248 (88.9%) ears and its superstructure was involved in 31 (11.1%) ears with CSOM. The presence of stapedial necrosis in all cases of CSOM was found to be less than that documented in former literature [1,5,7].

Our results showed that OCD is much more prevalent in cholesteatomous ears (69.3%) vs. in non-cholesteatomous CSOM ears (13.9%).

In non-cholesteatomous ears (230), incus was eroded in 31 ears (13.5%). Incus erosion was most frequently localized to the lenticular process in 35 (12.5%) ears followed by long process in 27 (9.6%) ears. Necrosis typically spared the body of the incus. Malleus handle was eroded in 2 (0.9%) ears; both of them had subtotal perforations. Stapes was eroded in 13 (5.7%) ears.

It is hypothesized that middle ear ossicles damage in CSOM is induced by an active phenomena of osteoclastic osseous resorption rather than by a passive avascular necrosis [8]. The suggested mechanism for bony erosion is excessive formation of inflammatory mediators in the tympanic cavity which induces osteoclast activation

and bony resorption resulting in ossicular destruction. The duration of the inflammatory process and its vicinity to the ossicular chain are factors which appear to be the most harmful for the ossicles [9,10].The factors that may explain that the incus lenticular and long processes being more vulnerable are possibly their tenuous blood supply, noticeable bone marrow, and their exposure to the external milieu especially in posterior perforations [11,12].

Resorption of malleus handle is more common in subtotal perforations where the handle is completely exposed to the external environment together with the cumulative effect of reduced blood supply from the drum.

The presence of cholesteatoma is associated with a higher prevalence of ossicular erosion. It is also associated with two or more ossicles being affected simultaneously. In our study, ossicular erosion in cholesteatomous eras was as follows: incus 65.3%, malleus 22.5%, and stapes 63.3%. In a study by Kurien et al. these figures were: incus 100%, malleus 67%, and stapes 67% [13]. In another study by Garap and Dubey, the figures were: incus 89%, malleus 32%, and stapes 41% [14].

In cholesteatomous ears, incudal erosion was most frequently localized to the lenticular process (32.6%) and the long process (30.6%).

Malleus erosion is a common occurrence in cholesteatoma (22.5%). Sade et al. reported erosion of malleus in around 26.0% in unsafe CSOM which correlates well with our finding [7]. Malleus erosion due to cholesteatoma was mostly localized to the head of the malleus which occurs most of the time in conjunction with erosion of the body of the incus due to attical extension of the cholesteatoma.

Stapes erosion occurred frequently in the presence of cholesteatoma, it was eroded in more than 60% of cholesteatomous ears. Stapedial necrosis numbers were found to be higher than reported by previous studies [7]. One possible explanation is that our patients were experiencing severe cholesteatoma since we are tertiary referral center and we manage more advanced stages of the disease.

The hypotheses of bone erosion in cholesteatoma ears involve several mechanisms including among others pressure induced erosion and enzymatic destruction by inflammatory products secreted by cholesteatoma matrix [15,16].

Despite the increased health awareness among the population of Qatar with easy access to government sponsored medical care, ossicular chain erosion remains to be a frequent and common complication of CSOM in Qatari population. We think that the patients are referred to tertiary care center for surgical treatment only in advanced stages of the disease. It is known that inflammation in the tympanic cavity is more damaging to middle ear ossicles the longer it stays [9,10].

Studying the frequency and the extent of OCD in CSOM is important as it helps surgeon to predict pre-operatively its probability according to the patient's disease. The presence of extensive OCD implies difficulty of restoring the hearing during a single procedure, and the possible need for revision surgery. So as Otolaryngologists we should be competent enough to do the ossicular chain reconstruction during surgery to give the best hearing results to our patients. Patients must therefore be fully informed and consented about these potential issues before surgery.

References

1. Anglitoiu A, Balica N, Lupescu S, Vintila R, Cotulbea S (2011) Ossicular chain status in the otological pathology of the Ent Clinic Timisoara. Medicine in Evolution 17: 344-351.

2. Iñiguez-Cuadra R, Alobid I, Borés-Domenech A, Menéndez-Colino LM, Caballero-Borrego M, et al. (2010) Type III tympanoplasty with titanium total ossicular replacement prosthesis: anatomic and functional results. Otol Neurotol 31: 409-414.

3. Yung M, Vowler SL (2006) Long-term results in ossiculoplasty: an analysis of prognostic factors. Otol Neurotol 27: 874-881.

4. Hosny S, El-Anwar M, Abd-Elhady M, Khazbak A, El Feky A (2014) Outcomes of Myringoplasty in Wet and Dry Ears. Int Adv Otol 10: 256-259.

5. Austin DF (1972) Ossicular reconstruction. Otolaryngol Clin North Am 5: 145-160.

6. Kartush JM (1994) Ossicular chain reconstruction. Capitulum to malleus. Otolaryngol Clin North Am 27: 689-715.

7. Sade J, Berco E, Buyanover D, Brown M (1981) Ossicular damage in chronic middle ear inflammation. Acta Otolaryngol 92: 273-283.

8. Krane SM, Dayer JM, Goldring SR (1977) Ossicular pathology. McCabe BF, Sadé J, Abramsow M. Cholesteatoma First International Conference. Birmingham.

9. Thomsen J, Jorgensen MB, Bretlau P, Kristensen HK (1974) Bone resorption in chronic otitis media. A histological and ultrastructural study. I. Ossicular necrosis. J Laryngol Otol 88: 975-981.

10. Sadé J, Berco E (1974) Bone destruction in chronic otitis media. A histopathological study. J Laryngol Otol 88: 413-422.

11. Tos M (1979) Pathology of the ossicular chain in various chronic middle ear diseases. J Laryngol Otol 93: 769-780.

12. Austin DF (1978) Sound conduction of the diseased ear. J Laryngol Otol 92: 367-393.

13. Kurien M, Job A, Mathew J, Chandy M (1998) Otogenic intracranial abscess: concurrent craniotomy and mastoidectomy--changing trends in a developing country. Arch Otolaryngol Head Neck Surg 124: 1353-1356.

14. Garap JP, Dubey SP (2001) Canal-down mastoidectomy: experience in 81 cases. Otol Neurotol 22: 451-456.

15. Ruedi L (1958) Cholesteatosis of the attic. J Laryngol Otol 72: 593-609.

16. Tumarkin A (1958) Attic cholesteatosis. J Laryngol Otol 72: 610-619.

22

Outcomes of Endolymphatic Shunt Surgery in Ménière's Disease Indicate Potential Contribution of Shear Stress Instead of Relieving the Endolymphatic Hydrops

Jing Zou[1,2*] and Ilmari Pyykkö[1]

[1]Hearing and Balance Research Unit, Field of Oto-laryngology, School of Medicine, University of Tampere, Tampere, Finland

[2]Department of Otolaryngology-Head and Neck Surgery, Center for Otolaryngology-Head & Neck Surgery of Chinese PLA, Changhai Hospital, Second Military Medical University, Shanghai, China

*Corresponding author: Zou J, Hearing and Balance Research Unit, Field of Oto-laryngology, School of Medicine, University of Tampere, Medisiinarinkatu 3, 33520 Tampere, Finland; E-mail: Jing.Zou@uta.fi

Abstract

Believing that the attack of Ménière's Disease (MD) resulted from overpressure of the endolymphatic fluid, Georges Portmann introduced a surgery on the endolymphatic sac for the control of vertigo through releasing the endolymphatic hydrops in 1927. Since then, different types of ES surgery have been sued to treat MD all over the world for more than 80 years and the endolymphatic shunt surgery by inserting drainage tubing into the ES became a standard procedure in treating MD. However, this therapeutic theory was challenged by a specifically designed study performed in Denmark. A recent temporal bone study of MD patients who underwent surgery showed that endolymphatic sac surgery did not relieve hydrops in patients with MD but did relieve vertigo in some patients.

In this review, we provided a novel hypothesis on the endolymphatic shunt surgery in MD, which is that potential shear stress induced by the endolymphatic shunt surgery in MD patients may modulate activities of the afferent system of the vestibular end organ, enhance plasticity of the vestibular system, and result in symmetric sensitivity in the vestibular system. TRPV may be involved in the molecular mechanism in endolymph cationic ion circulation affected by shear stress. Matrix maintenance in the vestibule may also be enhanced after shear stress. Shear stress-promoted differentiation of BMSC toward certain cell types may have beneficial effects on the vestibular system in MD.

Keywords: Ion channel; Menieres disease; Plasticity; Reactive oxygen species; Shear stress; Vestibular stimulation

Introduction

Ménière's disease (MD) is a symptom complex characterized by vertigo, fluctuating hearing loss, tinnitus, and aural fullness. MD significantly affects patients' quality of life and work performance. As a chronic illness, MD affects approximately 190 per 100,000 patients, according to a U.S. health claims database; however, population studies have shown a prevalence as high as 513 out of 100,000 [1]. The most descriptive pathologic feature of MD is endolymphatic hydrops, which can be observed in histopathology studies. Endolymphatic hydrops may be caused by endolymphatic malabsorption in endolymphatic duct and sac, with consequent dysfunction of the hydro-ionic homeostasis and disrupted endocochlear potential [2].

Endolymphatic hydrops can be visualized using gadolinium-enhanced MRI, which provides an objective diagnosis of MD [3,4]. Immune reactions, viral infections, inflammation, and vascular insufficiency are suspected to contribute to the progress of MD. Current therapy for MD includes betahistine, diuretics, corticosteroids, vasodilators, anti-inflammatory and antiviral medicines, intratympanic gentamicin injections (chemical vestibulectomy), the use of a MeniettR device, endolymphatic shunt surgery, and vestibular nerve section for untreatable MD.

The effect of endolymphatic shunt surgery on MD has been argued and no explanation was delivered. In this review, we provided a novel hypothesis on the endolymphatic shunt surgery in MD, which is that the shear stress potentially involved in the therapeutic effect according our previous studies. Since the inner ear including the vestibule is composed of nerve, vascular, and bone tissues, progresses in shear stress in these tissues were also reviewed.

Endolymphatic Shunt Surgery Relieves Vertigo but not Hydrops

The theory behind the endolymphatic shunt surgery for MD treatment is that an artificial endolymph opening is used to replace the nonfunctional endolymphatic sac and release the endolymphatic hydrops. After surgery, the vestibular end organ and Corti's organ regain function once normal or near normal hydrostatic pressure is restored. However, this therapeutic theory was challenged by a specifically designed study performed in Denmark [5]. In that study, the placebo effect was investigated by comparing the effect of a regular endolymphatic shunt with the effect of a placebo operation (regular mastoidectomy).

Thirty patients with typical MD participated in the study. They were selected for surgery because of unsuccessful medical treatment and were randomly assigned to a treatment group. The patients filled in daily dizziness questionnaires for 3 months before and 12 months after surgery, registering nausea, vomiting, vertigo, tinnitus, hearing impairment, and pressure in the ears. Minor differences between the active and placebo groups were found, but the greatest difference in symptoms was found when the pre- and postoperative scores were compared, and both groups improved significantly. Approximately 70% of the patients in both groups achieved lasting improvement, and no significant differences between the two groups were found during a 9-year follow-up [6]. The nonspecific effect of endolymphatic shunt surgery in MD treatment was supported by a study of the temporal bones of 15 MD patients who had undergone shunt surgery [7]. The surgery failed to expose the sac in 5 cases; nonetheless, 4 of these 5 patients had relief from vertigo. In 8 cases, the sac was exposed, but the shunt failed to reach the lumen; still, 4 of these 8 patients experienced relief from vertigo. The shunt was successfully placed within the lumen of the sac in 2 cases, but both cases failed to experience relief from vertigo.

Endolymphatic hydrops was present in all 15 cases. The authors concluded that while endolymphatic sac surgery does not relieve hydrops in patients with Ménière's syndrome, it does relieve vertigo in some patients; however, the mechanism of this relief is unknown [7]. We suspect that endolymphatic hydrops is not attributable to the attack of vertigo, which is supported by our recent MRI study showing that endolymphatic hydrops does not always accompany MD [8]. Drilling the mastoid itself instead of artificial endolymph opening may induce therapeutic effect on vertigo.

Shear Stress in the Inner Ear

On the interface of fluid and solid structures, there exists tangential force acting on the surface: the shear force. It produces, for example, shear stress (SS) on the endothelium when blood is flowing in the artery. The generated mechanical forces on the cells of the vascular wall are expressed in units of force / unit area (N/m^2 or Pascal [Pa] or $dyne/cm^2$). Abnormal SS often leads to atherosclerotic lesions [9,10]. The nature of fluid flow in the vessel is dependent on the velocity of flow and might be either laminar or oscillatory (turbulent) [9]. Laminar flow induces anti-atherogenic gene expression, whereas oscillatory flow results in a pro-atherogenic reaction [10,11].

In the auditory system, sound waves are transformed with the middle ear mechanisms from air media to fluid oscillation in the cochlear compartments, and the Corti organ converts the mechanical vibration into sensory inputs. The cochlear structures, especially the components in the Corti organ are always undergoing an oscillatory shear, which is a highly energy-demanding process [12-14].

Stimulation pattern in the vestibular system is different from that of the auditory system and no fluid oscillation is evoked at the static status. However, fluid oscillation occurs when the head motion is induced, i.e. the vestibular end-organs are stimulated to maintain the balance. Shear stress in the cochlea was first addressed by Zou et al. in 2005, which is that intensive hitting (a linear acceleration of 6 m/s^2) the bulla of the guinea pig at the bony external ear canal at 250 Hz for 15 min that is delivered from an electromagnetic shaker upregulated expressions of tumor necrosis factor-α (TNF-α) and vascular endothelium growth factor (VEGF) and receptors in the cochlea [15].

We hypothesize that shear stress may also occur in the vestibular system by drilling the temporal bone during the endolymphatic shunt surgery. The positive outcomes of endolymphatic shunt surgery in Menie`re's disease are potentially contributed by the shear stress instead of relieving the endolymphatic hydrops. The literature reports support that skull vibration stimulates the vestibular end organs. In

1973, Lucke reported the first clinical observation of nystagmus induced by bone vibration in unilateral vestibular lesions [16]. Hamann and Schuster observed a similar phenomenon in vestibular schwannomas [17]. Dumas et al. described Videonystagmography (VNG) recordings in patients with various vestibular diseases and studied the effect of the stimulus frequency on the response [18].

The frequency that elicited the strongest nystagmus was 100 Hz, which is the frequency to which muscular receptors are reportedly sensitive. Young et al. observed squirrel monkeys' peripheral vestibular neuron responses to head vibration and airborne sound at frequencies from 50 to 400 Hz. The responses were measured in terms of the phase-locking in discharge and changes in firing rate. The lowest phase-locking thresholds for vibration were -70 to -80 dB re 1 g, and the median values in the most sensitive frequency range (200 to 400 Hz) were -20 to -40 dB re 1 g; the minimum and median thresholds for sound were 76 and 120 to -130 dB SPL, respectively. The rate-change thresholds were 10 to 30 dB above the phase-locking thresholds. The squirrel monkey sacculus has no special sensitivity to vibration compared with the other vestibular end organs; the median phase-locking threshold to sound for the saccular neurons exceeded 100 dB SPL. Using extracellular single neuron recordings from a large number of primary vestibular neurons identified by their location and their response to natural stimulation, Curthoys et al. [19] found that there is a very clear preference for irregular otolith afferents to be selectively activated by bone-conducted vibration stimuli at low stimulus levels and that bone-conducted vibration stimuli activate some irregular utricular afferent neurons.

Manzari et al. observed ocular and cervical vestibular-evoked myogenic potentials for bone-conducted vibration in MD patients during quiescence vs. during acute attacks. The researchers found that during MD attacks, dynamic utricular function in the affected ear (as measured by the n10 wave of the ocular vestibular-evoked myogenic potential at 500 Hz) is enhanced, whereas dynamic saccular function in the affected ear (as measured by the p13 of the cervical vestibular-evoked myogenic potential to 500-Hz bone-conducted vibration) is reduced [20]. We hypothesize that the constant and intensive shear wave generated during temporal bone drilling overstimulates the vestibular end organs and raises the threshold of response in a similar way to a hearing threshold shift. When the thresholds of the oversensitive vestibular end-organs are raised to levels near those of the less-sensitive vestibular end-organs, vertigo in MD patients may be directly resolved. Meanwhile, the nonsensorineural cells of the vestibular end-organs undergo shear stress and gene transcriptions are modulated accordingly. The biological responses induced by vestibular shear stress may also modify the progress of MD, producing beneficial effects in patients.

Shear Stress-Induced Biological Responses in Different Tissues

Vessels

Krajnak et al. [21] assessed the frequency-dependent responses of the peripheral vascular system (rat tail) to repeated bouts of vibration using 62.5, 125, or 250 Hz vibrations (constant acceleration of 49 m/s^2) for 4 h/d for 10 d. Vascular responses indicative of dysfunction (e.g., remodeling and oxidative activity) became more pronounced as the frequency of the exposure increased. Vibration at frequencies >100 Hz that induced the greatest stress and strain on the tail [21]. The authors also investigated the effects of shear stress on vascular function using an animal model of metabolic syndrome (the obese Zucker rat).

The tails of lean and obese Zucker rats were exposed to vibration (125 Hz, 49 m/s² r.m.s.) or control conditions for 4 h/d for 10 d. Vibration exposure generally reduced the sensitivity of the rats' arteries to acetylcholine (ACh)-induced vasodilation. This decrease in sensitivity was most apparent in obese rats. Vibration also induced reductions in vascular nitric oxide (NO) concentrations and increases in vascular concentrations of ROS in obese rats. These results indicate that vibration interferes with endothelial-mediated vasodilation and that metabolic syndrome exacerbates these effects [22].

Nerves

Krajnak et al. [21] studied sensory nerve function in rats after acute exposure to vibration. They found decreased Aβ nerve fiber sensitivity in association with reduced expression of nitric oxide synthase-1 and a modest increase in calcitonin gene-related peptide (CGRP) transcript levels in tail nerves 24 h post-exposure to 4 h of continuous sinusoidal vibration at 125 Hz with a constant acceleration of 49 m/s² rms. These transient changes in sensory perception and transcript levels induced by acute vibration exposure may be indicators of more prolonged changes in peripheral nerve physiology [23].

In the inner ear, VEGF signaling was upregulated in the spiral ganglion cells and other cell populations' post-shear stress [15]. Shear stress-induced VEGF production in human adipose tissue mesenchymal stem cells has been reported to be mediated by NO. This response was partially inhibited by treatment with 5 mM of l-NAME, a nonspecific inhibitor of nitric oxide synthases (NOS), suggesting the participation of NOS enzymes (neuronal [nNOS], inducible [iNOS], or endothelial [eNOS]) [24].

The mechanism and significance of VEGF signaling modifications in the vestibular end-organs in response to shear stress need to be clarified. CGRP, choline acetyltransferase, and GABA are transmitters in the efferent pathways of the vestibular end organs. An animal model of transient bilateral vestibular input blockage with tetrodotoxin showed an obvious increase in the number of CGRP-immunoreactive fibers within the neurosensory epithelia of the maculae and cristae, indicating the plasticity of the impaired vestibular nervous system [25]. We suspect that CGRP in the vestibular end-organs might be upregulated by shear stress and could play an important role in MD rehabilitation.

Bone

Bacabac et al. [26] investigated bone cells' (MC3T3-E1 osteoblastic cells) responses to vibration at a wide frequency range (5 to100 Hz). NO release positively correlated with vibration, whereas prostaglandin E2 (PGE2) release negatively correlated with the maximum acceleration rate of the vibration. Cyclooxygenase2 (COX-2) mRNA expression increased in a frequency-dependent manner, which relates to the increased NO release at high frequencies [26]. Another study was performed on the same cell line, which was exposed to vibrational force originating from the NASA-designed amplifier-controlled shaker head that simulates the vibrations of a space shuttle launch (5 to 2,000 Hz). The mRNA levels of two growth-related protooncogenes, c-fos and c-myc, were upregulated significantly within 30 min after vibration, whereas those of osteocalcin and transforming growth

factor-1 decreased significantly within 3 h after vibration [27].

When exposed to low amplitude strain vibration with broad frequency components up to 50 Hz, the MC3T3-E1 cell line upregulated osteocalcin mRNA 2.6-fold after 7 d of sinusoidal strain combined with broad frequency vibration stimulation, and MMP-9 mRNA increased 1.3-fold after 3 d of vibration alone. The expression of adipogenic genes, such as PPAR-γ and C/EBP-α, markedly increased in response to SSV at 20 Hz and 30 Hz during maturation [28].

The proliferation of sarcoma osteogenetic-2 (SAOS-2) cells was slowed down, so the acceleration perceived by the cells' mechanosensors may change the cellular cycle by blocking duplication to differentiate the cells toward bone tissue. After microvibration treatment (magnitude: 0.3 ×g, frequency: 40 Hz, amplitude: ±50 μm, 30 min/12 h), bone marrow-derived mesenchymal stromal cell (BMSC) proliferation was decreased on Days 7 and 10; however, the numbers of genes and proteins expressed during osteogenesis, including Cbfa1, ALP, collagen I and osteocalcin, increased substantially. ERK1/2 activation was involved in microvibration-induced BMSC osteogenesis [29].

TRPV Is the Potential Molecular Sensor in Shear Stress in the Vestibule Induced By Endolymphatic Shunt Surgery

The Transient Receptor Potential (TRP) ion channel family consists of 28 ion channels. It can be divided into six subgroups based on the structure and activation characteristics of the channels. The TRP subfamilies are canonical (TRPC, seven channels), melastatin (TRPM, eight channels), ankyrin (TRPA, one channel), vanilloid (TRPV, six channels), polycystine (TRPP, three channels), and mucolipin (TRPML, three channels). The vertebrate TRPV channels have been shown to be sensitive to many forms of physical and chemical stimuli. All vertebrate TRPV members are calcium-permeable channels, with TRPV Groups 1 through4 characterized as moderately calcium-selective cation channels, while TRPV-5 and TRPV-6 are highly calcium-selective channels.

In the mouse inner ear, TRPV-1, -2, and -3 are coexpressed in the hair cells and supporting cells of the organ of Corti and in spiral ganglion cells, sensory cells in vestibular end organs, vestibular ganglion cells, and sensory nerve fibers. TRPV-2 has also been detected in the stria vascularis, dark cells, and endolymphatic sac. TRPV-4 is expressed in hair cells and the supporting cells of the organ of Corti and in the marginal cells of the stria vascularis, spiral ganglion cells, vestibular sensory cells, vestibular dark cells, vestibular ganglion cells, and the epithelial cells of the endolymphatic sac [29]. TRPV4 expression in the mouse inner ear is not influenced by vitamin D receptor knockout [30]. Hypotonic stimulation and 4-alpha-phorbol 12,13-didecanoate, a TRPV4 synthetic activator, increased the intracellular Ca(2+) concentrations in wild-type outer hair cells, whereas in TRPV4(-/-) mice, the outer hair cells failed to exhibit a Ca(2+) response to either stimulation. TRPV4 may function as an osmosensory and a mechanosensory receptor in the cochlea. TRPV4 was expressed predominantly in the apical membrane of mitochondria-rich cells, and cell volume regulation by TRPV4 was observed in a tissue culture of the rat endolymphatic sac. TRPV4 was also present in the endolymphatic sacs of patients with vestibular schwannomas and Ménière's disease.

TRPV4 is assumed to act as an osmoreceptor in cell and fluid volume regulation in the human endolymphatic sac [30]. At 8 weeks of age, TRPV4 knockout mice appeared normal, but at 24 weeks, they revealed significantly higher auditory brainstem response thresholds. TRPV4 knockout mice are more susceptible to noise exposure than TRPV4+/+ mice [31]. TRPV4 has a role in aminoglycoside uptake and retention in the cochlea. After kanamycin (KM) treatment, TRPV1 was significantly upregulated in both the spiral and vestibular ganglia, while TRPV4 was downregulated in the inner ear ganglia. As a therapeutic agent for MD, gentamicin treatment also upregulated TRPV1 and TRPV2 expression in sensory and ganglion cells of the inner ear, while TRPV4 expression in the stria vascularis and vestibular dark cells decreased [32]. Downregulation of TRPV4 in the inner ear may restore the Ca(2+) concentration in the endolymph. However, this hypothesis together with the impact of shear stress on TRPV expression and activities in the vestibule should be investigated in future research.

Conclusion

To summarize, potential shear stress induced by the endolymphatic shunt surgery in MD patients may modulate activities of the afferent system of the vestibular end organ, enhance plasticity of the vestibular system, and result in symmetric sensitivity in the vestibular system. TRPV may be involved in the molecular mechanism in endolymph cationic ion circulation affected by shear stress. Matrix maintenance in the vestibule may also be enhanced after shear stress. Shear stress-promoted differentiation of BMSC toward certain cell types may have beneficial effects on the vestibular system in MD.

References

1. Havia M, Kentala E, Pyykkö I (2005) Prevalence of Ménière's disease in general population of Southern Finland. Otolaryngol Head Neck Surg 133: 762-768.

2. Paparella MM, Djalilian HR (2002) Etiology, pathophysiology of symptoms, and pathogenesis of Meniere's disease. Otolaryngol Clin North Am 35: 529-545, vi.

3. Zou J, Pyykko I, Bjelke B, Bretlau P, Tayamaga T (2000) Endolympahtic hydrops is caused by increased porosity of stria vascularis? in Barany Society Meeting (Uppsala, Sweden).

4. Zou J, Pyykkö I, Bretlau P, Klason T, Bjelke B (2003) In vivo visualization of endolymphatic hydrops in guinea pigs: magnetic resonance imaging evaluation at 4.7 tesla. Ann Otol Rhinol Laryngol 112: 1059-1065.

5. Thomsen J, Bretlau P, Tos M, Johnsen NJ (1981) Ménière's disease: endolymphatic sac decompression compared with sham (placebo) decompression. Ann N Y Acad Sci 374: 820-830.

6. Bretlau P1, Thomsen J, Tos M, Johnsen NJ (1989) Placebo effect in surgery for Ménière's disease: nine-year follow-up. Am J Otol 10: 259-261.

7. Chung JW, Fayad J, Linthicum F, Ishiyama A, Merchant SN (2011) Histopathology after endolymphatic sac surgery for Meniere's syndrome. Otology & neurotology : official publication of the American Otological Society, American Neurotology Society [and] European Academy of Otology and Neurotology 32:660-664.

8. Shi H, Li Y, Yin S, Zou J (2014) The predominant vestibular uptake of gadolinium through the oval window pathway is compromised by endolymphatic hydrops in Meniere's disease. Otology & neurotology : official publication of the American Otological Society, American Neurotology Society [and] European Academy of Otology and Neurotology 35:315-322.

9. Chatzizisis YS, Coskun AU, Jonas M, Edelman ER, Feldman CL, et al. (2007) Role of endothelial shear stress in the natural history of coronary atherosclerosis and vascular remodeling: molecular, cellular, and vascular behavior. J Am Coll Cardiol 49: 2379-2393.

10. Cunningham KS, Gotlieb AI (2005) The role of shear stress in the pathogenesis of atherosclerosis. Lab Invest 85: 9-23.

11. Brooks AR, Lelkes PI, Rubanyi GM (2004) Gene expression profiling of vascular endothelial cells exposed to fluid mechanical forces: relevance for focal susceptibility to atherosclerosis. Endothelium 11: 45-57.

12. Billone M, Raynor S (1973) Transmission of radial shear forces to cochlear hair cells. J Acoust Soc Am 54: 1143-1156.

13. Furness DN, Zetes DE, Hackney CM, Steele CR (1997) Kinematic analysis of shear displacement as a means for operating mechanotransduction channels in the contact region between adjacent stereocilia of mammalian cochlear hair cells. Proceedings. Biological sciences / The Royal Society 264:45-51.

14. Wangemann P (2002) K+ cycling and the endocochlear potential. Hear Res 165: 1-9.

15. Zou J, Pyykkö I, Sutinen P, Toppila E (2005) Vibration induced hearing loss in guinea pig cochlea: expression of TNF-alpha and VEGF. Hear Res 202: 13-20.

16. Lucke K (1973) [A vibratory stimulus of 100 Hz for provoking pathological nystagmus (author's transl)]. Zeitschrift fur Laryngologie, Rhinologie, Otologie und ihre Grenzgebiete 52:716-720.

17. Hamann M (1999) [Ecological aspects between Contracaecum sp. (Nematoda, Anisakidae) and the host Serrasalmus spilopleura Kner, 1860 (Pisces, Characidae) in natural populations of northeastern Argentina]. Boletin chileno de parasitologia 54:74-82.

18. Dumas G, Michel J, Lavieille JP, Ouedraogo E (2000) [Semiologic value and optimum stimuli trial during the vibratory test: results of a 3D analysis of nystagmus]. Annales d'oto-laryngologie et de chirurgie cervico faciale : bulletin de la Societe d'oto-laryngologie des hopitaux de Paris 117:299-312.

19. Curthoys IS, Kim J, McPhedran SK, Camp AJ (2006) Bone conducted vibration selectively activates irregular primary otolithic vestibular neurons in the guinea pig. Experimental brain research 175:256-267.

20. Manzari L, Tedesco AR, Burgess AM, Curthoys IS (2010) Ocular and cervical vestibular-evoked myogenic potentials to bone conducted vibration in Meniere's disease during quiescence vs during acute attacks. Clinical neurophysiology : official journal of the International Federation of Clinical Neurophysiology 121:1092-1101.

21. Krajnak K, Miller GR, Waugh S, Johnson C, Li S, et al. (2010) Characterization of frequency-dependent responses of the vascular system to repetitive vibration. Journal of occupational and environmental medicine /American College of Occupational and Environmental Medicine 52:584-.

22. Krajnak K, Waugh S, Johnson C, Miller R, Kiedrowski M (2009) Vibration disrupts vascular function in a model of metabolic syndrome. Ind Health 47: 533-542.

23. Krajnak K, Waugh S, Wirth O, Kashon ML (2007) Acute vibration reduces Abeta nerve fiber sensitivity and alters gene expression in the ventral tail nerves of rats. Muscle & nerve 36(2):197-205.

24. Bassaneze V, Barauna VG, Lavini-Ramos C, Kalil J, Schettert IT, et al. (2010) Shear stress induces nitric oxide-mediated vascular endothelial growth factor production in human adipose tissue mesenchymal stem cells. Stem Cells Dev 19: 371-378.

25. Hara H, Takeno K, Shimogori H, Yamashita H (2005) CGRP expression in the vestibular periphery after transient blockage of bilateral vestibular input. ORL J Otorhinolaryngol Relat Spec 67: 259-265.

26. Bacabac RG, Smit TH, Van Loon JJ, Doulabi BZ, Helder M et al. (2006) Bone cell responses to high-frequency vibration stress: does the nucleus oscillate within the cytoplasm? FASEB journal : official publication of the Federation of American Societies for Experimental Biology 20: 858-864.

27. Tjandrawinata RR, Vincent VL, Hughes-Fulford M (1997) Vibrational force alters mRNA expression in osteoblasts. FASEB J 11: 493-497.

28. Oh ES, Seo YK, Yoon HH, Cho H, Yoon MY, et al. (2011) Effects of sub-sonic vibration on the proliferation and maturation of 3T3-L1 cells. Life Sci 88: 169-177.

29. Zhou Y, Guan X, Zhu Z, Gao S, Zhang C, et al. (2011) Osteogenic differentiation of bone marrow-derived mesenchymal stromal cells on bone-derived scaffolds: effect of microvibration and role of ERK1/2 activation. Eur Cell Mater 22: 12-25.

30. Kumagami H, Terakado M, Sainoo Y, Baba A, Fujiyama D, et al. (2009) Expression of the osmotically responsive cationic channel TRPV4 in the endolymphatic sac. Audiol Neurootol 14: 190-197.

31. Tabuchi K, Suzuki M, Mizuno A, Hara A (2005) Hearing impairment in TRPV4 knockout mice. Neurosci Lett 382: 304-308.

32. Ishibashi T, Takumida M, Akagi N, Hirakawa K, Anniko M (2009) Changes in transient receptor potential vanilloid (TRPV) 1, 2, 3 and 4 expression in mouse inner ear following gentamicin challenge. Acta Otolaryngol 129: 116-126.

23

Perineural Invasion of Skin Cancers in the Head and Neck: An Uncommon Phenomenon Revisited

Santhosh Gaddikeri[1]*, Amit Bhrany[2] and Yoshimi Anzai[1]

[1]Department of Radiology, University of Washington Medical Center, USA
[2]Department of Head and Neck surgery, University of Washington Medical Center, USA

Abstract

Objective: The purpose of this article is to describe the epidemiology, imaging findings, pathogenesis, and clinical impact of perineural invasion of skin cancers in the head and neck.

Conclusion: Perineural invasion in head and neck skin cancer can be microscopic disease discovered on pathology or gross perineural spread that can be predicted on imaging often accompanied with clinical symptoms. Physicians and radiologists should have high index of suspicion when evaluating with patient with skin cancer that is in close proximity to a cranial nerve. The advancement of imaging techniques has improved pre-operative detection of perineural invasion of skin cancer.

Keywords: Perineural invasion; Head and neck skin cancer; MRI

Introduction

Perineural Invasion (PNI) of tumor cells was first discovered by Cruveilhier in 1835, when he reported mammary carcinoma invading the facial nerve. In 1862, Neumann first described lower face skin cancer invading the mental nerve.

PNI describes a microscopic finding of tumor infiltration along a nerve, and is distinguished from Perineural Spread (PNS), which describes the presence of gross tumor growth along a nerve distinct from the main tumor mass on imaging. PNI is defined as cancer cell invasion in, around, and through nerves where tumor cells are seen within any of the layers (epineurium, perineurium, endoneurium) of the nerve sheath [1]. When tumor cells are not seen in the layers of nerve sheath, it can be difficult to differentiate it from tumor abutting on nerve.

PNI of tumor is a well-recognized mechanism of tumor dissemination. PNI from head and neck cancer is well-known disease entity, ranging from 27-82%, depending on histology and type of cancer [2]. Within the head and neck, adenoid cystic cancer has a high propensity for PNI, and squamous cell carcinoma can be often associated with PNI. Presence of PNI has a major negative impact on management and prognosis of patients with Hand N cancer. PNI from cutaneous malignancy is under-recognized and frequently overlooked clinically and radio graphically. Most common type of skin cancers with PNI are Squamous Cell Cancer (SCC), Basal Cell Cancer (BCC) and Neurotrophic Malignant Melanoma (NMM). The reported incidences of PNI in non-melanoma skin cancers are 0.18% to 10% in BCC and 2.5% to 14% in SCC [3,4]. The concept of "skip lesions" in PNI is controversial. One set of authors believe in the presence of so called skip lesions in PNI, although none of them provide a convincing evidence to prove the presence of this entity [5-8]. The other set of authors believe that the concept of skip lesions in PNI does not exist and is a misinterpretation which is being propagated in the medical literature by blind quoting of existing false information in the medical literature [9-11]. PNI should be differentiated from neural clinical manifestations that are due to gross extrinsic compression by a tumor on the nerve or direct tumor extension along the skull base foramina or fissures through different anatomical planes [10]. The cranial nerve most vulnerable for PNI from skin cancer is the trigeminal nerve due to its rich cutaneous innervation in the region of most UV exposed regions of the head and neck [12]. The facial nerve is also commonly involved with PNI, especially in cases of SCC that are metastatic to the parotid gland. Less commonly, greater auricular nerve from cervical plexus and nerves of extra-ocular movement (III, IV, and VI) can be involved.

Relevant Cranial Nerve Anatomy

Trigeminal nerve (V cranial nerve)

The trigeminal nerve is a mixed nerve with both motor and sensory components and is considered to be the largest of all cranial nerves. There are four cranial nerve V nuclei, mesencephalic nucleus (proprioception), main sensory (tactile sensation), main motor nucleus (motor innervation to the muscles of mastication) and the spinal nucleus (primitive sensations like pain and temperature), which span across the inferior midbrain to the upper cervical cord to the level of C2. The entry point of the cisternal segment of the nerve in the lateral aspect of pons is called 'root entry zone' (REZ). The nerve then relays in the gasserian ganglion located in the Meckel cave, which then divides in to V1 (Ophthalmic), V2 (Maxillary) and V3 (Mandibular) divisions. V1 and V2 divisions are pure sensory nerves and transit through the lateral wall of cavernous sinus and exit the cranial cavity through the superior orbital fissure (in to orbit) and foramen rotundum (in to pterygopalatine fossa), respectively. V1 and V2 divisions of trigeminal nerve innervate upper and mid 1/3rd of the face, respectively. The V3 division is a mixed nerve with motor innervation to the muscles of mastication and sensory to the lower 1/3rd of the face. It exits the cranial cavity through the foramen ovale in to the masticator space (Figure 1a).

*Corresponding author: Santhosh Gaddikeri MD, Department of Radiology, University of Washington Medical Center, 1959 NE Pacific Street, Box 357115, Seattle, WA- 98195-7115, USA; E-mail: sg272@uw.edu

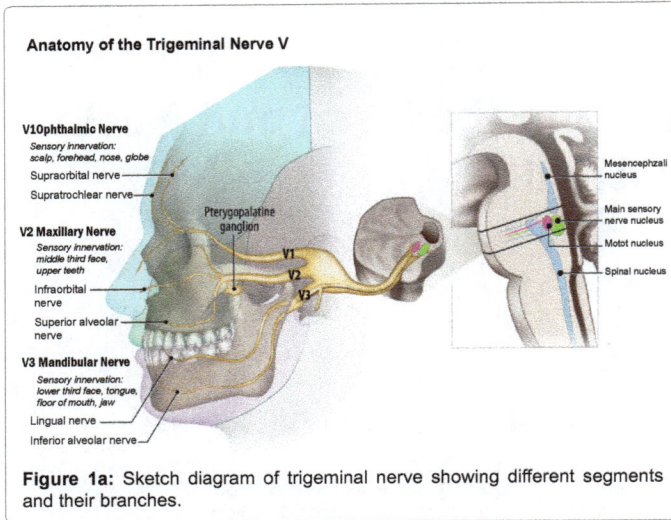

Figure 1a: Sketch diagram of trigeminal nerve showing different segments and their branches.

Facial nerve (VII cranial nerve)

The facial nerve is a mixed cranial nerve with motor, parasympathetic and taste sensory components in it. It has three nuclei (motor nucleus, superior salivatory and solitarius tract nucleus) located in the inferior pons antero-lateral to the abducens nucleus. The motor fibers arch around the ipsilateral abducens nucleus in the brainstem forming a bulge in the floor of IV ventricle called facial colliculus. The nerve then exits in to the cerebellopontine cistern at the pontomedullary junction and travels along the anterior and superior part of Internal Auditory Canal (IAC) to enter the petrous bone. The petrous portion of the nerve is divided into various segments such as labrynthine segment, geniculate ganglion, tympanic segment, and mastoid segments. The nerve then exits the skull base through stylomastoid foramen in to the parotid gland, which divides in to five major branches including temporal, zygomatic, buccal, marginal mandibular, and cervical (Figure 1b).

Pathogenesis

The biologic mechanism of PNI pathogenesis is not well understood, but a recent theory is that it relates to reciprocal signaling interactions and the (acquired) capacity of tumor cells to respond to signals within the peripheral nerve, which promote invasion. A number of neurotrophic agents have been identified as being of possible importance in PNI in other malignancies (prostate, pancreas) [13,14]. Some of these such as Nerve Growth Factor (NGF) have been shown to have increased expression in mucosal head and neck SCC demonstrating PNI [15]. The role of Neural Cell Adhesion Molecule (NCAM) in the pathogenesis of PNI in head and neck SCC is controversial. In 2000, Vural et al. [16] evaluated surgical specimens of 66 patients using monoclonal IgG antibody immuno peroxidase staining for NCAM and concluded that there was significant increase in the expression of NCAM in patients with PNI than in patients without PNI. In 2009, Solares et al. [17] reported that there was no expression of NCAM in all of the 18 patients with head and neck cutaneous SCC (including 14 patients with clinical PNI and 4 control patients without PNI). Previous theories proposing a mechanism of spread along low-resistance planes and endoneural lymphatic channels have now largely been discounted. Lymphatic channels do not penetrate the epineurium (the outer connective tissue layer binding fascicles within a single nerve).

The pathogenesis of PNI is unclear. Recently Liebig et al. [14] described PNI as a process resulting due to an active and reciprocal interaction between the nerve endings and the tumor cells. Tumor microenvironment plays a crucial role in the PNI of tumor cells (Figure 2). Few of the important molecular factors involved in this cross talk between the nerve endings and tumor cells include neurotropic factors

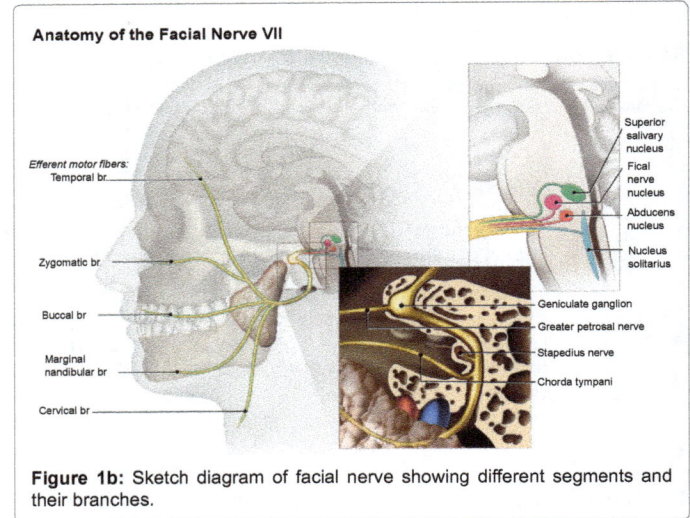

Figure 1b: Sketch diagram of facial nerve showing different segments and their branches.

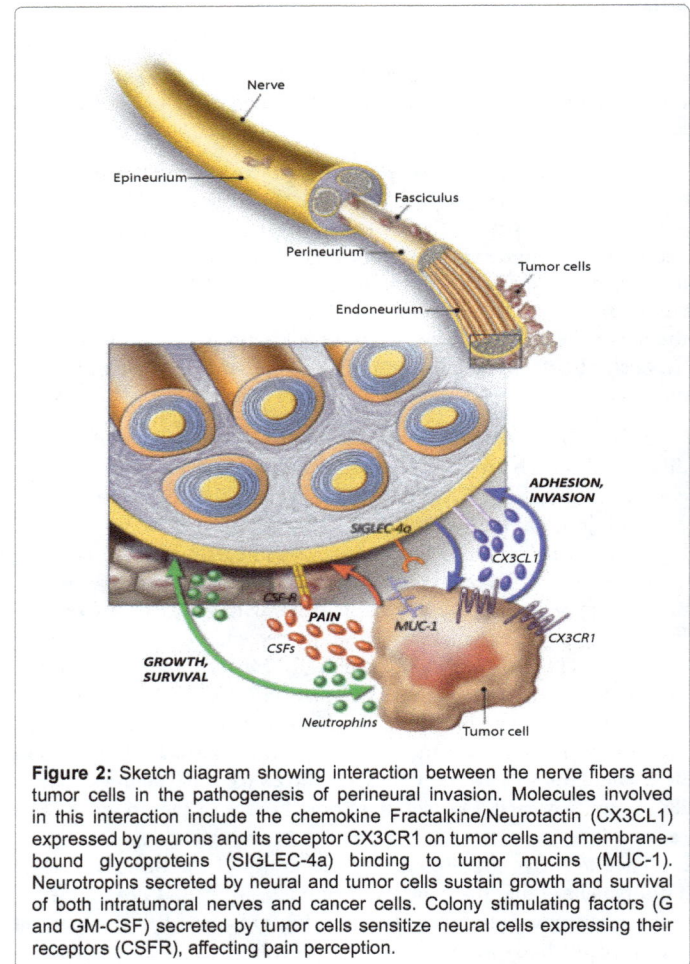

Figure 2: Sketch diagram showing interaction between the nerve fibers and tumor cells in the pathogenesis of perineural invasion. Molecules involved in this interaction include the chemokine Fractalkine/Neurotactin (CX3CL1) expressed by neurons and its receptor CX3CR1 on tumor cells and membrane-bound glycoproteins (SIGLEC-4a) binding to tumor mucins (MUC-1). Neurotropins secreted by neural and tumor cells sustain growth and survival of both intratumoral nerves and cancer cells. Colony stimulating factors (G and GM-CSF) secreted by tumor cells sensitize neural cells expressing their receptors (CSFR), affecting pain perception.

like Nerve Growth Factor (NGF), Brain Derived Nerve Growth Factor (BDNF), neurotropins (NT 3, 4 and 5), growth factors and axonal guidance molecules [18,19]. Neurotropins up regulate the tumor cells as well as the intratumoral nerves. Hematopoietic colony stimulating factors (G-CSF and GM-CSF) play a role in tumor-nerve interaction and most importantly tumor induced pain [20]. Myelin-associated glycoprotein (MAC, Siglec-4a) present on the nerve endings and laminin-5 on the tumor cells interact and facilitate PNI of tumor cells [21].

Diagnosis

PNI of head and neck skin cancer is often a misdiagnosed entity. The tumor cells in the initial stage invade the small peripheral cutaneous nerves which eventually spread centrally along the larger named nerves and can reach the brainstem if untreated. Depending on the presence or absence of clinical symptoms at the time of diagnosis, it can be classified in to two categories 'incidental PNI' and 'clinical PNI'. Factors predicting the PNI of skin cancer include type of tumor, size of the primary tumor, location, recurrent versus primary untreated tumor and tumor cell differentiation. The incidence of incidental PNI is more common in basal cell cancer as this represents the majority of non-melanoma skin cancer, whereas the clinical PNI is more common in patients with squamous cell cancer [3,22]. Tumors greater the 2 cm located in head and neck region particularly in the mid face and lip region due to rich cutaneous innervation are more vulnerable for PNI [6,23]. Recurrent skin cancers with prior resection and/or radiation therapy are more commonly associated with PNI than the primary untreated skin cancer and are usually of a higher histological grade (histologic grade 3 or 4) [24]. There is also increased incidence of PNI in male patients. Presence of PNI has been linked to increased incidence of regional lymph node, distant metastases and poorer prognosis [25-29].

PNI is definitively diagnosed upon histologic examination of a resected skin cancer or biopsy specimen. Most commonly, PNI is "incidental" or microscopic (mPNI); a pathological diagnosis made on specimen without the presence of preoperative symptoms suggestive of PNI. But PNI can clinically be suspected (clinical PNI, cPNI) when patients with cutaneous carcinomas manifest neural symptoms such as paresthesia, hypesthesia, pain in the distribution of a trigeminal nerve branch, or facial weakness. Early symptoms can be very subtle and often described as crawling of ants underneath the skin (formication) [30,31]. Early symptoms may go un-noticed, unless the clinician has a very high index of suspicion for PNI. If neglected, symptoms progress to pain, numbness and/or motor deficits along the distribution of the affected cranial nerve. Clinical symptoms may be erroneously ascribed to Bell palsy or trigeminal neuralgia which may further delay the diagnosis by 6 months to 2 years, but can be demonstrated radio graphically as described below [12].

Histologically, tumors cells are usually seen invading the nerve or may even extend along the length of the nerve. The tumor cells can spread retrograde toward central brain or brainstem or antegrade toward the distal nerve [32,33]. Occasionally, biopsy of the suspected cranial nerve may be necessary to confirm the diagnosis when clinically suspected preoperatively [34]. Such a biopsy is typically done at the time of resection of the cancer in attempts to confirm a clear margin of resection. Rarely, presence of concentric layers of fibrosis (peritumoral fibrosis) around the tumor cells or surrounded by the tumor cells can mimic PNI and make the diagnosis difficult [35].

Imaging

In patients with clinical symptoms suggestive of trigeminal or facial nerve involvement, imaging can be useful to confirm clinical suspicion and guide treatment planning. If neural involvement is confirmed or highly suggestive upon imaging, the extent of surgical resection to obtain a clear surgical margin, including sacrifice of portions of the facial and or trigeminal nerve, may be determined. If imaging demonstrates intracranial PNI or PNS, a lesion may be deemed to be surgically unresectable, and a primary radiation therapy treatment approach that encompasses the path of neural involvement may be considered. In addition, preoperative imaging can guide the extent radiotherapy required in the adjuvant setting. In patients with mPNI, imaging should be obtained if large nerve involvement is noted in the surgical specimen.

Contrast enhanced MRI is the best imaging study for the detection of PNS and also to assess the extent of disease spread along the cranial nerves. Subtle enhancement of nerve is difficult to diagnose on contrast enhanced CT until it creates a mass lesion. Hi-resolution focused gadolinium enhanced MRI or MR neurography are considered to be the most sensitive imaging for detection of PNI [31]. The MR imaging features that suggest PNI include obliteration of fat plane surrounding the cranial nerve, enhancement with or without enlargement of the nerve, mass in the cavernous sinus or Meckel cave and sometimes changes related to denervation of a group of muscles innervated by the affected cranial nerve suggest indirect signs of PNI (Figures 3-7). Although the accuracy of MR neurography is described as high as 83% in defining the extent of cranial nerve involvement [36], false negative MRI has been reported ranging from 22-47% of patients with clinical PNI in the early stages [31]. CT can detect foraminal widening and bony erosion in advanced cases [36-38] (Figure 8).

It is important to thoroughly evaluate cranial nerves that are suspected for invasion on MR imaging. Non contrast T1 weighted images often reveal loss of fat plane in pterygopalatine fossa or mandibular canal. Obliteration of Meckel's cave or infra orbital foramen also indicates presence of PNS. Asymmetric enhancement of nerve is better appreciated on post contrast MR images with fat suppression. Finally, indirect evidence of PNS can be seen as denervation changes of muscles that are supplied by the suspected cranial nerve (please find examples). In 2001, Williams et al. [39], described the zonal system (Table 1) to

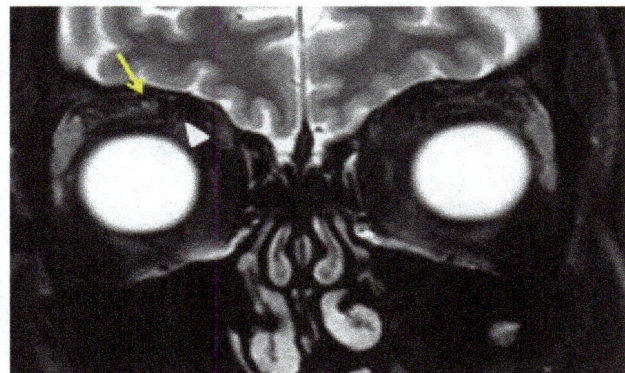

Figure 3a: 59 year old male patient with prior history of right forehead squamous cell cancer with new onset right forehead numbness and tingling sensation. A: STIR coronal image of orbit demonstrates thickening of the right V1 (ophthalmic) nerve (arrow) and also note the superior ophthalmic vein (SOV) flow void (arrow head).

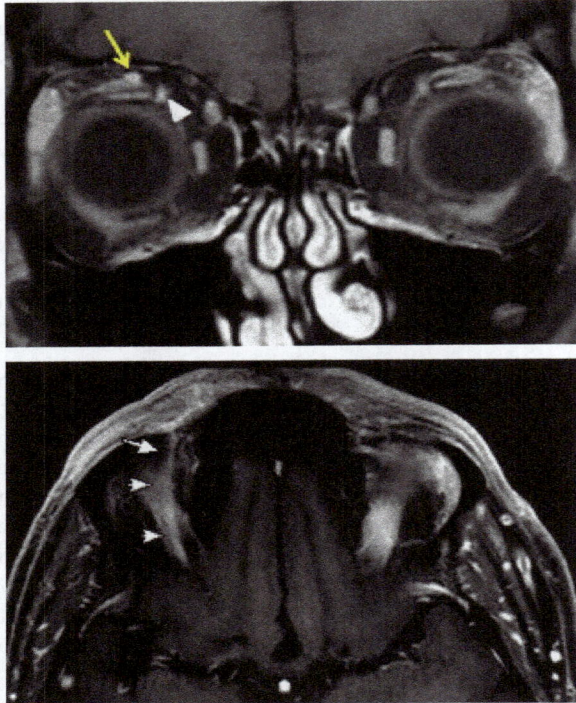

Figure 3b and c: Coronal and axial post Gad fat-suppressed T1WI demonstrates thickening and enhancement of the V1 nerve (arrow) suggesting perineural invasion. Enhancing SOV (arrow head) inferior to the superior rectus muscle.

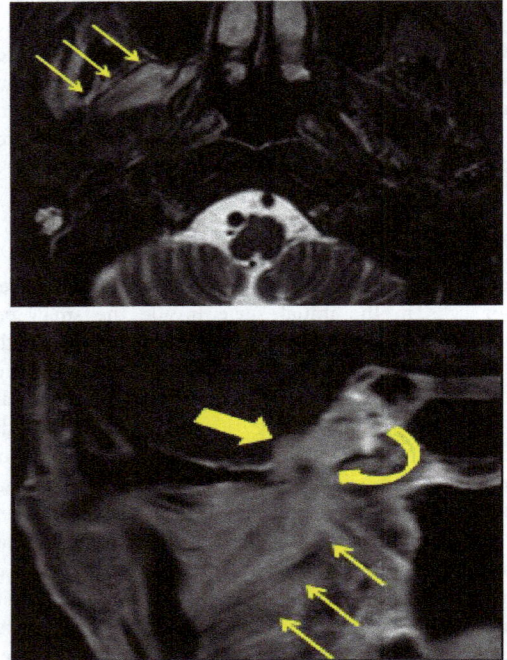

Figure 5: 45 year old female patient with history of right lower face metastatic melanoma. **A:** Coronal fat-suppressed post Gad T1WI demonstrates enlargement of right foramen ovale (curved arrow) with thickening and enhancement of the V3 (mandibular) nerve and right cavernous sinus mass (block arrow) due to perineural invasion. Also note diffuse enhancement of the masticator muscles (arrows) due to acute denervation. **B:** Axial STIR image showing increased T2 signal in the right masticator muscle due to acute denervation.

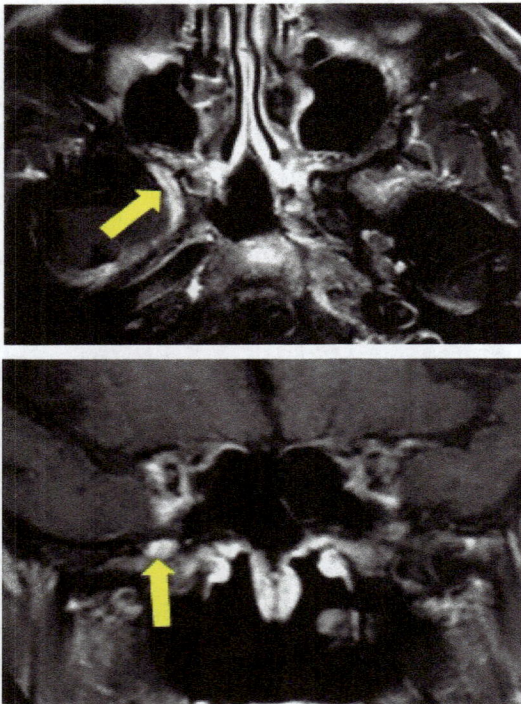

Figure 4: 72 year old male patient with right cheek squamous cell cancer. **A & B:** Axial and coronal post Gad fat-suppressed T1WI demonstrates thickening and enhancement of the right V2 (Maxillary) nerve (block arrow) at the foramen rotundum extending in to the cavernous sinus indicating perineural invasion.

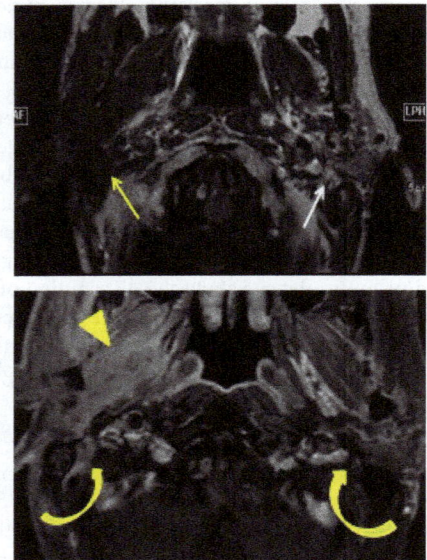

Figure 6: 65 year old male patient with past history of cutaneous squamous cell cancer in the right parotid region with intra-parotid recurrence. **A.** Axial T1WI demonstrate iso-intense mass in the right parotid region with loss of infiltration of fat in the right stylomastoid foramen (yellow arrow). Note the normal fat in left stylomastoid foramen (white arrow). **B.** Post Gad fat suppressed axial T1WI demonstrate enhancement in the right stylomastoid foramen suggesting perineural invasion along the VII (Facial) nerve and note the lack of enhancement in the normal left stylomastoid foramen (curved arrow). Infiltrating mass in the right masticator space (arrow head) which extended along the V3 nerve through the auriculotemporal nerve.

define the extent of the PNI along the cranial nerve to help guide the treatment options and correlate with the prognosis.

Treatment and Prognosis

PNI is most commonly diagnosed incidentally (mPNI), and thus almost all patients have had surgery for the primary tumor resection at the time of diagnosis. Patients with negative surgical margins and focal PNI in small cutaneous nerves (less than 0.1 mm) may be adequately followed clinically without any additional resection, radiation therapy or additional imaging to help determine if more proximal nerve involvement is present. But if patients have other risk factors such as large tumor size, chronic immunosuppression, lymphovascular invasion, large nerve (greater than 0.1 mm) involvement, MRI for to search for additional nerve involvement should be considered as should adjuvant radiation therapy to the primary site and draining nodal basins Since patients with PNI are at increased risk of nodal metastases up to 15% to 20% [31,40]. For patients with questionable positive PNI margins within the resected specimen, re-excision or adjuvant radiation therapy is recommended, and adjuvant radiation therapy should definitely be recommended in the setting of positive margins, gross residual disease and/or extensive PNI. Hyperfractionation therapy is often used to reduce the risk of radiation induced complications [41].

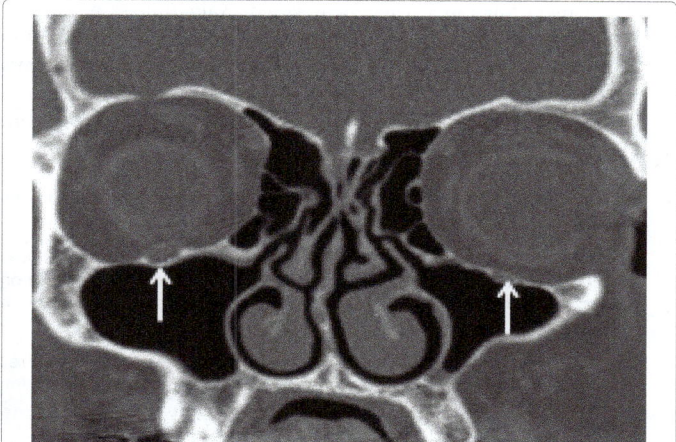

Figure 7A, B and C: Coronal and axial fat-suppressed post Gad T1WI of the Facial nerve in the previous patient demonstrates nodular thickening and enhancement of the right facial nerve (mastoid segment (MS), geniculate ganglion (GG), labyrinthine segment (LS) and fundus of IAC due to perineural invasion. Note right cavernous sinus mass (block arrow) due to perineural invasion along the V3 nerve.

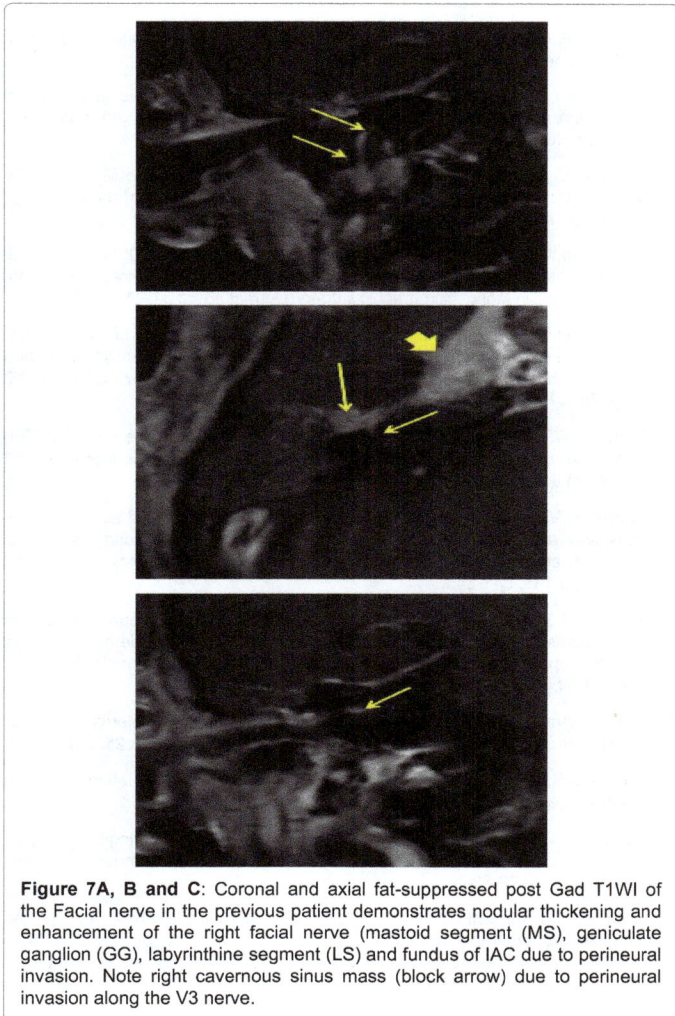

Figure 8: 72 year old male patient with right cheek squamous cell cancer. Coronal CT bone window image demonstrates asymmetric enlargement of the right inferior orbital canal on right when compared to left (arrow) due to perineural invasion along the inferior orbital nerve.

Grade	Zone involved	Zonal anatomy
PN 1	Clinical PNI imaging zone 1	V1: Up to superior orbital fissure, V2: Up to foramen rotundum, V3: Up to foramen ovale and VII: Up to stylomastoid bell or foramen
PN 2	Clinical PNI imaging zone 2	V1, V2 and V3: From zone 1 to Gasserian ganglion. VII: Zone 1 to lateral end of IAC including geniculate ganglion and labyrinthine segment of facial nerve
PN 3	Clinical PNI imaging zone 3	All nerves proximal to ganglion into the cisterns or into the brain stem

Table 1: Grading of Perineural Invasion (PNI) based on the zonal anatomy of the cranial nerve. Zone 2 and 3 are classified as T4 disease.

There is no proven benefit of adjuvant chemotherapy in clinical PNI for skin cancer [42].

In patients with cPNI, treatment depends on the resectability of the primary tumor which is determined with the aid of MR imaging. If the tumor is technically resectable then treatment is usually surgery followed by post-operative radiation. In 2012, Panizza B et al. [9] evaluated 21 patients with head and neck cutaneous SCC and concluded that surgical resection with negative margins in patients with disease extending up to Gasserian or geniculate ganglion provides best chance of cure.

Compared to patients without PNI, PNI is associated with a higher rate of recurrence and 5-year disease specific death. Jambusaria et al. [43] reported a 5-year disease specific survival of 84% in patients with PNI versus 96% in those without. Local site relapse is most common, and most relapses occur within two to four years after initial resection [43]. Clinical PNI patients have an increased rate of relapse compared to those with mPNI. Garcia-Serra et al, reported local control, cause specific survival and overall survival of 87%, 65% and 50% respectively over a 5-year follow up on 59 patients with mPNI compared to 55%, 59% and 55% on 76 patients with cPNI treated with surgery and postoperative radiotherapy[40]. Imaging positive cPNI patients have highest rates of local recurrence, 43% - 75% versus 24% and lower rates of disease-specific survival, 56% - 61% versus 100% compared to image negative patients [12].

Conclusion

The radiologist and the clinician should maintain a high index of suspicion of perineural involvement when evaluating skin cancers, particularly when they are recurrent and occur in close proximity with one or more cranial nerves in the head and neck region. Patients with skin cancers that exhibit PNI are more likely to exhibit local recurrence and have decreased disease-specific survival after treatment.

References

1. Ong CK, Chong VF (2010) Imaging of perineural spread in head and neck tumours. Cancer Imaging 10 Spec no A: S92-98.

2. Kurtz KA, Hoffman HT, Zimmerman MB, Robinson RA (2005) Perineural and vascular invasion in oral cavity squamous carcinoma: increased incidence on re-review of slides and by using immunohistochemical enhancement. Arch Pathol Lab Med 129: 354-359.

3. Leibovitch I, Huilgol SC, Selva D, Richards S, Paver R (2005) Basal cell carcinoma treated with Mohs surgery in Australia III. Perineural invasion. J Am AcadDermatol 53: 458-463.

4. Donaldson MJ, Sullivan TJ, Whitehead KJ, Williamson RM (2002) Squamous cell carcinoma of the eyelids. Br J Ophthalmol 86: 1161-1165.

5. Cottel WI (1982) Perineural invasion by squamous-cell carcinoma. J DermatolSurgOncol 8: 589-600.

6. Lawrence N, Cottel WI (1994) Squamous cell carcinoma of skin with perineural invasion. J Am AcadDermatol 31: 30-33.

7. Ratner D, Lowe L, Johnson TM, Fader DJ (2000) Perineural spread of basal cell carcinomas treated with Mohs micrographic surgery. Cancer 88: 1605-1613.

8. Veness MJ, Biankin S (2000) Perineural spread leading to orbital invasion from skin cancer. AustralasRadiol 44: 296-302.

9. Panizza B, Warren TA, Lambie D, Brown I (2012) The fallacy of skip lesions as an example of misinterpretations being propagated in the scientific literature. Oral Oncol 48: e33-34.

10. Panizza B, Warren T (2013) Perineural invasion of head and neck skin cancer: diagnostic and therapeutic implications. Curr Oncol Rep 15: 128-133.

11. Matorin PA, Wagner RF Jr (1992) Mohs micrographic surgery: technical difficulties posed by perineural invasion. Int J Dermatol 31: 83-86.

12. Mendenhall WM, Amdur RJ, Hinerman RW, Werning JW, Malyapa RS, et al. (2007) Skin cancer of the head and neck with perineural invasion. Am J ClinOncol 30: 93-96.

13. Ayala GE, Wheeler TM, Shine HD, Schmelz M, Frolov A, et al. (2001) In vitro dorsal root ganglia and human prostate cell line interaction: redefining perineural invasion in prostate cancer. Prostate 49: 213-223.

14. Liebig C, Ayala G, Wilks JA, Berger DH, Albo D (2009) Perineural invasion in cancer: a review of the literature. Cancer 115: 3379-3391.

15. Kolokythas A, Cox DP, Dekker N, Schmidt BL (2010) Nerve growth factor and tyrosine kinase A receptor in oral squamous cell carcinoma: is there an association with perineural invasion? J Oral Maxillofac Surg 68: 1290-1295.

16. Vural E, Hutcheson J, Korourian S, Kechelava S, Hanna E (2000) Correlation of neural cell adhesion molecules with perineural spread of squamous cell carcinoma of the head and neck. Otolaryngol Head Neck Surg 122: 717-720.

17. Solares CA, Brown I, Boyle GM, Parsons PG, Panizza B (2009) Neural cell adhesion molecule expression: no correlation with perineural invasion in cutaneous squamous cell carcinoma of the head and neck. Head Neck 31: 802-806.

18. Chédotal A, Kerjan G, Moreau-Fauvarque C (2005) The brain within the tumor: new roles for axon guidance molecules in cancers. Cell Death Differ 12: 1044-1056.

19. Chilton JK (2006) Molecular mechanisms of axon guidance. DevBiol 292: 13-24.

20. Schweizerhof M, Stösser S, Kurejova M, Njoo C, Gangadharan V, et al. (2009) Hematopoietic colony-stimulating factors mediate tumor-nerve interactions and bone cancer pain. Nat Med 15: 802-807.

21. Anderson TD, Feldman M, Weber RS, Ziober AF, Ziober BL (2001) Tumor deposition of laminin-5 and the relationship with perineural invasion. Laryngoscope 111: 2140-2143.

22. Ballantyne AJ (1984) Perineural invasion by SCC. J DermatolSurgOncol 10: 502-504.

23. Goepfert H, Dichtel WJ, Medina JE, Lindberg RD, Luna MD (1984) Perineural invasion in squamous cell skin carcinoma of the head and neck. Am J Surg 148: 542-547.

24. Veness MJ (2000) Perineural spread in head and neck skin cancer. Australas J Dermatol 41: 117-119.

25. Jennings L, Schmults CD (2010) Management of high-risk cutaneous squamous cell carcinoma. J ClinAesthetDermatol 3: 39-48.

26. Clayman GL, Lee JJ, Holsinger FC, Zhou X, Duvic M, et al. (2005) Mortality risk from squamous cell skin cancer. J ClinOncol 23: 759-765.

27. Moore BA, Weber RS, Prieto V, El-Naggar A, Holsinger FC, et al. (2005) Lymph node metastases from cutaneous squamous cell carcinoma of the head and neck. Laryngoscope 115: 1561-1567.

28. Cassarino DS, Derienzo DP, Barr RJ (2006) Cutaneous squamous cell carcinoma: a comprehensive clinicopathologic classification. Part one. J CutanPathol 33: 191-206.

29. Cassarino DS, Derienzo DP, Barr RJ (2006) Cutaneous squamous cell carcinoma: a comprehensive clinicopathologic classification--part two. J CutanPathol 33: 261-279.

30. Balamucki CJ, Dejesus R, Galloway TJ, Mancuso AA, Amdur RJ, et al. (2013) Impact of Radiographic Findings on For Prognosis Skin Cancer With Perineural Invasion. Am J ClinOncol .

31. Galloway TJ, Morris CG, Mancuso AA, Amdur RJ, Mendenhall WM (2005) Impact of radiographic findings on prognosis for skin carcinoma with clinical perineural invasion. Cancer 103: 1254-1257.

32. Nemec SF, Herneth AM, Czerny C (2007) Perineural tumor spread in malignant head and neck tumors. Top MagnReson Imaging 18: 467-471.

33. Parker GD, Harnsberger HR (1991) Clinical-radiologic issues in perineural tumor spread of malignant diseases of the extracranial head and neck. Radiographics 11: 383-399.

34. Esmaeli B, Ahmadi MA, Gillenwater AM, Faustina MM, Amato M (2003) The role of supraorbital nerve biopsy in cutaneous malignancies of the periocular region. OphthalPlastReconstrSurg 19: 282-286.

35. Hassanein AM, Proper SA, Depcik-Smith ND, Flowers FP (2005) Peritumoral fibrosis in basal cell and squamous cell carcinoma mimicking perineural invasion: potential pitfall in Mohs micrographic surgery. DermatolSurg 31: 1101-1106.

36. Gandhi, M.R., B. Panizza, D. Kennedy (2011) Detecting and defining the anatomic extent of large nerve perineural spread of malignancy: comparing "targeted" MRI with the histologic findings following surgery. Head Neck 33: 469-575.

37. Nemzek WR, Hecht S, Gandour-Edwards R, Donald P, McKennan K (1998) Perineural spread of head and neck tumors: how accurate is MR imaging? AJNR Am J Neuroradiol 19: 701-706.

38. Hanna E, Vural E, Prokopakis E, Carrau R, Snyderman C, et al. (2007) The sensitivity and specificity of high-resolution imaging in evaluating perineural spread of adenoid cystic carcinoma to the skull base. Arch Otolaryngol Head Neck Surg 133: 541-545.

39. Williams LS, Mancuso AA, Mendenhall WM (2001) Perineural spread of cutaneous squamous and basal cell carcinoma: CT and MR detection and its impact on patient management and prognosis. Int J RadiatOncolBiolPhys 49: 1061-1069.

40. Garcia-Serra A, Hinerman RW, Mendenhall WM, Amdur RJ, Morris CG, et al. (2003) Carcinoma of the skin with perineural invasion. Head Neck 25: 1027-1033.

41. Hulyalkar R, Rakkhit T, Garcia-Zuazaga J (2011) The role of radiation therapy in the management of skin cancers. DermatolClin 29: 287-296, x.

42. Mendenhall WM, Amdur RJ, Williams LS, Mancuso AA, Stringer SP, et al. (2002) Carcinoma of the skin of the head and neck with perineural invasion. Head Neck 24: 78-83.

43. Jambusaria-Pahlajani A, Miller CJ, Quon H, Smith N, Klein RQ, et al. (2009) Surgical monotherapy versus surgery plus adjuvant radiotherapy in high-risk cutaneous squamous cell carcinoma: a systematic review of outcomes. DermatolSurg 35: 574-585.

24

Pilot Study to Evaluate the Prevalence of Hearing Loss in a Rural Community Using Dp Oae Screener

Lingamdenne Paul Emerson*

Department of ENT, Arogyavaram Medical Centre, Madnapalle, Andhra Pradesh, India

*****Corresponding author:** Lingamdenne Paul Emerson, M.S (ENT), Department of ENT, Arogyavaram Medical Centre, Madnapalle, Andhra Pradesh, India;
E-mail: paulecmcvellore@gmail.com

Abstract

Hearing impairment is a leading cause of disease burden, yet population-based studies that measure hearing impairment are rare. In a developing country where most of the population live in rural areas this disability causes educational and emotional disability in children and economic and social disability in adults. A Pilot study was conducted for screening for hearing loss in a rural community using Dp OAE screener. A total number of 1117 rural and tribal populations between age groups of 6 months to 70 years were screened. Pure tone audiometry was done simultaneously. It was found that the prevalence of hearing loss in the community does not correlate with the symptoms expressed by the population with 63.31% failing the test (refer) which was confirmed by Pure Tone Audiometry. It was found that among patients with "refer" there was disabling hearing loss in adults (>80%; 40dB HL and above).This model envisages the use of Oto acoustic emissions which are sensitive to both sensorineural and conductive hearing loss, to be an cost effective screening tool in a rural community.

Keywords DpOAE; Hearing loss; Pure tone audiometry; Community screening; Population studies

Introduction

There are 360 million persons in the world with disabling hearing loss (5.3% of the world's population) and 32 (9%) million of these are children [1] and the estimated prevalence is 6.3% in Indian population, yet population-based studies that measure hearing impairment are rare. The most commonly used model to date has been a hospital based screen employing a team of dedicated screeners measuring otoacoustic emissions (OAE) in neonates in the maternity unit before discharge and using audiometry and various questionnaires in combination for adults [2]. In a survey of the current status of Neonatal hearing screening program in India it was found to be less than adequate and there was a problem of following up identified children [3,4]. In a developing country where most of the population live in rural areas , due to the stigma and traditional practices this disability is neglected leading to educational, emotional trauma in children and economic disability in adults in addition to being discriminated. Thus the need of the study arose to use a sensitive hearing screening device which can be operated by anyone and is accurate in a rural community with low literacy rates and awareness.

Oto-acoustic emissions (OAEs) can be defined as the audio frequency energy which originates in and is released from the cochlea, transmitted through the ossicular chain and tympanic membrane and measured in the external auditory meatus. They can occur either spontaneous or in response to acoustic stimulation. Oto-acoustic emissions are vulnerable to a variety of agents such as acoustic trauma [5], hypoxia [6] and oto-toxic medication [7] that cause hearing loss by damaging outer hair cells. Taking into account estimates of amplification provided by outer hair cells, complete destruction of OHC'S alone could result theoretically, in a hearing loss of 60 dB. Early investigations in to OAE'S proved that they are not present when the

sensorineural hearing loss exceeds 40-50 dB. It has been established that DPOAEs are reduced or eliminated by compromise of middle ear conduction pathway and can also be used to confirm the presence of any middle ear pathology. OAEs only occur in a normal cochlea and if hearing is at least 30 dB or better. Otoacoustic emissions are never found when hearing loss at 1000 Hz exceeds 40 dB hearing level and when the mean audiometric hearing loss (at 500, 1000, 2000 and 4000 Hz) exceeds 45 dB hearing level [8,9]. DPOAEs measures have shown excellent intra-subject test reliability which allows monitoring of dynamic changes of cochlear function [10]. Because OAE are sensitive to both sensorineural and conductive hearing loss, they were found to have the potential to be an effective screening tool across all populations, including children [11]. Sensitivity and specificity of OAE testing for hearing impairment ranges from 76.9-98% and 90% respectively [12-14]. The test procedure typically takes less than 2 minutes for both ears. It is non-invasive and does not require sedation for the patient. In order to PASS, OAEs must be present and be at least 5 dB above the background noise at 3 out of 4 frequencies. The Ero-ScanTM noise rejection algorithm is the most effective allowing for reliable testing in up to 70 dBSPL of background noise [15].

Aim

To identify Hearing loss in the community Using Portable Dp OAE SCREENER.

Methodology

This study was conducted in the rural and tribal areas of Vellore district where most are labourers living in quiet environments and lack of noise pollution.

Inclusion criteria

All residents aged 6 months and above.

Exclusion criteria

Meatal atresia, anomalies of external ear where probe insertion was not possible. Otitis media, otitis externa, discharge and wax in external auditory canal.

Christian medical college, Vellore Institutional Review Board (IRB) gave approval for the study.

A door to door survey of population was done in rural areas and tribal areas of Jawadhu hills in Vellore District. The team comprised of ENT specialist, audiologist and community workers. An informed consent (Tamil) was taken and the procedure was explained. A brief questionnaire was filled up by the community workers. The community workers were trained to operate Maico-ero scan DpOAE instrument. Screening for hearing loss was done in the community in an area where the noise level was <60 dB (verified by Noise level meter) after evaluation by ENT specialist. Pure tone audiometry was simultaneously done by the audiologist by a portable audiometer. A Screening DPOAE with fixed protocol (4 s) with Frequencies: 2–5 kHz was followed with an Intensity: 65/55 dB with a sound noise ratio of 6 dB the criteria for pass was: 3 out of 4 frequencies .Results were referred as "Pass"/"Refer". Refer patients (Adults) were further evaluated in the community by Pure tone Audiometry. Children (<16 years) were referred to tertiary centre for further evaluation.

Initially a pilot study was undertaken to compare the results of using the OAE SCREENER in the community and in a audiometric booth which were similar.

Classification

1. Group A–6 months to 3 years (Children at home)

2. Group B–3-5 years (Pre-school)

3. Group C–5-16 years (School)

4. Group D–Above 16 Years (Adults)

Statistical methods

All the data was entered into Microsoft excel format and SPSS software. Prevalence and age associated hearing loss was analysed using chi-square statistics. The sample size was calculated assuming an average prevalence rate of 10% [16].

Results

In our study a total number of 1117 were screened over a period of six months in both tribal areas and rural areas around Vellore district. 50.6% were females. From the brief questionnaire symptoms of hearing loss were reported by 3 (<16 years) and 34 (>16 years) persons respectively. The most common findings were chronic suppurative otitis media (36), wax completely occluding was seen in 16 persons and acute otitis media was seen in 13 persons. There was almost similar prevalence among Rural and tribal population (Rural 40.8%; Tribal 48.8%). Male to female prevalence was also similar. Hearing loss was mostly bilateral (Table-1).

Prevalence of hearing loss: Figure 1 and Table 2

Group A–6 months to 3 years (Children at home): A total of 311(n) children were screened for hearing loss. Acute otitis media was seen in 2 children. DpOAE could not be done in two children.

Pass score was obtained in 281 (90.9%).

Group B–3-5 years (Pre-school): A total of 38(n) children were screened of which 4 (1%) were "refer".

Group C–5-16 years (School): A total of 280(n) children were screened of which 62 (22.14%) had "refer". This group are being evaluated at the tertiary care centre.

Group D–Above 16 years (Adults): A total of 488(n) persons were screened of which refer was found in 309 (63.31%).

Hearing Loss In % age		Pearsons Chi Square	p Value
Rural-40.87	Tribal-48.82	2.817	0.093
Male-40.17	Female-44.58	1.74	0.187

Table 1: Prevalence of hearing loss.

	GROUP A (6 months to 3 years)	Group B 3-5 years	Group C 5-16 years	Group D above 16 years
"Refer"	29	4	62	309

Table 2: Patients who failed the Dp OAE test.

Pure tone audiometry revealed hearing loss in 42.4% in "refer" and in 16% (70) who "passed" the test.Moderate hearing loss in 46.3%, Moderately severe in 30.9%, severe in 17.8% and profound in 5% was found in the patients (Figure 2).

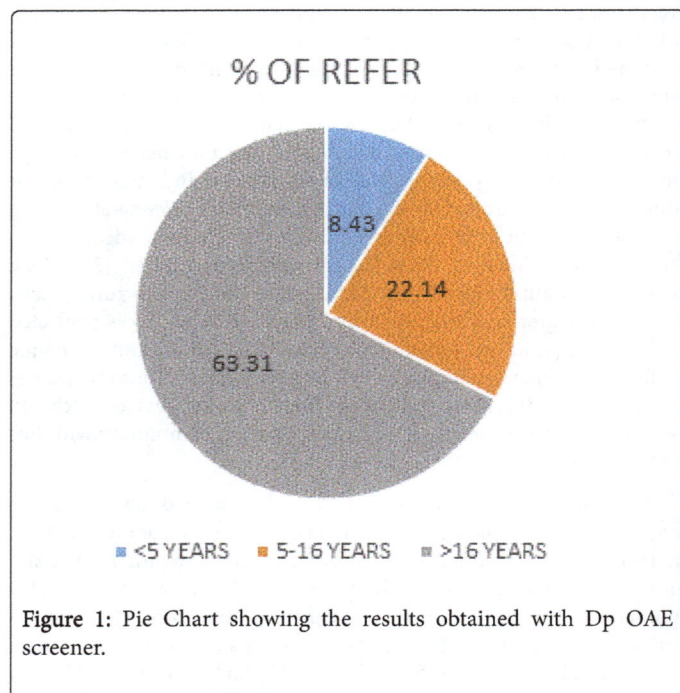

Figure 1: Pie Chart showing the results obtained with Dp OAE screener.

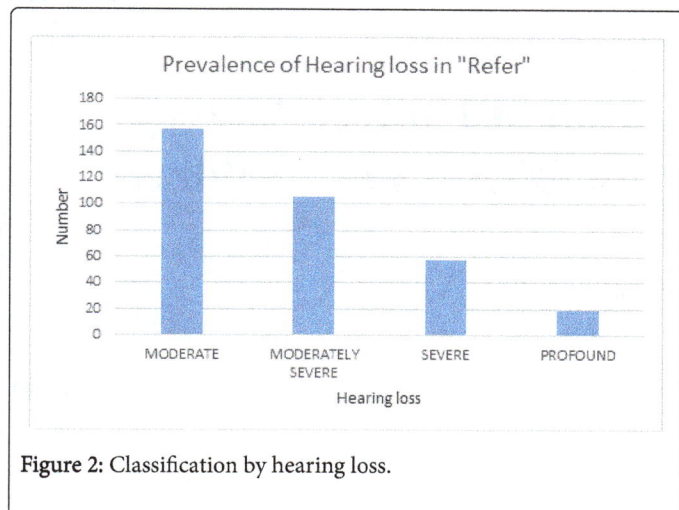

Figure 2: Classification by hearing loss.

Discussion

A review of literature revealed few population based studies in the Asia. Even though neonatal hearing screening is becoming mandatory, there are no comprehensive programmes for screening of children and adults. In this study 63.31% failed the test and among them more than 80% adults had disabling hearing loss (Moderate and above) which was confirmed by Pure Tone Audiometry.

Hearing loss is a significant problem which goes undetected and unrecognized because of the lack of awareness about the rehabilitative options available. People do not find it to interfere with their daily life because of lack of noise pollution and quiet environments they live in. Thus the exact prevalence of hearing loss is not known. This was also demonstrated in the study as the prevalence of hearing loss in the community does not correlate with the symptoms expressed by the population The use of trained community workers using an OAE screener which is non-invasive, does not depend on the subjects response (Pure tone Audiometry) gives us a definitive picture of the prevalence of this disability in the community and is better than questionnaire methods in a developing country where majority of people live in rural and tribal regions.

Conclusion

This study demonstrates the need for hearing screening at primary level in a rural community. Early detection of hearing loss is a cost effective and easily operable model is the need of the hour. Oto-acoustic emission testing is one which is easy to use reliable and can be used to screen large numbers. This model of identifying hearing loss using an OAE screener will lead to further evaluation and management at an early stage and can be implemented in developing and low income countries.

References

1. WHO (2015) Deafness and hearing loss.

2. Yueh B, Shapiro N, MacLean CH, Shekelle PG (2003) Screening and management of adult hearing loss in primary care: Scientific review. JAMA 289: 1976-1985.

3. Kumar S, Mohapatra B (2011) Status of newborn hearing screening program in India. Int J Pediatr Otorhinolaryngol 75: 20-26.

4. Augustine AM, Jana AK, Kuruvi Ila KA, Danda S, Lepcha A, et al.(2014) Neonatal hearing screening experience from a tertiary care hospital in southern India . Indian Pediatr 51: 179-183.

5. Hamernik RP, Ahroon WA, Lei SF (1996) The cubic distortion product otoacoustic emissions from the normal and noise-damaged chinchilla cochlea. J Acoust Soc Am 100: 1003-1012.

6. Rebillard G, Lavigne-Rebillard M (1992) Effect of reversible hypoxia on the compared time courses of endocochlear potential and 2f1-f2 distortion prod ucts. Hear Res 62: 142-148.

7. Ress BD, Sridhar KS, Balkany TJ, Waxman GM, Stagner BB, et al.(1999) Effects of cis-platinum chemotherapy on oto-acoustic emissions. The development of an objective screening protocol. Otolaryngol Head Neck Surg 121: 693-701.

8. Collet L, Gartner M, Moulin A, Kauffmann I, Disant F, et al.(1989) Evoked otoacoustic emissions and sensorineural hearing loss. Arch Otolaryngol Head Neck Surg 115: 1060-1062.

9. Gorga MP, Neely ST, Ohlrich B, Hoover B, Redner J, et al. (1997) From laboratory to clinic: A large scale study of distortion product otoacoustic emissions in ears with normal hearing and ears with hearing loss. Ear Hear 18: 440-455.

10. Rupa V (2001) Clinical utility of distortion product oto-acoustic emissions. Indian Journal of Otolaryngology Head and Neck Surgery 54: 88-90.

11. Kei J, Brazel B, Crebbin K, Richards A, Willeston N (2007) High frequency distortion product otoacoustic emissions in children with and without middle ear dysfuncti on. Int J Pediatr Otorhinolaryngol 71: 125-133.

12. Davis A, Bamford J, Wilson I, Ramkalawan T, Forshaw M, et al. (1997) A critical review of the role of neonatal hearing screening in the detection of congenital hearing impairment. Health Technology Assessment 1: 1-176.

13. Llanes EGDV, Chiong CM (2004) Evoked otoacoustic emissions and auditory brainstem responses: Concordance in hearing screening among high -risk children. Acta Oto-Laryngologica 124: 387-390

14. Thompson DC, McPhillips H, Davis RL, Lieu TA, Homer CJ, et al.(2001) Universal newborn heari ng screening. JAMA: The Journal of the American Medical Association 286: 2000-2010.

15. http://www.maico-diagn ostics.com/products/oae/eroscan/

16. Mishra A, Verma V, Shukla GK, Mishra SC, Dwivedi R (2011) Prevalence of hearing impairement in the distri ct of Lucknow, India. Indian J Public Health 55: 132-134.

25

Preliminary Study on the Application of Upper: Airway Model Construction with 3DMIA in OSAHS of Children

Dabo Liu[1*], Chao Cheng[2], Jiahui Pan[3] and Susu Bao[3]

[1]*Department of otorhinolaryngology, Guangzhou Women and Children's Medical Center, Guangzhou, China*

[2]*Pediatric Center, Southern Medical University Zhujiang Hospital, Guangzhou, China*

[3]*School of Computer Science, South China Normal University, Guangzhou, China*

*****Corresponding author:** Dabo Lium, Department of otorhinolaryngology, Guangzhou Women and Children's Medical Center, Address: No.318 Renmin Zhong Road, Guangzhou, 510120, China; E-mail: gzdaboliu@163.com

Abstract

Objective: To investigate the applicability of 3DMIA[1] software to upper airway modeling in children with obstructive sleep apnea hypopnea syndrome (OSAHS).

Methods: A total of 30 children diagnosed with OSAHS by polysomnography were included in this study. Data regarding upper airway structure were collected via spiral CT while sleeping and awake, from which a three-dimensional model of the upper respiratory tract from the nasopharynx to the supraglottic region using 3DMIA software was constructed. The upper airway olume and airway minimum cross-sectional area were measured employing software algorithms.

Results: The upper airway volume and airway minimum cross-sectional area of the 30 children during sleep were significantly less than while awake ($P < 0.01$).

Conclusions: 3DMIA software modeling and software algorithm measurement were more objective than traditional radiology (e.g. Fujioka) with respect to evaluation of the extent of the upper airway narrowing in OSAHS children, and showed good applicability to studying upper airway morphology and function in children with OSAHS.

Keywords: Obstructive Sleep Apnea Hypopnea Syndrome (OSAHS); Computer; Modeling; Children

Introduction

Obstructive Sleep Apnea Hypopnea Syndrome (OSAHS) affects multiple systems and multiple organs of children, and it is a syndrome which combines multiple subjects with its own specific etiological factor, pathology, physiology, clinical features and therapy. At present, those basic studies on OSAHS of children are limited on its influences on sleep structure, incretion and the neural development during the growing process of children. However, as a sleep apnea disease featuring at upper respiratory tract obstruction, upper airway structure and morphous factor is publically regarded as one of those important morbidity factors for OSAHS. So, to accurately acquire the data of the upper airway structure and the function condition is the foundation to choose appropriate treatment for OSAHS patients. On the above basis, accurate location of the upper airway stegnosis of the OSAHS patients is necessary to guide the surgery. Since this subject was established in January of 2011, we have conducted 3-dimensional model construction study of the CT data of those children who were diagnosed with OSAS by PSG with 3DMIA software to discuss the possibility of acquiring more accurate upper airway morphous of OSAS children by using software to construct models of upper airway.

Materials and Methods

General data

We chose 30 OSAHS children (18 boys and 12 girls, age of 5-14 years old, average age of 9.5 years old) in our hospital (from 2011-01 to 2012-01). Those OSAHS children were diagnosed according to the Diagnosis standard of OSAHS of children, 2005 made by Stephen et al[1] those children were monitored and observed by PSG, and the diagnosis standard included: apnea hypopnea time>2 respiratory cycle, OAI (Obstructive Apnea Index)>1/h, AHI (apnea hypopnea index) ≥ 5/h, LSa02(Lowest Oxygen Saturation)< 92%; among those children, 30 cases were detected with OAI 1.4-15/h,AHI 7.3-422/h,LSaO$_2$64%-91%;

---

[1] Software Specifications: the 3-dimensional reconstruction software adopted in this research was 3DMIA, automatically developed by the Computer School of South China Normal University (the code number of software copyright: 2008SR18799, 2008SR18798). The software could be used in the following areas: registering, segmentation (level set, region growing), volume-rendering, 3-dimensional reconstruction (including the adjustments of window width and window level) and surface rendering 3-dimensional reconstruction. Each part of the model could be used to observe the tissue. The tissue could be grouped randomly to be observed and be randomly amplified or diminished. Transparent observation could be set randomly. The produced document was in the form of STL, and could be opened and viewed with 3DMAX and other ordinary 3-dimensional production software but could not be measured.

all cases were observed with snore during sleep, buccal respiration, wheeze and oppression.

Methods to collect CT data

We used **brilliance ct 256-channel scanner** to conduct scanning. Scanning method: the patient was set in the dorsal position (The body part below the neck was wrapped by clothing made of lead) and the head of the patient was sent into the scanner first; the patient should hold the breath; the line connecting the external auditory foramen and the inferior border of nasal wing on the same side was set as the basal line; data of the volume of the respiratory passage from nasopharynx to the area above glottis; we used double window presentation, and the width of the soft tissue window was 200Hu with the window position of 40Hu, while the width of the bone window was 1200Hu with the window position of 600Hu; digital images were acquired (for detailed scanning parameters see Table 1). After we adjusted the patient's position, we suggested the patient to take eupnea and we performed spiral CT scanning. After the scanning was finished, we administrated chloral hydrate to the patient for oral use. After the patient was asleep, we adjusted his or her position and at the same time, performed CT scanning quickly to ensure that this CT scanning was performed during sleep cycle of the patient. Informed consents were obtained from the relatives of all children enrolled in this investigation. This research was approved by the Ethic Committee of our hospital.

Cases	Upper airway volume mm^3		Minimum cross section areas of air duct(mm^2)		Cases	Upper airway volume mm^3			Minimum cross section areas of air duct(mm^2)	
	Awake	Asleep	Awake	Asleep			Awake	Asleep	Awake	Asleep
1	18	15	43	22	16	26		18	66	38
2	25	20	57	24	17	30		23	116	88
3	25	17	59	27	18	14		10	64	51
4	13	9	63	45	19	17		14	39	25
5	13	12	66	29	20	22		17	70	39
6	25	23	63	29	21	16		13	122	108
7	21	12	74	46	22	33		24	147	103
8	31	19	132	48	23	11		8	59	49
9	15	10	118	102	24	13		9	87	45
10	21	19	66	44	25	25		20	67	34
11	27	16	155	75	26	21		15	78	32
12	12	10	60	31	27	22		18	92	75
13	24	15	55	19	28	15		10	82	71
14	29	21	97	76	29	23		20	72	48
15	27	15	201	188	30	29		15	101	77

Table 1: Scanning Parameters

Method to establish model

When we constructed the model of upper airway, we adopted the 3DMIA software automatically developed by the Computer School of South China Normal University (the code number of software copyright: 2008SR18799, 2008SR18798). We inserted the data sequence which was consistent with DICOM standard to the automatically developed medical imaging processing software 3DMIA, and used the software to perform important procedures such as imaging division, 3-dimensional reconstruction, and data measuring, etc. We performed imaging division of the CT data by using progress division as a dynamic self-adaptation region developing method [2]. We performed 3-dimensional surface rendering to those divided imaging by the Marching Cubes method. The free edge of soft palate, staphyle, the free edge of tip of the epiglottis and glottis were taken as identification markers. We identified the following parts as the key parts of the upper airway model: the postzone of soft palate, the staphyle zone, the postzone of tongue, the postzone of epiglottis and air tube. After we identified those key parts, we extracted centrage in appropriate region chosen in the upper airway 3-dimensional model mentioned above. Without changing the topology of upper airway, we simplified the 3-dimensional information to the central axis of upper airway to make it convenient to automatically calculate the cross section area along the centrage. By doing the above, we could offer references to analyze and estimate the stegnosis or the obstruction of the upper airway [3]. Through the above calculation method, we extracted from the model the upper airway volume and the minimum air duct cross section area of those children before and after they fell asleep respectively. We used traditional A/N method to acquire A/N ratio: a tangent line was made in the basilar clivus out of the skull, and the most prominent point of the adenoid B was taken to make a vertical line to the tangent line with A being the crossover point; the distance of A and B was measured as the value of A; AB line was prolonged and reached the juncture C in the pars palatalis through pharyngonasal cavity and air passage; the distance of AC was measured as the value of N (Figure 1).

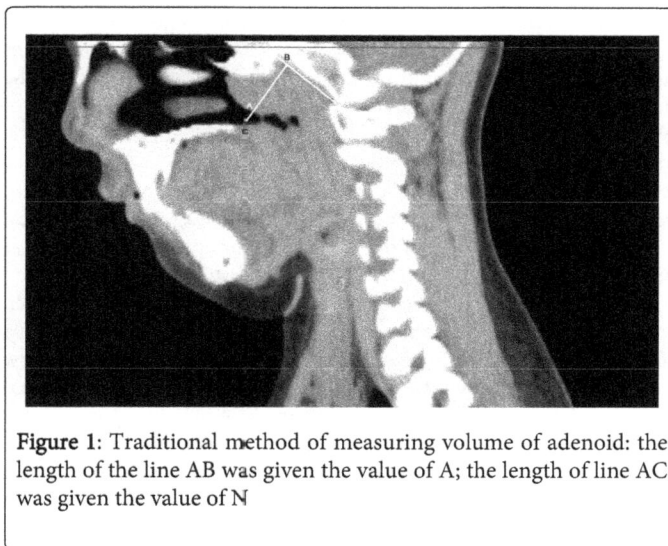

Figure 1: Traditional method of measuring volume of adenoid: the length of the line AB was given the value of A; the length of line AC was given the value of N

Statistical method

We used SPSS 11.0 to conduct statistical analysis; we used t-test of paired samples for measurement data; $P < 0.01$ meant statistical significance.

Results

We completely collected the upper airway CT volume data of those 30 children and successfully finished 3DMIA software model construction. We also acquired the upper airway volumes and the minimum cross section areas of those children before and after falling asleep respectively by the calculation method of the software. The results showed that: the upper airway volumes and the cross section areas of those children when they were asleep were significantly lower than when they were awake and the differences showed statistical significance (t=9.392, P<0.01; t=9.256, P<0.01, Table 2). The average A/N ratio was 0.67, and there were 14 patients whose A/N ≥ 0.67, accounted for 0.47% among all children with the disease.

kV	mAs	Thickness	HP	Width of the reconstructed layer	S-F0V
120	75	0.3×32	21	2~3mm	S

Table 2: Showing statistical significance.

Discussion

At present, studies on OSAHS of children are limited on its influences on sleep structure, incretion, the neural development and other aspects during the growing process of children. In clinical, there still existed some doubts and confusions about it, for example: most scholars took PSG as the golden standard for the diagnosis of OSAHS children, however, as researches on the sleep mechanism and OSAHS went deeper, we found it difficult for sleep monitoring to reflect the sleep parameter of OSAHS children at normal times; except for some children showing more obvious First Night Effect (FNE), most children couldn't adapt to the complex sleep monitoring device and relatively uncomfortable sleep progress, thus leading to the distortion of monitoring results; besides, some children had high risks factors such as obesity, jaw facial deformity and so on, these children were too little and had so many complications, so if we performed sleep monitoring to this type of children, the risks would increase significantly and at the same time, the whole progress couldn't be completed mostly. If we could acquire more diagnosis parameter through noninvasive imaging data to act as subsidiary way for the diagnosis of the above children, we would increase the diagnosis of OSAHS of children to a new high. For the treatment of the disease, operations to relieve local blockage was taken as the first choice publically. However, for OSAHS which was a sleep-respiratory disease featuring at blockage of upper airway, operation to relieve anatomical abnormity was publically known as an important principle to treat OSAHS [4]. However in clinical practices, we could often observe that some children could show clinical features and physical signs which were not in consistent with the blockage degree described in books. To study the reasons, according to many clinical studies [5-7], the airflow obstruction planes included multiple planes such as nasopharynx, oropharynx, laryngopharynx and so on. The whole upper airway above the glottis was almost included. So, to acquire more accurate data of upper airway morphous and function condition and to precisely locate the upper airway stagnosis of OSAHS children to provide reference for operation were necessary conditions to further optimize operation plan and choose reasonable treatment method for OSAHS patients.

At present, there are many methods in clinical to evaluate patients' local stegnosis of upper airway.. All of the above examination methods have their own advantages and disadvantages respectively and the

information they acquire show different emphasizes. In recent years, with the widely used computer simulation technology, powerful calculation capacity of computers and leading in of finite element analysis, we could reconstruct the airway structure and morphous with volume data collected by CT. Using related software to perform accurate data comparison and measurement of the model was more and more used in the studies on the morphous and functions of upper airway. In this study, the imaging data were obtained by 256-slice CT. The dosage of X-ray was decreased by 60% to 80% compared with that used by previous equipments and the potential clinical ethic issue was properly avoided. Software 3DMIA adopted in this study was a medical image processing software with great functions automatically developed by the Computer School of South China Normal University, it could be used to progress various plane images, reconstruct 3-dimensional model and measure data of multiple medical image data. The produced 3-dimensional model in STL form could act as the foundation for continuous studies. Semi-auto calculation of the minimum cross section area of upper airway could accurately and quickly find the stegnosis in multiple planes of the patients. By using this 3-dimensional visualization method, we could analyze the 3-dimensional anatomical structures of OSAHS children before operation, and in the aspects of operation value concerns, risk evaluation and other aspects, this methods had more significant advantages than those methods adopted in other related studies. (Figure 2)

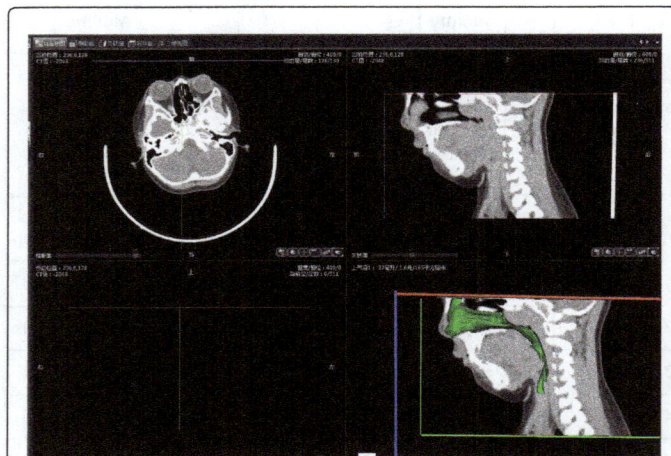

Figure 2: Operating interface for constructing a 3-dimensional model of the upper airway by 3DMIA software. A complete 3-dimensional model was reconstructed by integrating the data of these three plane volumes

At present, studies on this aspect were mostly based on the plane image measurement by X-ray, CT and etc. As for this point, Major and other scholars [8] pointed out in the study that children's upper airways were complex 3-dimensional structure; for children with OSAHS, with the influences left by diseases, their morphous of upper airways had variations to some extent, so when turned to 2-dimensional images, some information would be lost. In this study, we used software to perform 3-dimensional model construction and could acquire relatively accurate data of upper airway morphous and the relative correlation between each anatomical structure. Compared with those current studies based on data collected by CT, our study processed the data by surface-rendering, and the 3-dimensional model we produced were totally with complete virtual physical characteristics and space information other than the volume-rendering model acquired by adjusting CT value. In the models we established, through the specific functions of software, we could, within a specific space range, perform local maximization, rotation, transition and other operations to the model, which was beneficial to identify specific morphous, range and direction of upper airway stegnosis and this was the advantage other domestic studies didn't have.

In identifying the stegnosis location of airways of children with OSAHS, most studies were concentrated in cavum nasopharyngeum and taking the size of adenoid as the study direction. Conventional tests, such as nasopharyngeal X-ray from a lateral view have been adopted to measure the size of adenoid in children, as an evaluation criterion for the degree of the upper airway stenosis. However, there are various limitations and disadvantages including magnification error caused by varying focus-slice distance and measurement error resulting from inaccurate selection of measurement point. Meantime, nasopharyngeal X-ray from a lateral view displays an overlap image, easily intervened by the ascending branch of mandible. In addition, it fails to display the structures of nose and nasopharynx in details.

In our study, we adopted the centrage extraction calculation method of the software, located the minimum cross section area of pars nasalis pharyngis with computer and measured in 3-dimensional vision. We found that among those 30 OSAHS children, when they were asleep, only 11 children showed that the most prominent point of pars nasalis pharyngis, namely the point with biggest A value, was in the same plane with the minimum cross section area of pars nasalis pharyngis along the centrage of airway, accounted for 37% of the total. The other 63% children showed that, the narrowest position of pars nasalis pharyngis was not in the same plane with the most prominent point of adenoid. So we might not correctly identify the stegnosis degree of children's upper airways according to the traditional A/N ratio. As for the reasons, we analyzed and thought that, from the 3-dimensional morphous view, the morphous of OSAHS children's upper airways in pars nasalis pharyngis were often in wedge cube or trapezoid cube shape; although at most times, the anteroposterior diameter between the most prominent point of adenoid and pars palatalis was the narrowest, the left-to-right diameter namely the distance between the left and right lateral pharyngeal wall might not be the narrowest, so the area was not the smallest (Figure 3, Figure 4). We haven't got a relatively public received method or standard in evaluating the stegnosis degree of OSAHS children's upper airways till now, but if we see the trend, we will find that it is accepted by most scholars step and step that we should evaluate the relative volume of stegnosis tissue to upper airway volume other than only evaluate the absolute volume of soft tissue [9]. By using fluid mechanics theories, Powell et al. [10] had proved among adults that in narrow and irregular upper airways, the air current shear stress born by stegnosis tissue significantly increased. This process might cause progressive injuries to the mechanics recipients of upper airway and other recipients that coordinated the contraction of diaphragmatic muscle and respiratory muscles. So, we thought that there existed some defects in our traditional way of evaluating the illness stage and operation indications of OSAHS children by simply measuring the volume of adenoid. Using 3DMAX software to construct model to evaluate the morphous of children's complete upper airways, and measuring the minimum airway area through computer would be more beneficial to make objective diagnosis to the illness of OSAHS children.

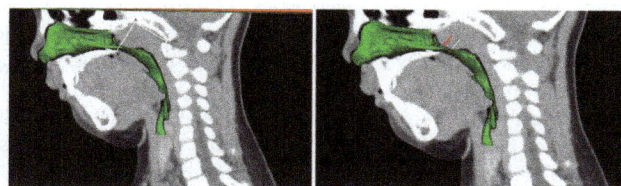

Figure 3: B in left was the most prominent point. Same point in right indicated by red arrowhead was not the narrowest point measured by computer, indicated by white arrowhead was

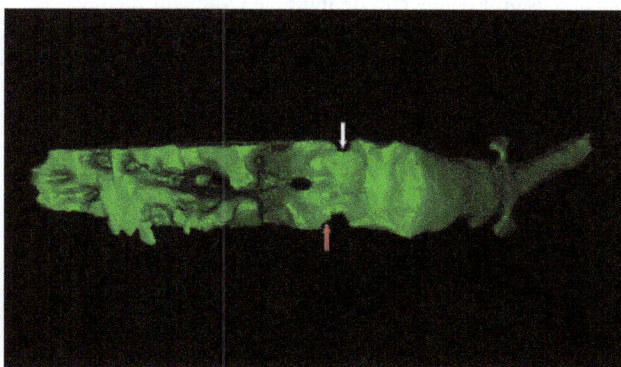

Figure 4: Relative correlation is more obvious in this axial view of the model (red arrowhead was the most prominent point while white arrowhead was the narrowest point of air way)

During quantitative study on the constructed model we found that most OSAHS children's upper airway stegnosis appeared in multiple planes from choana narium along laryngopharynx and formed a discontinuous stegnosis, and the narrowest part often located in the nasopharynx or oropharynx plane (Figure 5). This morphous characteristic was not mentioned in other domestic studies, and this was the advantage brought by 3-dimensional model which could provide more information than traditional 2-dimensional image. Besides, compliances change of upper airways was also regarded as an important morbidity factor for OSAHS. On the basis of constructing model, we measured and compared the upper airway volumes and found that upper airway volume of children was significantly bigger when they were awake breathing than they were asleep breathing, and the minimum cross section area of airway was also larger than they were asleep. Differences showed statistical significance. However, when normal individuals were breathing, the upper airway distension muscular tension was in a dynamic balance with pharyngeal cavity negative pressure to ensure the openness and smoothness of pharyngeal cavity. Result of this study could indicate that the compliance of pharyngeal wall of OSAHS children increased which would easily lead to collapse and obstruction when the children inspired air. This change could reflect the difference of upper airway compliances of airways when the children were awake and asleep to some extent, and could objectively reflect the position, range and extent of the stegnosis and the collapse. In the past, we often diagnosed severe cases of OSAHS children by clinical symptoms and sleep monitoring in clinical practice, but we were lack of good methods to pre-judge the specific stegnosis or the illness degree. This 3-

dimensional model method would provide more anatomical references for the diagnosis of severe cases. As for treatment, for those severe cases of OSAHS children, operation was still the major treatment method. However, as those OSAHS children often had stegnosis in multiple planes, if we performed operation to solve the problem in only one plane we couldn't achieve satisfactory results. And for these patients, the operation was more difficult, anaesthesia status was difficult to control, complication rate during the perioperative process was high, post-operation outcomes were not quite satisfactory, so to choose a correct interference method was always the challenge we had to face in clinical practice. By 3-dimensional model construction, we could precisely locate the stegnosis and collapse point, the range and extent of the children's upper airways. By comprehensively judging and evaluating these factors and appropriately choose multiple treatment methods such as CAPA, we could improve the therapeutic outcomes of those severe cases of OSAHS children. In this regard, the 3-dimensional reconstruction of upper airways and volume measurement had unique advantages.

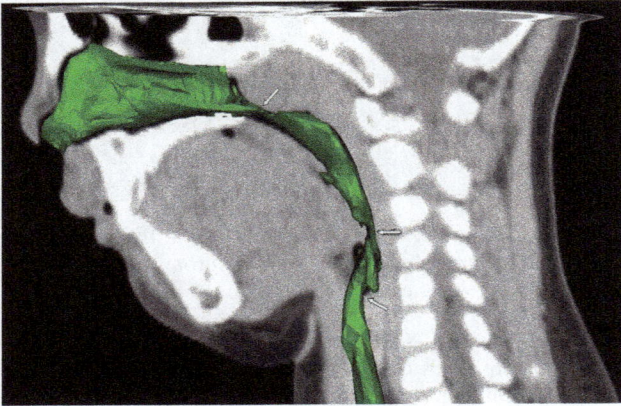

Figure 5: By 3D reconstruction, it was clear that the point indicated by white arrowhead in image was the narrowest point, and a noncontiguous obstruction was present near the laryngeal pharynx segment

With our measurement by using 3-dimensional model construction technology, we could directly reflect the airway volume changes of airway compliances, observe the position, range, extent and direction of the stegnosis and collapse of upper airway, and could study the morphous and functional features of upper airways of OSAHS children. The maneuverability and effectiveness were primarily proved in this study and this method was a relatively good way to study on the morphous and function of upper airway. In the following studies, we would enlarge the sample size and add control groups to make more systematical and exquisite studies on the morphous and functions of upper airways of OSAHS children.

References

1. Stephen H. Sheldon, Richard Ferber, Meir H. Kryger (2005) Principles and Practice of Pediatric sleep medicine. Elsevier Science Health Science div. 207.

2. Jiahui Pan, Chao Cheng, Susu Bao, Dabo Liu, Jianping Ye (2013) Study of Computer-aided Diagnosis Method of Childhood Obstructive Sleep Apnea Syndrome. J Comput Biol 9: 5837- 5844.

3. Jiahui Pan, Susu Bao (2010) One Biliary Tract Virtual Surgery Simulation System; Application Research of Computers (02) .

4. Section on Pediatric Pulmonology, Subcommittee on Obstructive Sleep Apnea Syndrome American Academy of Pediatrics. (2002) Clinical practice guideline: diagnosis and management of childhood obstructive sleep apnea syndrome. Pediatrics 109: 704-712.

5. Redline S1, Tishler PV, Schluchter M, Aylor J, Clark K, et al. (1999) Risk factors for sleep-disordered breathing in children. Associations with obesity, race, and respiratory problems. Am J Respir Crit Care Med 159: 1527-1532.

6. Morales-Angulo C, Gallo-Terán J, Azuara N, Rama Quintela J (2006) [Otorhinolaryngo logical manifestations in patients with Down syndrome]. Acta Otorrinolaringol Esp 57: 262-265.

7. Erler T, Paditz E (2004) Obstructive sleep apnea syndrome in children: a state-of-the-art review. Treat Respir Med 3: 107-122.

8. Major MP, Flores-Mir C, Major PW (2006) Assessment of lateral cephalometric diagnosis of adenoid hypertrophy and posterior upper airway obstruction: a systematic review. Am J Orthod Dentofacial Orthop 130: 700-708.

9. Ruoff CM, Guilleminault C (2012) Orthodontics and sleep-disordered breathing. Sleep Breath 16 : 271-273.

10. Powell N, Guilleminault C (2009) Abnormal pharyngeal airflow in obstructive sleep apnea using computational fluid dynamics: Feasibility study. Proceeding of the 9th World Congress on Sleep. Apnea (Seoul, Korea).

Prevalence of Hearing Loss among First Grade School Children in Tirana, Albania

Suela Sallavaci[1*], Ervin Toci[2], Ylli Sallavaci[3] and Gentian Stroni[4]

[1,3]Service of Otorhinolaryngology, University Hospital Center "Mother Teresa", Tirana, Albania

[2]Department of Epidemiology and Health Systems, Institute of Public Health, Tirana, Albania

[4]Service of Infectious Diseases, University Hospital Centre "Mother Teresa", Tirana, Albania

*Corresponding author: Dr. Suela Sallavaci, Prof Assoc, Service of Otorhinolaryngology, University Hospital Center "Mother Teresa", Tirana, Albania; E-mail: sallavacis@hotmail.com

Abstract

Background: Hearing Loss (HL), which affects disproportionally children in low income countries, is increasing worldwide. HL could be associated with a range of speech, language and cognitive problems in children. In Albania the information about this condition is largely outdated. In this context, the aim of this paper was to assess the prevalence of HL among first grade school children in Tirana, the capital city of Albania.

Methods: A cross-sectional survey was carried out for three consecutive years during 2008-2011, in 163 schools of Tirana. In total 15,163 first-grade pupils were screened in order to detect those with a high probability of HL, which were later invited to undergo definitive diagnosis procedures. During the first year of study a hearing threshold of ≥ 35 dB for the better ear was used as a cut-off whereas a threshold of ≥30 dB was used for the two remaining study waves.

Results: In total, the prevalence of any suspected hearing impairment was 4.4%. The 3-year prevalence of total diagnosed conductive and sensorineural HL was 3.61% and 0.09%, respectively, with no clear trends across the study years. The total prevalence of Otitis Media with Effusion and Chronic Otitis Media was 1.36% and 0.17%, respectively.

Conclusions: Hearing loss prevalence among children aged 6-7 years in Albania during 2008-2011 was relatively low. However, in absolute numbers, around 3,000 children would benefit from the early detection of such condition.

Keywords: Albania; Hearing Impairment; School-age children; Prevalence

Introduction

Hearing loss is becoming an issue of increasing importance worldwide. For instance, WHO world estimations of people living with hearing difficulties have risen steadily from 120 million in 1995 [1], to 250 million in 2000 [2] whereas in 2011 there were about 360 million living with disabling hearing loss of which 32 million were children aged 0-14 years [3]. Increasing trends of hearing impairment were observed among youngsters as well: among adolescents aged 12-19 years it was observed an increasing prevalence of any hearing loss between 1988-1994 (14.9%) and 2005-2006 (19.5%) [4]. The global prevalence of hearing loss among children aged 0-14 years old was 1.7% in 2011, and substantially higher in low income countries compared to high-income ones [5].

Hearing impairments during childhood might have negative effects as they could delay the development of speech, language and cognitive skills of the affected children often resulting in poorer school performance compared to children with normal hearing capabilities [3]. For instance, a study among 1228 school children found that 3rd grade children with hearing impairment had significantly lower scores for reading vocabulary, language mechanics, word analysis and spelling as well as lower scores on a range of functional tests whereas no differences were observed among 6th and 9th graders [6]. Other studies have suggested relationships between hearing impairment in children with worse school performance and language skills among children aged 0-18 years [7], 11 years [8] and 6-12 years [9]. In addition, children with hearing impairments showed persistent low school performance even after individualized education plan efforts [10,11]. There is evidence that the earlier the hearing impairments are detected and addressed the better the outcomes in terms of improvements of language and comprehension skills [12]. In children under 15 years of age, disabling hearing impairment is defined as permanent unaided hearing threshold for the better ear of ≥ 31 dB calculated as the average hearing threshold level at four frequencies 0.5, 1, 2 and 4 kHz whereas for adults the average threshold is ≥ 41 dB [13].

The prevalence of hearing impairment among school aged children has been assessed in both developed and developing countries, but the results vary substantially due to different kinds and degrees of hearing impairment assessed and different age-groups included. Globally, the prevalence of hearing impairment defined by a threshold of ≥ 35 dB in the better ear was 1.4% among children 5-14 years old in 2008 [14]. In developed countries, the prevalence of any hearing impairment and mild sensorineural hearing loss among school aged children was 11.3% and 5.4%, respectively, among 1228 US children in grades 3, 6 and 9 [6]. A large study including more than 6000 children aged 6-19 years reported that 14.9% of them had some kind of hearing impairment [15], a study among 6581 grade 1 and grade 5 children in Australia found that the prevalence of slight/moderate bilateral sensorineural hearing loss was 0.88% [16] whereas a UK study suggested that 2.05% of children aged 9-16 years had permanent hearing impairment [17]. In developed countries, the prevalence of hearing impairments among primary school children ranged from 8.8% in Iran [18], 15% in Malasyia [8] but 2.4% in Zimbabwe [19].

In Albania the information about the prevalence of hearing impairment in the general population as well as in the community of children is scarce. Some screening efforts date back to 1980 and were carried out by the professionals of Mother Teresa University Hospital Center in Tirana (UHCT), the only tertiary hospital in the country. Therefore, there is immediate need to update the figures about hearing impairment prevalence among children in this South-European country. In this context, the aim of the present paper is to provide the scientific community with updated information about the prevalence of hearing impairment among first grade school children of Tirana in order to shed light upon this largely under researched area in Albania.

Methods

Study population and sampling

This project was carried out during 2008-2011 under the technical and scientific responsibility of the otorhinolaryngology service, University Hospital of Tirana [20]. A specific component of this exercise included the screening of hearing impairment among school-age children of Tirana aiming to collect epidemiological data on prevalence of hearing impairment in the group of children in order to educate and raise the awareness of pedagogical staff regarding the childhood hearing problems.

The cross-sectional survey was repeated three times consecutively during the 2003-2004, 2004-2005 and 2005-2006 academic years. The sampling framework included all primary schools in urban Tirana. Among those we selected randomly and proportional to size around 20% of these schools at each academic year under study, thus resulting in 55 schools sampled during the first wave of the survey, 53 schools during the second wave and 55 schools during the third wave of the survey, for a total of 163 schools surveyed. In all the selected schools we examined all the first grade pupils. From 16,229 first grade pupils in all surveyed schools during the 3-years study period we examined 15,163 pupils or 93.4% of the target sample. More detailed information about the percentage of the sample covered during each of the study years is presented in (Table 1).

Academic year	No of schools	No of children	No of 1st grade children	Examined children	Children with suspected hearing impairment	Showed up for stage 2 diagnosis	Didn't show up for level 2 diagnosis
2003-2004	55	49471	5622	5392 (95.9) *	152 (2.8) †	123	29
2004-2005	53	49413	5459	5077 (93.0)	257 (5.1)	239	18
2005-2006	55	49244	5148	4694 (91.2)	262 (5.6)	224	38
Total	163	148,128	16,229	15,163 (93.4)	671 (4.4)	586	85

* Proportion of examined children among all 1st grade children.

† Proportion of children with suspected hearing impairment among examined children.

Table 1: Distribution of screened children according to academic study year and prevalence of suspected hearing impairment, Tirana, Albania

Data collection

The screening process comprised of two stages. During the first stage, the screening process aimed to detect children who had a high probability of experiencing any kind of hearing impairment and defined in this paper as "suspected cases". In the second stage, the suspected cases identified during the first stage, were then invited to undergo specialized diagnostic tests in order to confirm the diagnosis and the potential cause.

In the first stage of the screening program, four Otolaryngology Trainees near the premises of Otorhinolaryngology Service at UHC "Mother Teresa" were trained about the use of screening tools thus enabling them to master the basic screening techniques. Each selected school was contacted and the school director was explained the aim of the study thus ensuring excellent cooperation with the pedagogical staff. Simple questionnaires were distributed to parents and teachers with the aim to detect severe cases of hearing impairment prior to screening efforts. Pupils were retrieved in small groups of 4-5 children and examined and then they were sent back to their respective class thus allowing for the other children to be examined without interfering with the pedagogical process. To detect children who might suffer from any hearing impairment, tonal audiometry was used. During the first academic year under survey (2003-2004) a hearing threshold for the better ear of ≥ 35 dB was used as a cut-off for diagnosing any hearing impairment (suspected cases) whereas during the two subsequent academic years under survey the threshold used was ≥ 30 DB. On average each tonal audiometry examination lasted about 10 minutes.

Every case suspected by the examiners to have any hearing impairment during the first stage of screening was then invited to undergo a second level examination in the Audiology Section of the Service of Otorhinolaryngology in the UHC "Mother Teresa" in Tirana where the final diagnosis was set. A letter was sent to the respective parent of suspected cases explaining that their children might suffer some kind of hearing impairment and inviting them to accompany their children to the premises of the Service of Otorhinolaryngology in the UHC "Mother Teresa" for a free of charge final diagnosis of the problem. From 671 suspected cases, only 586 children underwent second stage total diagnostic examination. For the 85 children detected with potential hearing impairment during the first stage of screening process, the reasons for not showing up for further diagnostics examinations was the reluctance of their parents about the "free-of-charge" nature of the medical visit as well as their negligence.

During the second stage, a series of procedures were used in order to set the final diagnosis. An extended Otorhinolaryngological medical visit was carried out for the thorough examination of nose, ear and throat in order to detect any problem that might have affected the hearing process. This was done for every child suspected to have any hearing impairment and detected during the first stage of screening. To set the final diagnosis we used the tympanometry, stapedial reflex and tonal audiometry examinations.

Based on the results of Otorhinolaryngological visit, potential causes of hearing impairment were diagnosed. These events included the Otitis Media with Effusion, Chronic Otitis Media, earwax, etc. In addition, hearing loss was categorized into sensorineural hearing loss and conductive hearing loss which comprised also children with Otitis Media with Effusion and Chronic Otitis Media.

Free of charge specialized care and support was offered for cases diagnosed with hearing impairment. Those cases diagnosed with Otitis Media with Effusion or Chronic Otitis Media were treated free of charge for the respective conditions. Cases diagnosed with sensorineural hearing loss were equipped with hearing aid devices when appropriate. Cases diagnosed with conductive hearing loss were treated for their primary (adenoids, tonsils, etc.) and secondary conditions.

Calculation of prevalence rates

In order to calculate the yearly prevalence rate of conductive or sensorineural hearing loss and the prevalence rate of Otitis Media with Effusion and Chronic Otitis Media we divided the respective number of children diagnosed with a specific condition by the number of children screened in each of the academic years under study. To calculate the total prevalence of these conditions we divided the total cases with a specific event by the total population of children screened. Prevalence rates were expressed per 100 children. Absolute numbers and respective percentages were calculated and reported.

Results

The number of schools, number of children, 1st grade children and the number of examined children are presented in (Table 1). In each academic year under study more than 90% of eligible 1st grade children were screened, whereas during the three-year period of the study 93% of all 1st graders were screened. The prevalence rates of any suspected hearing impairment showed an increasing trend from 2.8% during 2003-2004 academic years to 5.1% and 5.6% during the two other academic years under study. In total, the prevalence of any suspected hearing impairment was 4.4%. Table 2 presents the results of final examination of children detected during the first stage of the screening program and who showed up for further examination of their problem. Among children who showed up, 25 of them resulted to have normal hearing (3 at 1st year, 8 at 2nd year and 14 at the 3rd year of study) after thorough ORL examination. The cause of their suspected hearing impairment resulted to be of mechanical nature, such as earwax, after the removing of which the hearing was restored (Table 2).

Academic year	Screened children	Stage 2 children	Conductive hearing loss			Total conductive hearing loss	Sensorineural hearing loss	Normal hearing†
			Tympanic effusion	Chronic otitis media	Conductive hearing loss			
2003-2004	5392	123	37 (0.69) *	6 (0.11) *	73 (1.35) *	116 (2.15) *	4 (0.07) *	3
2004-2005	5077	239	89 (1.75)	7 (0.14)	130 (2.56)	226 (4.45)	5 (0.10)	8
2005-2006	4694	224	80 (1.70)	13 (0.28)	112 (2.39)	205 (4.37)	5 (0.11)	14
Total	15,163	586	206 (1.36)	26 (0.17)	315 (2.08)	547 (3.61)	14 (0.09)	25

* Absolute number and prevalence rate expressed per 100 screened children (in parenthesis)

† These cases were suspected to have any hearing impairment during the first stage but after further examination their hearing resulted normal. For example, they had earwax which was removed.

Table 2: Prevalence of various diagnoses after specialized medical diagnostic procedures

The 3-year prevalence of total conductive hearing loss (comprising Otitis Media with Effusion, Chronic Otitis Media and conductive hearing loss diagnoses) was 3.61% whereas the prevalence of sensorineural hearing loss was 0.09% during the same period of time. The prevalence of total conductive hearing loss was lower during the first year under study (2.15%) and then showed inconsistent trend during the two other years under study (4.45% and 4.37%, respectively). The total 3-year prevalence of Otitis Media with Effusion and Chronic Otitis Media was 1.36% and 0.17%, respectively. Regarding Otitis Media with Effusion, its prevalence was very low during the first year of screening (0.69%) and then more than doubled in the subsequent years. Whereas the prevalence of Chronic Otitis Media increased monotonically over the years from 0.11% in 2008-2009 academic year, to 0.14% in 2009-2010 academic year and 0.28% in 2010-2011 academic year (Table 2).

Discussion

This is the first large scale screening effort aiming to detect the prevalence of hearing loss among primary school children in Albania. Our findings suggest that hearing loss has a relatively low prevalence among children aged 6-7 years. The prevalence of total conductive and sensorineural hearing loss was 3.61% and 0.09%, respectively, during the 3-year study period. Therefore, the prevalence of any hearing loss (conductive+sensorineural) was 3.70% in this large sample of 1st grade children. We found an extremely low prevalence of sensorineural hearing loss of only 0.09%. The prevalence of other causes of conductive hearing loss such as Otitis Media with Effusion and Chronic Otitis Media was 1.36% and 0.17%, respectively.

The prevalence of conductive or sensorineural hearing loss was more or less stable during the three years under study. We think that the lower prevalence detected at the 1st year under study for these two types of hearing loss are attributed to the higher threshold used in the first year of study ($\geq$ 35 dB) compared to a threshold of $\geq$ 30 dB used in two remaining study years. A higher threshold means that fewer pupils will be suspected as having a hearing impairment and this subsequently affects the prevalence rates.

The especially low prevalence of sensorineural hearing loss might be attributed to several factors which are present in the Albania population. The most important factors contributing to this low prevalence is the mentality of the parents in Albania: they consider a child with hearing impairment as handicapped or disabled and therefore they send these children to special schools in order to avoid the judgment from the society. This is a pity since these children could benefit from the right interventions and the use of hearing aid devices.

Despite the low prevalence of hearing loss impairment, the findings could have important implications. The prevalence of 3.70% is translated into 561 children in our study population and, taking into account that we surveyed only about 20% of schools in Tirana, the absolute number of children aged 6-7 years who could benefit from different interventions could be approximately 3,000 for the 3-years under study. As we explored in the introduction of this paper, hearing impairment among school children could affect their language and social skills as well as their school performance [3,6-9]. For example, Otitis Media with Effusion (OME), which might affect 9 out of 10 pre-school aged children [21], could be an important treatable cause of hearing loss. Furthermore, in up to 40% of cases this condition might become recurrent and in 10% of cases it lasts longer than 1 year [22] thus increasing the risk of hearing loss if untreated. A study found that 1 in 4 school children aged 7 years had some degree of Otitis Media with Effusion [23]. However, routine screening for OME is not recommended because the evidence of more benefits from early detection is lacking [24]. The low prevalence of Otitis Media with Effusion in our study and other studies is due to the different aims of each study: we aimed to detect the hearing impairment and selected only children who showed such signs on tonal audiometry whereas other studies physically examined all children for signs of Otitis Media with Effusion and thus reported much higher prevalence [23]. Otitis Media with Effusion often accompanies conductive hearing loss [25] and if the disease persists then the child could exhibit adverse school or developmental effects [26-28].

There is evidence that Chronic Otitis Media is the commonest cause of hearing loss among children in low and middle income countries [29-31]. However, this condition was not very prevalent (0.17%) in our group of children possibly because Chronic Otitis Media thrives due to overcrowding, poor hygiene control and nutrition and lack of medical care conditions which are not prevalent in Albania as compared to some African countries [30,31].

Our results are in concordance with previous studies which have found that conductive hearing loss is more prevalent than sensorineural one among school children [8,18]. The prevalence of unilateral sensorineural hearing loss among school-children is reported to be 3%-5% [6,15]. Children with sensorinueral hearing loss often required extra educational plans and efforts [7].

Apart from academic and developmental problems, hearing loss among children constitutes a financial burden as well. For example, in USA the total costs of OME, a common cause of hearing loss, amount up to 4$ billion dollars each year [32]. If the hearing problems are left untreated then the costs of hearing impairment could be very high. For example, in Europe the annual cost of mild, moderate and severe/ profound hearing impairment per person were 2,200, 6,600 and 11,000 Euros, respectively, whereas the total cost of hearing impairment in Europe would be around 300 billion Euros including all costs related to this condition [33].

In this context, the detection and appropriate treatment of children with hearing impairments in Albania should be given the appropriate priority among other health services as it can save future individual disabilities and societal costs.

In summary, this paper has provided with recent information about the prevalence of hearing impairment among school children in Albania based on screening efforts. The prevalence of hearing loss among children in this South-Eastern European country is relatively low compared to other reports. However, the consistent findings during the three consecutive waves of the survey suggest that the information is robust. However, further cross-sectional surveys are needed in order to confirm the trends observed in our study.

References

1. Smith AW (1998) The World Health Organisation and the prevention of deafness and hearing impairment caused by noise. Noise Health 1: 6-12.

2. Mathers C, Smith A, Concha M. Global Burden of hearing loss in the year 2000. Geneva.

3. World Health Organization, 2000.

4. World Health Organization. Millions of people in the world have hearing loss that can be treated or prevented. World Health Organization, WHO/NMH/PBD, 2013.

5. Shargorodsky J, Curhan SG, Curhan GC, Eavey R (2010) Change in prevalence of hearing loss in US adolescents. JAMA 304: 772-778.

6. Duthey B (2013) Background paper 6.21 Hearing loss. Update on 2004 background paper. World Health Organization.

7. Bess FH, Dodd-Murphy J, Parker RA (1998) Children with minimal sensorineural hearing loss: prevalence, educational performance, and functional status. Ear Hear 19: 339-354.

8. Lieu JE (2004) Speech-language and educational consequences of unilateral hearing loss in children. Arch Otolaryngol Head Neck Surg 130: 524-530.

9. Khairi Md Daud M, Noor RM, Rahman NA, Sidek DS, Mohamad A (2010) The effect of mild hearing loss on academic performance in primary school children. Int J Pediatr Otorhinolaryngol 74: 67-70.

10. Lieu JE, Tye-Murray N, Karzon RK, Piccirillo JF (2010) Unilateral hearing loss is associated with worse speech-language scores in children. Pediatrics 125: e1348-1355.

11. Lieu JE, Tye-Murray N, Fu Q (2012) Longitudinal study of children with unilateral hearing loss. Laryngoscope 122: 2088-2095.

12. Lieu JE (2013) Unilateral hearing loss in children: speech-language and school performance. B-ENT Suppl 21: 107-115.

13. Yoshinaga-Itano C, Apuzzo ML (1998) Identification of hearing loss after age 18 months is not early enough. Am Ann Deaf 143: 380-387.

14. World Health Organisation (2001) Deafness and Hearing Impairment Survey. Report of consultative meeting of principal investigators, WHO Project ICP DPR 001.

15. Stevens G1, Flaxman S, Brunskill E, Mascarenhas M, Mathers CD, et al. (2013) Global and regional hearing impairment prevalence: an analysis of 42 studies in 29 countries. Eur J Public Health 23: 146-152.

16. Niskar AS1, Kieszak SM, Holmes A, Esteban E, Rubin C, et al. (1998) Prevalence of hearing loss among children 6 to 19 years of age: the Third National Health and Nutrition Examination Survey. JAMA 279: 1071-1075.

17. Wake M, Tobin S, Cone-Wesson B, Dahl HH, Gillam L, et al. (2006) Slight/mild sensorineural hearing loss in children. Pediatrics 118: 1842-1851.

18. Fortnum HM, Summerfield AQ, Marshall DH, Davis AC, Bamford JM (2001) Prevalence of permanent childhood hearing impairment in the United Kingdom and implications for universal neonatal hearing screening: questionnaire based ascertainment study. BMJ 323: 536-540.

19. Absalan A, Pirasteh I, Dashti Khavidaki GA, Asemi Rad A, Nasr Esfahani AA, et al. (2013) A Prevalence Study of Hearing Loss among Primary School Children in the South East of Iran. Int J Otolaryngol 2013: 138935.

20. Westerberg BD, Skowronski DM, Stewart IF, Stewart L, Bernauer M, et al. (2005) Prevalence of hearing loss in primary school children in Zimbabwe. Int J Pediatr Otorhinolaryngol 69: 517-525.

21. Nika D Hearing impairment among Albanian children and the contribution of MAGIS in-between medical therapy and social integration. MAGIC, Cooperazione Italiana allo Sviluppo. Tirana, Albania (In Albanian).

22. Paradise JL, Rockette HE, Colborn DK, Bernard BS, Smith CG, et al. (1997) Otitis media in 2253 Pittsburgh-area infants: prevalence and risk factors during the first two years of life. Pediatrics 99: 318-333.

23. Williamson IG, Dunleavy J, Baine J, Robinson D (1994) The natural history of otitis media with effusion - a three-year study of the incidence and prevalence of abnormal tympanograms in four South West Hampshire infant and first schools. J Laryngol Otol 108:930-934.

24. Lous J, Fiellau-Nikolajsen M. (1981) Epidemiology of middle ear effusion and tubal dysfunction. A one-year prospective study comprising monthly tympanometry in 387 non-selected seven-year-old children. Int J Pediatr Otorhinolaryngol 3:303-317.

25. [No authors listed] (2001) Screening for otitis media with effusion: recommendation statement from the Canadian Task Force on Preventive Health Care. CMAJ 165: 1092-1093.

26. Joint Committee on Infant Hearing (2000) Year 2000 position statement: principles and guidelines for early hearing detection and intervention programs. Am J Audiol 9: 9-29.

27. Gravel JS1, Wallace IF, Ruben RJ (1995) Early otitis media and later educational risk. Acta Otolaryngol 115: 279-281.

28. van Cauwenberge P, Watelet JB, Dhooge I (1999) Uncommon and unusual complications of otitis media with effusion. Int J Pediatr Otorhinolaryngol 49 Suppl 1: S119-125.

29. Casby MW (2001) Otitis media and language development: a meta- analysis. Am J Speech Lang Pathol 10:65-80.

30. World Health Organization (WHO) (1986) Report by the Director General. Prevention of deafness and hearing impairment. Document A39/14. Geneva: WHO.

31. World Health Organization (WHO) (2004) Chronic Suppurative Otitis Media: Burden of Illness and Management Options. Geneva.

32. Smith AW, Bradley AK, Wall RA, McPherson B, Secka A, et al. (1988) Sequelae of epidemic meningococcal meningitis in Africa. Trans R Soc Trop Med Hyg 82: 312-320.

33. Shekelle P, Takata G, Chan LS, et al. (2003) Diagnosis, natural history, and late effects of otitis media with effusion. Evidence Report/Technology Assessment No. 55. AHRQ Publication No. 03 E023. Rockville, MD: Agency for Healthcare Research and Quality.

34. Shield B (2006) Evaluation of the social and economic costs of hearing impairment. A report for HEAR-IT.

27

P. [V27i; E114g] Compound Heterozygous State in Gjb2 Gene Could Be an Indicator of the Severity of Congenital Hearing Loss

Tufan T*, Erkoc MA, Yilmaz MB, Comertpay G and Alptekin D

Department of Medical Biology, University of Cukurova, Adana, Turkey

*Corresponding author: Tufan T, Department of Medical Biology, University of Cukurova, Adana, Turkey; E-mail: t.turantufan@gmail.com

Abstract

Hearing loss (HL) is the most common sensory disorder, affecting all age groups, ethnicities, and genders. Several genes responsible for hearing loss are related to ion recycling and homeostasis in the inner ear. Mutations in GJB2 gene, the gene encoding gap junction protein connexin26 (Cx26), are most common detected in patients with congenital, recessively inherited, nonsyndromic HL in humans. In order to investigate the molecular etiology of patients with congenital, recessively inherited, and nonsyndromic HL and healthy individuals as control in a family, they were included in this study. Thus, exons of GJB2 gene were amplified by polymerase chain reaction (PCR) and sequenced. In this family, V27I missense mutation and V27I + E114G compound heterozygosity were detected in the results of sequence analysis. The V27I mutation was found in patient with severe HL and healthy individuals. The V27I + E114G compound heterozygosity was detected only in deaf patients. Based on our data, V27I mutations could be considered as a polymorphism not leading to HL. Since V27I + E114G compound heterozygosity was found only in deaf patients, it could be considered as a contributor of HL severity.

Keywords: GJB2 gene; Hearing loss; Sequencing; Missense mutation

Introduction

Hearing loss is the most common congenital sensory impairment worldwide [1], which affects approximately 3% of the population [2]. In most of these cases, the inheritance pattern is autosomal recessive (75-80%), although autosomal dominant (20%), X-linked (2-5%) and mitochondrial (<1%) inheritance also occur [3]. 30% of cases of prelingual hearing loss disorders are classified as syndromic, in cases where additional physical findings lead to HL; the remainders are non-syndromic [4].

Hearing loss affects approximately 70 million people worldwide. Environmental causes, account for 50-60% of cases, can range from neonatal insults, such as prematurity, jaundice, or prenatal infection to iatrogenic causes. The genetic etiologies, account for 40-50% of cases, can be inherited as either syndromic or non-syndromic forms, or have a spectrum of inheritance patterns [2,5]. Non-syndromic deafness accounts for 60-70% of inherited hearing impairment and involves more than 100 different genes with autosomal dominant (DFNA), autosomal recessive (DNFB), X-linked (DFN), and maternal inheritance. The most common cause of non-syndromic autosomal recessive hearing loss is mutations in Cx26, a gap junction protein encoded by the GJB2gene which is located at chromosome 13 q11-12 [6]. Expression of GJB2 has been well documented in a variety of cells and tissues. In the cochlea, it is believed that GJB2 plays a critical role in the recycling of K+ by ferrying K+ away from the hair cells during auditory transduction [7].

Autosomal recessive nonsyndromic sensorineural hearing impairment (ARNSHI) comprises 80% of familial HL cases. Mutations in the GJB2, the gene encoding gap junction protein Cx26, are the largest genetic etiologic contributor to ARNSHI [7]. To date, more than 100 mutations either leading or contributing to HL have been reported in literature. The most common mutation in Europe, North America, and the Mediterranean is a deletion of 6 guanine nucleotides referred to as 35delG [2]. The V37I and V27I are other GJB2 variants, which are much discussed in literature and usually considered as a genetic risk-indicator of HL and a determinant of severity of disease [8].

It has been well documented that GJB2 mutations diverge largely among different ethnic groups. 35delG is commonly seen in Caucasians [4], although 167delT has high prevalence in the Ashkenazi Jewish population [9]. This present study was performed to determine GJB2 gene variants of a Turkish family with autosomal recessive nonsyndromic congenital HL.

Materials and Methods

Subjects and molecular genetic analysis

A familial HL patients with autosomal recessive nonsyndromic congenital HL and their healthy family members were included in this study if the following criteria were met

(1) There exist hearing-impaired siblings.

(2) There exist healthy control sibling at least one.

(3) There is no evidence of any obvious syndrome. The family with hearing loss consists of 4 deaf patients and 2 healthy persons.

Genomic DNA was extracted from peripheral blood using Qiagen DNA extraction kit (Qiagen, Hilden, Germany) and coding sequences of GJB2 gene were amplified by polymerase chain reaction (PCR) using GML Sequence Primers followed by Big-Dye Terminator 3.1 Cycle Sequencing kit (Applied Biosystems, Inc., Foster City, CA). The sequence results were analyzed using Sanger sequencing machine.

Results

A familial HL case showing autosomal recessive non-syndromic sensorineural hearing impairment was included in present study as a case report shown in (Figure 1). Their hearing losses were nonprogressive and were either congenital or prelingual in onset. Cases' disease severities are indicated in (Table 1).

Patient and Control Numbers	Genotype	Disease Severity
II:1	V27I + E114G / wt	Deaf
II:2	V27I + E114G / wt	Deaf
II:3	wt / wt	Severe
II:4	V27I / wt	Severe
II:5	V27I / wt	Healthy
II:6	V27I + E114G / wt	Deaf
I:1	V27I / wt	Healthy

Table 1: Genotype and disease severity in patients and controls.

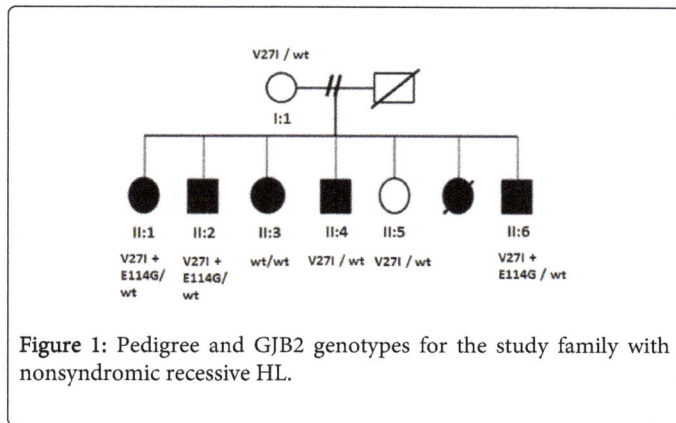

Figure 1: Pedigree and GJB2 genotypes for the study family with nonsyndromic recessive HL.

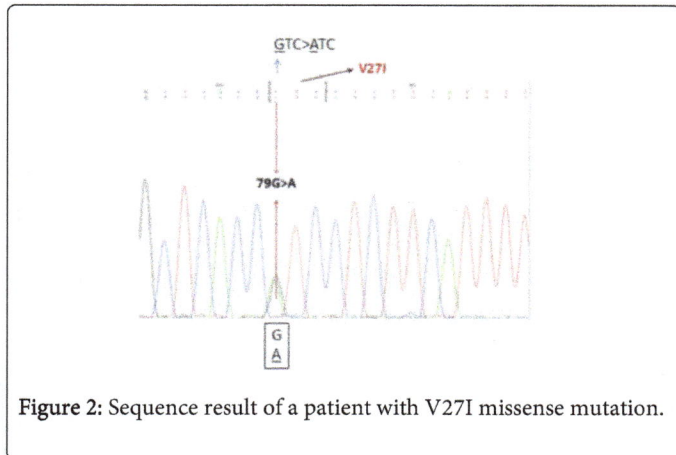

Figure 2: Sequence result of a patient with V27I missense mutation.

Results of GJB2 sequence analysis in the present study showed that V27I mutation shown in Figure 2 was found in both healthy individuals and patients with severe HL. Previous studies have indicated that V27I mutation is usually considered as a noncausative mutation when it is seen alone [10,11]. The V27I mutation was also detected in a compound heterozygous state with E114G mutation, the Glu to Gly at amino acid position 114 shown in (Figure 2), in only completely deaf patients.

In autosomal recessive single gene disorders, the allelic configurations of detected variants play a key role both in determining correct molecular diagnosis and in disease treatment [12]. V27I +E114G heterozygous state in cis markedly devastated the function of the gap junctions that have crucial role in hearing process and it has been shown that E114G mutation was always detected on the same chromosome that carries the V27I variant [13]. So the heterozygous state found in present study could be considered as contributor to disease severity (Figure 3).

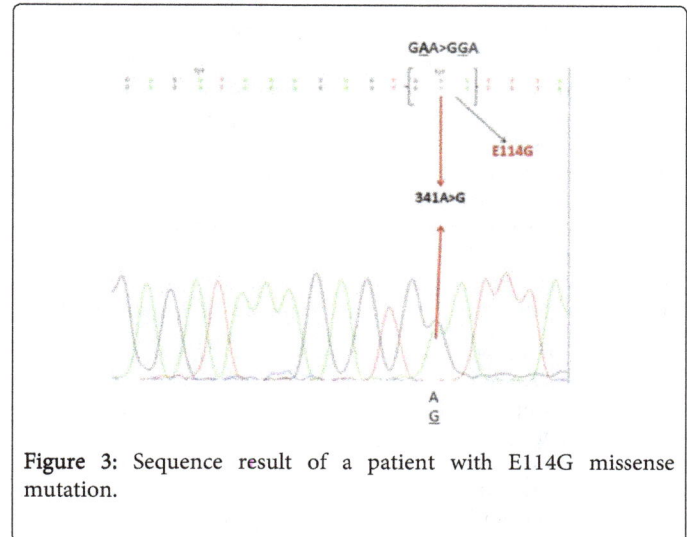

Figure 3: Sequence result of a patient with E114G missense mutation.

Discussion

To date, over 20 different genes associated with recessive deafness have been identified. GJB2 gene, which is largely expressed in the cochlea, is involved in both syndromic and nonsyndromic HL with a dominant or recessive inheritance pattern. Mutation of the GJB2 gene is the major contributor to autosomal recessive HL and, to a small percentage, autosomal dominant HL. The molecular genetic analyses of the GJB2 gene in a family that consist of both HL patients and healthy individuals showed various variants depending on the severity of the disease. As can be seen in (Figure 1) showing the molecular genetic results of the family, V27I missense mutation in both patients with mild to severe HL and healthy members was identified, although V27I+E114G compound heterozygote was detected only in deaf patients.

The V27I mutation is very often found in patients with HL and it has been considered as a polymorphism not leading to HL [10,11]. Since V27I, the sequence change of the Val to Ile at amino acid position 27, was also detected in healthy individuals in the present study, it cannot be regarded as causative mutation of HL. It might be thought as a contributor because of being located in transmembrane protein domain. The V27I mutation was also detected in a compound heterozygous state with E114G mutation, the Glu to Gly change at amino acid position 114. In autosomal recessive single gene disorders, the allelic configurations of detected variants play a key role in determining correct molecular diagnosis and in disease treatment. Depending on whether these changes are on the same (in cis) or on opposite (in trans) chromosomes, they can be considered as a causative or noncausative [12].

Previous results of in vitro functional studies on the Xenopus oocyte system demonstrated that [13]. It has been found that the V27I and E114G variants are appeared very often in both deaf probands and hearing controls and the E114G variant is always in cis with the V27I variant. Although in vitro experiments suggest a pathogenic role for the complex allele, the equal distribution of p.[V27I; E114G] in deaf probands and hearing controls makes it a less likely cause of profound congenital deafness [14] Pandya et al. suggested that when these two variants are shown together in cis-configuration, homozygous V27I +E114G or compound heterozygote with another mutation could cause hearing loss [13]. Choi et al. used in-vitro assay and population study to examine the pathogenesis of V27I and E114G variants and indicated that E114G variant is deleterious but V27I+E114G represent a nonpathogenic polymorphism and suggesting that only E114G homozygote or compound heterozygote carrying E114G type with other mutations may cause HL [15]. Also, V27I+E114G/wt genotype was found as the cause of hearing loss in a family involved in a previous study [16]. Two polymorphisms (V27I and E114G) detected in GJB2 gene were not pathogenic variants causing inherited deafness which had been described in a previous study [17]. Moreover, while p.V27I mutation is not leading to HL, V27I + R75W compound heterozygous state was reported as a disease causative mutation [18].

Based on our data, V27I missense mutation and V27I + E114G compound heterozygote detected in GJB2 gene involved in a familial HL case are nonpathogenic variants. Our study indicates that these mutations are not the main causative mutations associated with HL in this family. However, since V27I + E114G compound heterozygous state in our study was found in only deaf patients, it could be thought that these variants impair the function of gap junctions and play a role in increasing the severity of HL. This information will be valuable in considering HL cases or early diagnosis.

References

1. Mehl AL, Thomson V (2002) The colorado newborn hearing screening project, 1992–1999: On the threshold of effective population-based universal newborn hearing screening. Pediatrics 109: e7.

2. Zhong LX (2013) Non-syndromic hearing loss and high-throughput strategies to decipher its genetic heterogeneity. Journal of Otology 8: 6-24.

3. Smith RJ, Bale JF Jr, White KR (2005) Sensorineural hearing loss in children. Lancet 365: 879-890.

4. Denoyelle F, Marlin S, Weil D, Moatti L, Chauvin P, et al. (1999) Clinical features of the prevalent form of childhood deafness, DFNB, due to a connexin-26 gene defect: implications for genetic counselling. Lancet 353: 1298-1303.

5. Morton NE1 (1991) Genetic epidemiology of hearing impairment. Ann N Y Acad Sci 630: 16-31.

6. Bitner-Glindzicz M1 (2002) Hereditary deafness and phenotyping in humans. Br Med Bull 63: 73-94.

7. Kikuchi T, Kimura RS, Paul DL, Adams JC (1995) Gap junctions in the rat cochlea: immunohistochemical and ultrastructural analysis. Anat Embryol (Berl) 191: 101-118.

8. Gallant E (2013) Homozygosity for the V37I GJB2 mutation in fifteen probands with mild to moderate sensorineural hearing impairment: Further confirmation of pathogenicity and haplotype analysis in Asian populations. American Journal of Medical 161: 2148-2157.

9. Ben-Yosef T, Friedman TB (2003) The genetic bases for syndromic and nonsyndromic deafness among Jews. Trends Mol Med 9: 496-502.

10. Kelley PM, Harris DJ, Comer BC, Askew JW, Fowler T, et al. (1998) Novel mutations in the connexin 26 gene (GJB2) that cause autosomal recessive (DFNB1) hearing loss. Am J Hum Genet 62: 792-799.

11. Prasad S, Cucci RA, Green GE, Smith RJ (2000) Genetic testing for hereditary hearing loss: connexin 26 (GJB2) allele variants and two novel deafness-causing mutations (R32C and 645-648delTAGA). Hum Mutat 16: 502-508.

12. Chen N, Schrijver I (2011) Allelic discrimination of cis-trans relationships by digital polymerase chain reaction: GJB2 (p.V27I/p.E114G) and CFTR (p.R117H/5T). Genet Med 13: 1025-1031.

13. Pandya A, Arnos KS, Xia XJ, Welch KO, Blanton SH, et al. (2003) Frequency and distribution of GJB2 (connexin 26) and GJB6 (connexin 30) mutations in a large North American repository of deaf probands. Genet Med 5: 295-303.

14. Tekin M, Xia XJ, Erdenetungalag R, Cengiz FB, White TW, et al. (2010) GJB2 mutations in Mongolia: complex alleles, low frequency, and reduced fitness of the deaf. Ann Hum Genet 74: 155-164.

15. Choi SY, Lee KY, Kim HJ, Kim HK, Chang Q, et al. (2011) Functional evaluation of GJB2 variants in nonsyndromic hearing loss. Mol Med 17: 550- 556.

16. Davarnia B, Babanejad M, Fattahi Z, Nikzat N, Bazazzadegan N, et al. (2012) Spectrum of GJB2 (Cx26) gene mutations in Iranian Azeri patients with nonsyndromic autosomal recessive hearing loss. Int J Pediatr Otorhinolaryngol 76: 268-271.

17. Han SH, Park HJ, Kang EJ, Ryu JS, Lee A, et al. (2008) Carrier frequency of GJB2 (connexin-26) mutations causing inherited deafness in the Korean population. J Hum Genet 53: 1022-1028.

18. Dalamón V, Béhèran A, Diamante F, Pallares N, Diamante V, et al. (2005) Prevalence of GJB2 mutations and the del (GJB6-D13S1830) in Argentinean non-syndromic deaf patients. Hear Res 207: 43-49.

28

Risk of Developing Sudden Sensorineural Hearing Loss in Patients with Acute Otitis Media

Mehmet Akdag*, Ismail Onder Uysal, Salih Bakir, Fazıl Emre Ozkurt, Suphi Muderris, Ediz Yorgancılar and Ismail Topcu
Department of Otolaryngology, Faculty of Medicine, Dicle University, Turkey

Abstract

Objective: The aim of the study was to determine the etiology of Sudden Sensorineural Hearing Loss (SSHL) and to call attention to Acute Otitis Media (AOM) with SSHL.

Study Design and Setting: We conducted a retrospective, multicenter analysis of SSHL. We were used spearman correlation matrix test for correlations between all variables. One hundred twelve patients with SSHL were evaluated.

Results: A total of 112 patients (62 males, 50 females) ranging in age from 17 to 70 years (average male 40.21 ± 14.04, average female 40.26 ± 11.16) were included. Fourteen of these had AOM. The majority of patients had moderate hearing loss. Flat and down-sloping types of audiogram were also observed ($P<0.05$). There was a positive relationship between SSHL and AOM, SOM, cardiac pathology as hypertension. No significance was established in terms of age or sex ($p>0.05$). Otoscopic examination was consistent with AOM. SSHL occurred as mixed-type hearing loss. Tympanometry was observed as type A.

Conclusion: In the treatment and follow-up periods, AOM patients should be checked and treated for the presence (if any) of early hearing loss.

Keywords: Acute otitis media; Sudden sensorineural hearing loss; Hearing loss; Sensorineural hearing loss; Otitis media; Pure-tone audiogram; Tympanometry

Introduction

Acute Otitis Media (AOM) is one of the most common ear diseases. It is an inflammation within the middle ear cleft, located behind an intact tympanic membrane. Patients with AOM may exhibit symptoms and signs specific to ear disease, including pain, fever, bulging tympanic membrane, middle ear effusion, otorrhea and hearing loss [1]. Uncommon symptoms and signs of AOM include hearing loss, tinnitus, vertigo, and nystagmus. Although both diagnosis and treatment of AOM have improved enormously, serious complications are still common albeit less frequent now than in the past. However, non-life-threatening complications, such as hearing loss, frequently trouble many patients and have led to controversy regarding the importance and management of such complications [2].

Hearing loss may occur in the form of Sudden Sensorineural Hearing Loss (SSHL). SSHL is defined as a decrease in hearing greater than 30 dB over at least three contiguous frequencies, occurring in a total of 72 h or less. The incidence is equal in men and women, while individuals of all ages can be affected; however, the peak incidence is in the fourth or fifth decades [3].

Features associated with disorders underlying hearing loss need to be check-listed. However, the etiopathogenesis of SSHL in AOM is still controversial. Temporary sensorineural hearing impairment is generally attributed to the effect of increased tension and stiffness of the Round Window (RW). Aggressive middle ear infections may result in the release of infection, involving the round or oval windows [4]. Today, widespread use of antimicrobial agents in the management of Otitis Media (OM) has significantly reduced the incidence of hearing loss or complications such as labyrinthitis [5,6]. SSHL may occur as labyrinthitis and may result from various diseases, but is mostly idiopathic.

The main problem still consists of understanding both the etiopathogenesis and etiology of SSHL. The diagnosis and treatment of SSHL is considered a medical emergency. Delay in the diagnosis and treatment of SSHL may result in temporary or permanent sensorial hearing loss. SSHL can be caused by AOM or one of its complications or sequelae.

This study focused, in particular, on AOM cases with SSHL, since the diagnosis of SSHL in AOM cases has been neglected.

Materials and Methods

The study was approved by the Dicle university medical ethics committee (11.06.2012/592) and was carried out in accordance with the Declaration of Helsinki as amended in 2008. We reviewed the medical records of 112 patients between these dates that 1996-1998 and 2010-2012 with SSHL treated in the Department of Otorhinolaryngology-Head and Neck Surgery in the medical hospitals at Dicle and Cumhuriyet universities and the private Akademi ENT surgery center in Turkey. We were observed SSHL that will be appear after AOM frequently in first ten days most of our medical records.

We excluded subjects with a history of acoustic trauma, head trauma, barotrauma, ototoxic drug use or otological surgery, and those with any other otological diseases such as otosclerosis, Meniere's disease or suppurative labyrinthitis, since all of these may involve

*Corresponding author: Mehmet Akdag, Department of Otolaryngology, Faculty of Medicine, Dicle University, 21280 Diyarbakir, Turkey; E-mail: drmehmetakdag@hotmail.com

changes in the inner ear. After reviewing the medical records of these patients retrospectively, 112 cases were identified and medical records of patients who had undergone evaluation for AOM with SSHL were selected then they were reevaluated for their last visit during the study period (62 male; 55.4%, 50 females; 44.6%). Of these, 14 patients had AOM, 18 had secretory otitis media, 16 had upper respiratory diseases, 14 had systemic disease and 50 were idiopathic.

Following ear, nose and throat examinations, all patients underwent pure-tone audiogram, tympanometry, Speech Recognition Threshold (SRT), Word Recognition Score (WRS), biochemical and microbiological tests.

Pure tone audiometry was performed on all participants in sound-proofed booths for objective hearing assessment following the guidelines of the American Speech-Language-Hearing Association (ASHA) [7]. Pure-tone air-conduction thresholds were determined for each ear at 500, 1,000, 2,000, 3,000, 4,000, 6,000 and 8,000 Hz. Bone-conduction thresholds were measured at two frequencies at 500, 1000,2,000, and 4,000 Hz. The presence of hearing loss was defined as a Pure-Tone Average (PTA) of thresholds at 500, 1,000, 2,000 and 4,000 Hz greater than 15 dB HL (decibel hearing level). Pure-Tone Average (PTA) was calculated at the hearing thresholds 0.5, 1.0, 2.0, and 4.0 kHz (arithmetic mean). Pure-tone and speech audiometry were performed using a diagnostic audiometer (Madsen OB 822 Clinical Audiometer). A TDH-39 standard headset was used for air conduction thresholds and speech tests. Measurements were made using an ascending-descending technique, at 5-dB steps at all frequencies. If a patient made two or more responses to a set of three stimuli, he/she was deemed to have heard the sound. We were differentiated between AOM and SOM by otoscopic examination and tympanometric test. Tympanometric measurements were performed using a TDH-39 headset and middle ear analyzer (Clinical Middle Analyzer AZ 26, Interacoustic). Severity of SSHL was classified as slight, 16-25; mild, 26-40; moderate, 41-55; moderately severe, 56-70; severe, 71-90; or profound, over 90 dB HL. The duration, side (unilateral or bilateral), severity, and type of auditory impairment were all recorded. Audiometry was performed at the initial clinic visit and was then repeated after the treatment regimen.

We selected temporal bone tomography or magnetic resonance imaging for cases with unilateral AOM or that remained resistant to treatment.

Statistical Analysis

Statistical analyses were carried out using SPSS 15.0 (SPSS. Inc. Chicago, IL, USA) for Windows. All of the data in this study was evaluated descriptive statistics analyses as mean ± Standard Deviation (SD). We were used spearman correlation matrix test. This test is symmetric and gives the correlations between all variables. We analyses between SSHL and acute otitis media, serous otitis media, cervical pathology, hypertension, diabetes mellitus, gentel, age and idiopatic.

Results

One hundred twelve patients, ranging in age from 17 to 70 years (male average 40.21 ± 14.04, female average 40.26 ± 11.16) were enrolled. Sixty-two (55.4%) right and 50 (44.6%) left ears were affected. SSHL distribution was statistically equal between the genders. Peak incidence was in the fourth decade. No significance was observed in terms of age or sex (p>0.05). Details obtained during the diagnosis of patients are shown in Figure 1.

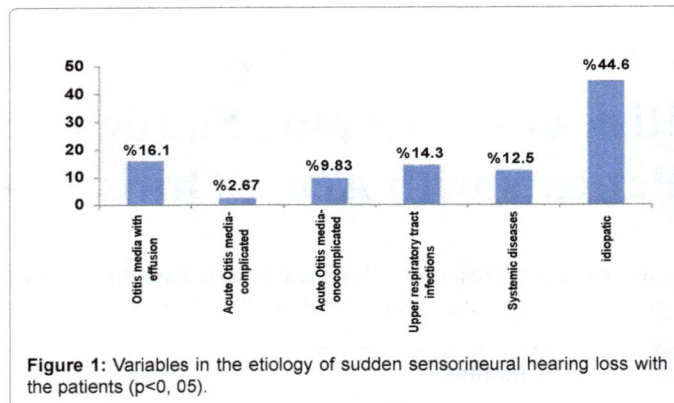

Figure 1: Variables in the etiology of sudden sensorineural hearing loss with the patients (p<0, 05).

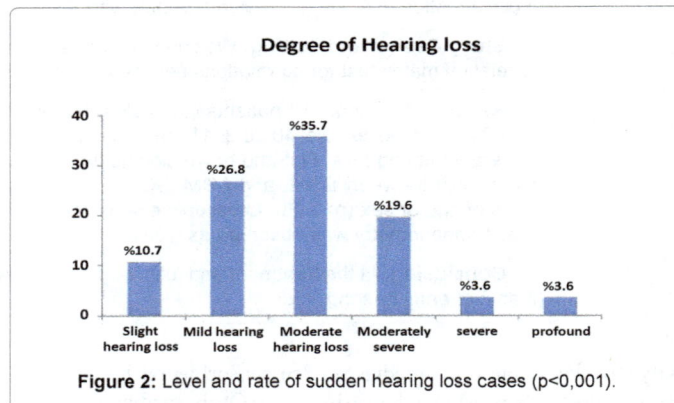

Figure 2: Level and rate of sudden hearing loss cases (p<0,001).

Patients with concurrent AOM and mixed hearing loss were selected. Fourteen patients with AOM were identified. Eight presented with hearing loss alone and six experienced dizziness or tinnitus together with hearing loss. Otoscopy revealed a thickened, hyperemic or bulging tympanic membrane in all the patients, while none exhibited nystagmus, signs of meningeal irritation or neurological deficits. All 14 patients had audiometrically confirmed, SNHL and decreased SRT and WRS at initial presentation, ranging from slight hearing impairment to profound hearing loss (Figure 2). Audiograms revealed mixed hearing loss in all patients. Hearing loss was at a minimum of three consecutive frequencies or more (the most common being 500- 1000- 2000 Hz) for SSHL. Audiometric tests were performed, and sensorineural hearing loss was identified as mixed-type hearing loss. In terms of the audiometric configuration of SSHL, the majority of audiogram shapes were flat (7 cases, 50%), followed by downsloping (4 cases, 28.5%), upsloping (1 case, 7.1%), cookie-bite (1 case, 7.1%) and inverse cookie-bite (1 case, 7.1%). PTA was 43.2 dB in flat shape, 41.0 dB in downsloping, 35.9 dB in upsloping, 33.5 dB in cookie-bite and 32.9 dB in inverse cookie-bite. Tympanometry was type A.

We were analyses between SSHL and acute otitis media, serous otitis media, cervical pathology, hypertension, diabetes mellitus, gentel, age and idiopatic. From this analyses; SSHL were positively correlated with acute otitis media, serous otitis media, cervical pathology, hypertension, and diabetes mellitus.

Tympanocentesis was performed in two patients due to a bulging tympanic membrane accompanied by severe pain and bullous myringitis.

Virological and microbiological tests for herpes virus,

cytomegalovirus (CMV IgM and IgG), Epstein-Barr virus (EBV IgM and IgG), infection and syphilis (FTA-ABS) were negative in all patients. At complete blood count, five patients exhibited a slight elevation in white blood cell count. Other laboratory values did not reveal the specific cause of SSHL in any patient.

If the symptoms of tinnitus and hearing loss did not resolve after oral or parenteral antibiotic, antivirals, topical steroids, systemic steroid treatment or tympanocentesis then we performed CT or MRI. Temporal CT identified three patients with a minimal decrease in aeration in the mastoid and middle ear cavities (Figure 5). Temporal MRI identified two patients with a minimal enhancement in the inner ear cavities (Figure 4). However, no specific pathology was detected at CT or MRI for patients AOM with SSHL. Eleven of the 14 patients with AOM responded to medical treatment. However, hearing loss and tinnitus persisted in the other three, representing 12.5% of all patients; 9.82% of these were temporary, while 2.67% represented permanent hearing loss.

Apart from AOM, there are various other etiologies leading to SSHL (Figure 1). There was a positive relationship between SSHL and AOM, SOM, cardiac pathology as hypertension (Table 1). Eighteen patients

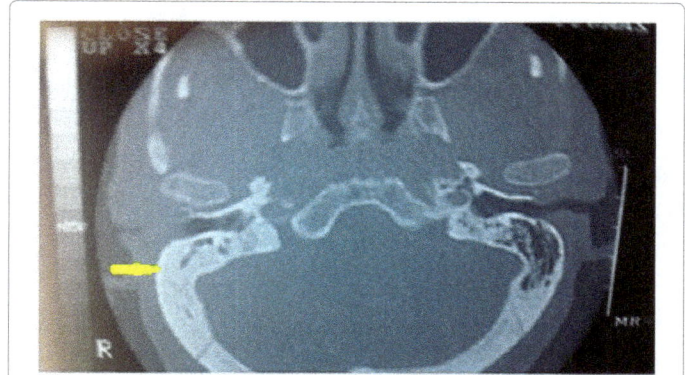

Figure 5: There is decrease aeration in the right mastoid area one of our patients (arrow).

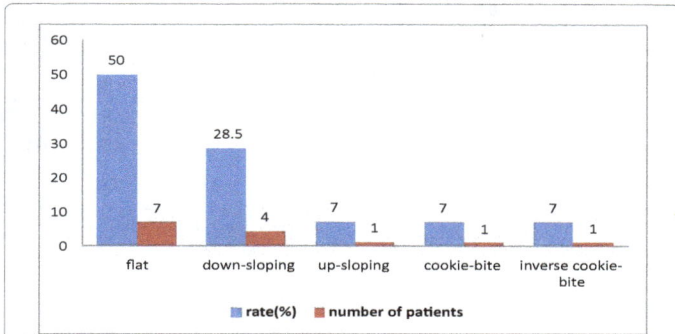

Figure 3: Rate and mean distribution and shape of audiogram in patients with sudden hearing loss.

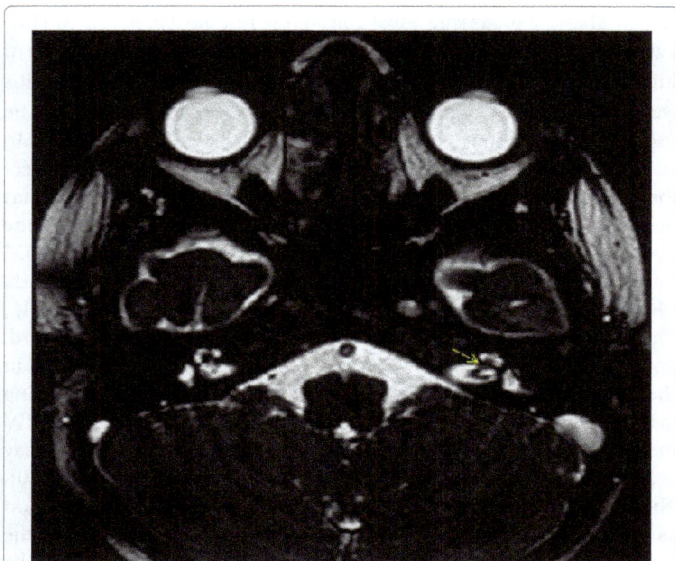

Figure 4: There is minimal enhancement at the left cochlear nerve one of our patients (arrow).

had serous otitis media. Such patients are characterized by mixed-type hearing loss at audiometry and by type B at tympanometry. Fourteen patients had systemic etiologies. The foramina of the cervical vertebrae were narrow in six of these. Of the remaining eight patients, three had complications of diabetes and five had cardiovascular diseases. The characteristics of the cardiac population wasn't different other patients. Another group of 16 patients presented with upper respiratory diseases. In this group, no hyperemia or other symptoms of AOM were observed in the tympanic membrane, and tympanometry showed type A. However, only the sensorineural type was identified in audiograms, compatible with upper respiratory diseases. The remaining 50 patients, who only had hearing loss and tinnitus with normal otoscopy and showed no evidence of any systemic disease, were deemed idiopathic.

Discussion

There are different theories have attempted to explain the pathogenesis of SSHL. These infectious, traumatic, neoplastic, autoimmune, toxic, circulatory, neurological and metabolic [8]. Endothelial function and cardiovascular factors is current cause of SSHL and speciality idiopathic sudden hearing loss [9].

This study concentrated on AOM and SSHL. AOM with accompanying SSHL has rarely been reported over the last few decades, and the literature on the subject is insufficient. AOM may be involved in the unknown etiologies of hearing loss and tinnitus. The aim of the study was to call physicians' attention to AOM with SSHL. Audiograms have been compared and discussed on the basis of their shapes in many previous studies. Our statistical analysis revealed that the most common audiogram shape was flat, followed by downsloping (Figure 3). Cookie-bite, upsloping and inverse cookie-bite shapes was relatively uncommon. There was no improvement in subjects with tinnitus and a downsloping audiogram. Tinnitus at presentation with SHL has been identified as a negative prognostic indicator [10].

Additionally, imaging using CT and MRI was performed in the three patients resistant to therapy and those with unilateral AOM. We did not arrange imaging for all patients, since CT scanning has potential significant adverse events, including radiation exposure and side-effects of intravenous contrast, while offering no useful information that would improve initial management except in the event of a history of trauma, or chronic ear disease. CT can be used in situations where MRI is not possible, such as patients with pacemakers or severe claustrophobia, or even due to financial constraints [11]. CT or MRI revealed no anomalies in our patients' middle or inner ear pathways. A decrease in mastoid

			AOM	SOM	UR TI	DM	H pr	Servical path	Idiopatic	Gentel	Age	control
Spearman rho	AOM	Correlation coefficient	1,000	-,165	-,154	-,063	-,063	-,090	-,352 (**)	-,189	-,053	.
		Sig. (2-tailed)	.	,081	,104	,511	,511	,346	,000	,045	,581	.
		N	112	112	112	112	112	112	112	112	112	112
	SOM	Correlation coefficient	-,165	1,000	,238 (*)	,078	,073	,328 (**)	-,359 (**)	-,470 (**)	,365 (**)	.
		Sig. (2-tailed)	,081	.	,011	,414	,447	,000	,000	,000	,000	.
		N	112	112	112	112	112	112	112	112	112	112
	UR TI	Correlation coefficient	-,154	,238 (*)	1,000	,406 (**)	-,068	,243 (**)	-,380 (**)	-,336 (**)	,099	.
		Sig. (2-tailed)	,104	,011	.	,000	,478	,010	,000	,000	,298	.
		N	112	112	112	112	112	112	112	112	112	112
	DM	Correlation coefficient	-,063	,078	,406 (**)	1,000	-,028	-,039	-,154	,044	,037	.
		Sig. (2-tailed)	,511	,414	,000	.	,773	,679	,104	,648	,700	.
		N	112	112	112	112	112	112	112	112	112	112
	H pr	Correlation coefficient	-,063	-,073	-,068	-,028	1,000	-,039	-,154	,154	-,233 (*)	.
		Sig. (2-tailed)	,511	,447	,478	,773	.	,679	,104	,104	,013	.
		N	112	112	112	112	112	112	112	112	112	112
	Servical path	Correlation coefficient	-,090	,328 (**)	,243 (**)	-,039	-,039	1,000	-,221 (*)	-,256 (*)	,083	.
		Sig. (2-tailed)	,346	,000	,010	,679	,679	.	,019	,007	,385	.
		N	112	112	112	112	112	112	112	112	112	112
	Idiopatic	Correlation coefficient	-,352 (**)	-,359 (**)	-,380 (**)	-,154	-,154	-,221 (*)	1,000	,328 (**)	-,031	.
		Sig. (2-tailed)	,000	,000	,000	,104	,104	,019	.	,000	,747	.
		N	112	112	112	112	112	112	112	112	112	112
	Gentel	Correlation coefficient	-,189 (*)	-,470 (**)	-,336 (**)	,044	,154	-,256 (**)	,328 (**)	1,000	-,321 (**)	.
		Sig. (2-tailed)	,045	,000	,000	,648	,104	,007	,000	.	,001	.
		N	112	112	112	112	112	112	112	112	112	112
	Age	Correlation coefficient	-,053	,365 (**)	,009	,037	-,233 (*)	,083	-,031	-,321 (**)	1,000	.
		Sig. (2-tailed)	,581	,000	,298	,700	,013	,385	,747	,001	.	.
		N	112	112	112	112	112	112	112	112	112	112
	control	Correlation coefficient	.	.	.	.	.	.	.	.	.	.
		Sig. (2-tailed)	.	.	.	.	.	.	.	.	.	.
		N	112	112	112	112	112	112	112	112	112	112

** Correlation is significant at the 0.01 level (2-tailed).
* Correlation is significant at the 0.05 level (2-tailed).

Table 1: The data of used in sperman correlation test.

aeration at CT may suggest labyrinthitis, from serous to purulent. There was association between lack of aeration and permanent sensorineural hearing loss [12]. However, this result is not statistically reliable due to the small sample sizes involved. MRI is not used in routine situations except in the case of retrocochlear pathology unresponsive to medical therapy. Thickening of the nerve localization was determined in only two patients. In addition, there was no apparent evidence in serological tests, except for systemic disease such as diabetes mellitus. In our study, the results of audiological-4 examinations other than diagnostic tests were consistent with the criteria set out in Robert et al. guidelines recently announced as a result of numerous studies [13].

Tympanogenic labyrinthitis or SHL is a rare intratemporal complication of otitis media. The decline in its incidence is partly due to earlier diagnosis, the development of better antibiotics, and greater awareness of the complications of otitis media among medical staff [14]. The etiopathogenesis of SSHL in AOM is still controversial. Viral infection is important in the pathogenesis of AOM, although it may be followed by bacterial colonization. AOM should therefore be primarily considered a bacterial infection. Many studies, using tympanocentesis, have identified Streptococcus pneumonia (up to 40%), Haemophilus influenzae (25-30%) and Moraxella catarrhalis

(10-20%) as the organisms most commonly responsible for AOM [14]. Labyrinth irritation is induced by bacterial toxins or other mediators of inflammation [4]. Until recently, diagnosis of tympanogenic labyrentitis was made on clinical grounds. The presence of labyrinthitis may be suggested only if bone conduction loss co-exists with otitis media. In such a case, the toxins have presumably penetrated the RW to affect the cochlea, resulting in hearing loss. Acute purulent otitis media has been thought to cause temporary and permanent SSHL in the same way as chronic otitis media [15-18]. Engel et al. [17] investigated AOM in which streptolysin D damaged RW permeability, leading to SSHL. Morgolis and Nelson [19] published a case report of AOM with SSHL. The RW is probably more important than the oval window in this regard. The RW membrane is often thin and more susceptible to invasion in the nonchronically infected ear [19]. Additionally, the risk to hearing loss may be greater in acute than in chronic infection, since the RW membrane is demonstrably thicker in the latter condition, and pus may accumulate under pressure when the tympanic membrane is intact [20]. The RW is permeable to many biological substances and may function as a point of entry for harmful materials from the middle ear into the inner ear, leading to pathological changes in the latter [21,22]. The middle ears in the rat and humans exhibit numerous similar structural characteristics. It has recently been established that the reaction of the rat middle ear to S. pneumonia bears a close resemblance to that of the human middle ear [23]. On the basis of animal experiments, it may be suggested that RW response and penetrability to middle ear inflammatory conditions can vary according to the different stages of AOM [24].

Paparella et al. [25-27] indicated that proinflammatory molecules and mediators, along with bacteria and bacterial components, can pass through the RW into the inner ear and cause structural damage and hearing loss. Loss of outer hair cells at the base of the cochlea has been noted in otitis media. Accordingly, the infectious and inflammatory processes that occur in the middle ear, such as AOM, may result in cochlear or vestibular symptoms such as hearing loss or vertigo. Song et al. [28] described several patients with asymmetric SNHL and decreased SRS secondary to AOM.

In our study, we investigated the otoscopic and clinical characteristics of AOM in patients diagnosed with SSHL. The fact that the literature is compatible with our study may confirm the association between AOM and SSHL. We determined a 2.67% incidence of permanent SSHL in complicated AOM.Our scan of the literature revealed one study of the adult rate of SSHL with AOM. Swart [29] reported an incidence of SSHL with AOM of 8%. It was therefore impossible to perform a comparative discussion of the rate of SSHL with AOM, although, based on circumstantial evidence, both transient and permanent SHL can result from AOM. Margolis et al. [30] reported SHL that was more pronounced at higher frequencies (4,000 to 8,000 Hz) in two adults with documented purulent middle ear effusions. They also noted that children who have recovered from otitis media have significantly poorer hearing in the extended high-frequency range compared to children without significant histories of otitis media. Although our diagnostics from those of Morgolis, we identified four adult patients whose higher frequency hearing (down-sloping) loss was resistant to therapy in AOM. One developed permanent tinnitus. The remaining three patients recovered fully at all frequencies in the auditory pathway. Also Chul Ho et al. [4] also reported a case of tympanogenic labyrinthitis complicated by AOM.

The limitation of our study is that it is retrospective. There was few data and clinical trials in the world. In agreement with the literature, this study revealed that follow-up is essential for patients with AOM since they are likely to develop sudden hearing loss.

Conclusion

It is important to remember that SSHL can also develop in AOM cases. Following diagnosis, such patients should be examined audiometrically and treated promptly for the presence of early hearing loss, if identified.We think the further, more detailed studies on the subject are now required.

References

1. Richard A (1993) Acute otitis media and otitis media with effusion. In: Cummings CW (Edr.) Otolaryngology-Head & Neck surgery. (2nd Edn.), Mosby-Year Book Missour, p: 2808-2886.

2. Margaret A (1993) Otitis media with Effusion. In: Byron J. Bailey (Edr.) Head and Neck Surgery-Otolaryngology Kenna B. Lippincott company, Philadelphia, p: 1592.

3. Shikowitz MJ (1991) Sudden sensorineural hearing loss. Med Clin North Am 75: 1239-1250.

4. Jang CH, Park SY, Wang PC (2005) A case of tympanogenic labyrinthitis complicated by acute otitis media. Yonsei Med J 46: 161-165.

5. Rappaport JM, Bhatt SM, Burkard RF, Merchant SN, Nadol JB Jr (1999) Prevention of hearing loss in experimental pneumococcal meningitis by administration of dexamethasone and ketorolac. J Infect Dis 179: 264-268.

6. Morizono T, Giebink GS, Paparella MM, Sikora MA, Shea D (1985) Sensorineural hearing loss in experimental purulent otitis media due to Streptococcus pneumoniae. Arch Otolaryngol 111: 794-798.

7. American Speech–Language–Hearing Association (2005) Guidelines for manual pure-tone threshold audiometry.

8. Stew BT, Fishpool SJ, Williams H (2012) Sudden sensorineural hearing loss. Br J Hosp Med (Lond) 73: 86-89.

9. Ciccone MM, Cortese F, Pinto M, Di Teo C, Fornarelli F, et al. (2012) Endothelial function and cardiovascular risk in patients with idiopathic sudden sensorineural hearing loss. Atherosclerosis 225: 511-516.

10. Kuhn M, Heman-Ackah SE, Shaikh JA, Roehm PC (2011) Sudden sensorineural hearing loss: a review of diagnosis, treatment, and prognosis. Trends Amplif 15: 91-105.

11. American College of Radiology (ACR). Expert Panel on Neurologic Imaging: Turski PA, Wippold FJ II, Cornelius RS, Brunberg JA, Davis PC et al. (1996) ACR appropriateness criteria, vertigo and hearing loss (last review date: 2008).

12. Robert J Stachler, Sujana S Chandrasekhar, Sanford M Archer, Richard M Rosenfeld, Seth R Schwartz, et al. (2012) Otolaryngology- Head and Neck Surgery 146(1S) S1– S35.

13. Tos M, Stangerup SE (1985) Secretory otitis and pneumatization of the mastoid process: sexual differences in the size of mastoid cell system. Am J Otolaryngol 6: 199-205.

14. Schuknecht HF (1993) Infections: labyrinthitis. In: Pathology of the ear. Lea & Febiger, Pennsylvania, p: 211-216.

15. Philip D Yates (2004) Otitis Media Current Diagnosis & Treatment in Otolaryngology. Head & Neck Surgery: 695.

16. Cureoglu S, Schachern PA, Paparella MM, Lindgren BR (2004) Cochlear changes in chronic otitis media. Laryngoscope 114: 622-626.

17. Engel F, Blatz R, Kellner J, Palmer M, Weller U, et al. (1995) Breakdown of the round window membrane permeability barrier evoked by streptolysin O: possible etiologic role in development of sensorineural hearing loss in acute otitis media. Infect Immun 63: 1305-1310.

18. Mokhtar Bassiouni, Michael M Paparella (1984) Labyrinthitis. Volume II: Otology and Neuro-Otology Section 3: Diseases of the Ear Part 4: Inner Ear Chapter 42: 2.

19. Margolis RH, Nelson DA (1993) Acute otitis media with transient sensorineural hearing loss. A case study. Arch Otolaryngol Head Neck Surg 119: 682-686.

20. Ludman H (1987) Complications of suppurative otitis media In: Kerr AG (Edr.) Scott- Brown's Otolaryngology. (5th Edn.), Butterworths, London, P: 264-291.

21. Carpenter AM, Muchow D, Goycoolea MV (1989) Ultrastructural studies of the human round window membrane. Arch Otolaryngol Head Neck Surg 115: 585-590.

22. Nagahara K, Yoza T, Naito Y, Ogino F (1985) Oxygenation through the round window membrane and the inner ear function. Auris Nasus Larynx 12 Suppl 1: S120-122.

23. Hermansson A, Emgård P, Prellner K, Hellström S (1988) A rat model for pneumococcal otitis media. Am J Otolaryngol 9: 97-101.

24. Ikeda K, Sakagami M, Morizono T, Juhn SK (1990) Permeability of the round window membrane to middle-sized molecules in purulent otitis media. Arch Otolaryngol Head Neck Surg 116: 57-60.

25. Huang M, Dulon D, Schacht J (1990) Outer hair cells as potential targets of inflammatory mediators. Ann Otol Rhinol Laryngol Suppl 148: 35-38.

26. Schachern PA, Paparella MM, Hybertson R, Sano S, Duvall AJ 3rd (1992) Bacterial tympanogenic labyrinthitis, meningitis, and sensorineural damage. Arch Otolaryngol Head Neck Surg 118: 53-57.

27. Schachern PA, Paparella MM, Goycoolea M, Goldberg B, Schlievert P (1981) The round window membrane following application of staphylococcal exotoxin: an electron microscopic study. Laryngoscope 91: 2007-2017.

28. Song JE, Sapthavee A, Cager GR, Saadia-Redleaf MI (2012) Pseudo-sudden deafness. Ann Otol Rhinol Laryngol 121: 96-99.

29. Swart SM, Lemmer R, Parbhoo JN, Prescott CA (1995) A survey of ear and hearing disorders amongst a representative sample of grade 1 schoolchildren in Swaziland. Int J Pediatr Otorhinolaryngol 32: 23-34.

30. Margolis RH, Saly GL, Hunter LL (2000) High-frequency hearing loss and wideband middle ear impedance in children with otitis media histories. Ear Hear 21: 206-211.

29

Role of CT and MRI in the Follow-Up of Operated Middle Ear Cholesteatoma

Myriam Jrad*, Farouk Graiess, Selma Behi, Rym Bachraoui, Ghazi Besbes and Habiba Mizouni

Department of Radiology, La Rabta Hospital, Jabberi 1017, Tunis, Tunisia

*Corresponding author: Myriam Jrad, MD, Clinical Chief, Departement of Radiology, La Rabta Hospital, Jabberi 1017, Tunis, Tunisia; E-mail: myriamjrad@gmail.com

Abstract

Background: Recurrence is the main risk that may occur during the follow-up of operated middle ear cholesteatoma. Imaging plays an important role in its diagnosis, leading to avoid surgical second look when it is not mandatory. The aim of our study was to evaluate postoperative CT and MRI in patients who had undergone middle ear cholesteatoma surgery.

Methods: Retrospective study from June 2010 to June 2015 including operated patients for middle ear cholesteatoma whom follow-up was made in the ENT department of Rabta hospital and who had postoperative CT and/or MRI in the imaging department. Comparison of radiological and second look surgical findings was made with analysis of sensitivity, specificity, PNV, PPV for each type of imaging exam.

Results: Forty ears included (36 patients, median age=38. 5, sex-ratio=1.1). Thirty four ears had CT showing well aerated middle ear cleft (n=1), total opacification (n=7), partial soft-tissue opacity with convex margins (n=11), pearl-shaped lesion (n=7) and concave margins opacity (n=8). CT was not able to further characterize these opacities (specificity 20%) but it was efficient in the evaluation of ossicular and bony walls lysis. Twenty five ears had MRI showing recurrent cholesteatoma (n=15), scar tissue (n=8) and aerated postoperative cavity with alteration of the labyrinth T2 signal (n=2). MRI specificity was about 25%. 100% PNV allowed excluding recurrence when MRI was showing no soft tissue mass. PPV of diffusion weighted imaging (DWI) and delayed post contrast T1 weighted imaging was respectively 83.3% and 71.4%. A hypersignal on DWI and no contrast uptake were highly in favor of cholesteatoma.

Conclusion: CT is insufficient for the diagnosis of recurrent cholesteatoma. MRI contribution is hindered by false negatives due to too small lesions to be detected.

Keywords: CT scan; MRI; Cholesteatoma; Middle ear; Tympanoplasty

Abbreviations: CT scan: Computed Tomography Scan, MRI: Magnetic Resonance Imaging

Introduction

Middle ear cholesteatoma is defined by the presence, in the tympanic cavity, of keratizing squamous epithelium [1]. It isn't a neoplasic tumor despite its destructive properties [2]. It can be removed using two techniques depending on the size of the cholesteatoma and the damage done to the ossicular bones, the eardrum and the posterior wall of the ear canal [3]. The closed technique, opposed to the open technique, is usually preferred. Post-operative surveillance is based on the CT scan, which used to be the gold standard in the detection of recurrent cholesteatoma [4] and the MRI showing better results due to different imaging sequences.

The purpose of our study is to illustrate the imaging findings in the follow-up of operated middle ear cholesteatoma and to evaluate their performance is detecting recurrent cholesteatoma.

Material and Methods

We conducted a retrospective study of the charts of 36 patients (40 ears) who had undergone a surgery for middle ear cholesteatoma in the Departement of Otolaryngology of Rabta hospital, between June 2010 and 2015 and who had a postoperative CT and/or MRI in the Imaging department.

CT scan of the temporal bone was performed for almost all patients. The protocol consisted on a spiral acquisition with a slice plan parallel to the lateral semicircular canal with multiplanar reconstruction in coronal and sagital plans and a slice thickness of 0.6 mm. The injection of X-ray contrast medium was used only in cases when infectious or thrombo-embolic complications were suspected. The MRI was conducted with axial and coronal views on T1, T2 weighted, echo-planar diffusion-weighted (when available on the machine) and contrast enhanced images. We compared the radiological findings with those of the second look surgery to evaluate the performance of each type of imaging exam.

Results

The number of patients reviewed in this study was 36 including 19 males (53%) and 17 females (47%), aged from 16 to 70 years (mean 38.5).

Clinical findings

Four patients (11%) had cholesteatoma in both ears, while 22 (61%) had their left ear operated and 10 (28%) had the right ear operated. For the initial surgery, 17 ears had a closed technique, 10 had an open technique and for the rest of the patients the surgical findings were missing. These were patients who didn't undergo surgery in our hospital.

The post-operative symptoms were otorrhea in 20 ears, worsening of hearing loss in 5 ears, vertigo in 5 years and otalgia in 5 ears. Twenty patients only noted the fact that they didn't get any better. The recurrence of cholesteatoma was certain for seven ears after the otoscopic examination.

Radiologic findings

CT scan

For the 40 operated ears, 34 had a post-operative CT scan showing a well-aerated cleft (n=1) (Figure 1), total opacification (n=7) (Figure 2), partial soft-tissue opacity with convex margins (n=11) (Figure 3), pearl-shaped lesion (n=7) (Figure 4) and concave margins opacity (n=8) (Figure 5). Newly appeared ossicular erosion, when comparing to the initial surgical findings concerned the incus bone (n=10), the malleus (n=6) and the stapes (n=5). In most case the erosion consisted in a total loss of the bone. Erosion of the middle ear cleft walls was observed most frequently in the outer attic wall (n=30), this erosion didn't match the initial surgery findings for 4 ears. The other walls were damaged in 5 cases concerning the tegmen tympani and also in 5 cases concerning the other walls of the middle ear cleft. CT scan showed also destruction of facial nerve canal (n=7), erosion of the lateral SCC (n=2), erosion of the upper SCC (n=1), labyrinthitis (n=1) and mastoiditis (n=1).

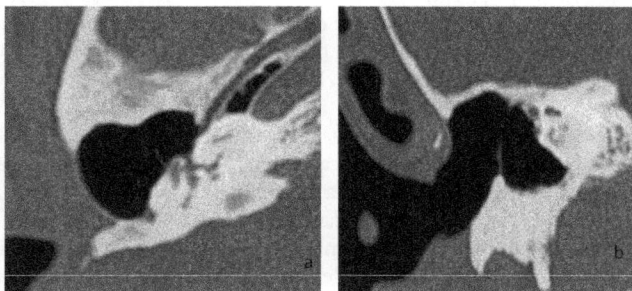

Figure 1: Axial (a) and coronal (b) computed tomography of the right temporal bone showing a well-aerated cleft (arrow).

MRI

Among the 40 ears included in this study, 25 had an MRI of the temporal bone. Nineteen of those had already a post-operative CT scan. In 15 cases, the MRI concluded to a recurrent cholesteatoma (Figure 6). On standard T1-weighted sequence, 12 (80%) had an intermediate signal intensity when compared with the brain gray matter, two (13.3%) had hypointense signal intensity and one (6.7%) had hyperintense signal intensity.

On standard T2-weighted sequence, 12 (80%) had a hyperintense signal intensity and three (20%) had intermediate signal intensity. Late

post-gadolinium T1-weighted sequence was performed for 14 ears and there were no enhancement in all cases. The DWI was performed for eleven ears showing a marked hyperintense signal in 7 cases and it was not specific in the others cases. In 8 cases, the MRI concluded to fibrous tissue (Figure 7). It was described as intermediate signal intensity in T1-weighted imaging in 7 cases and all cases had hyperintense signal in T2-weighted sequence as well as an enhancement in late post-gadolinium T1-weighted sequence. The DWI didn't show marked hyperintense signal in all cases. The two left MRI exams were performed to confirm a labyrinthine abnormality.

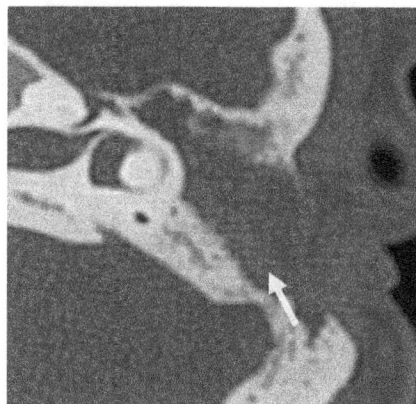

Figure 2: Axial computed tomography of the right and left temporal bone showing a total opacification (Arrow) of the middle ear cleft.

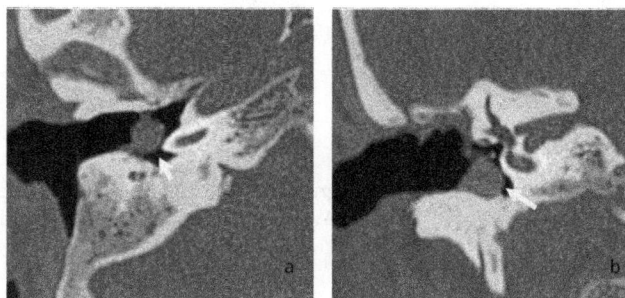

Figure 3: Axial (a) and coronal (b) computed tomography of the right temporal bone showing a partial opacification (arrow) of the middle ear cleft with convex margins.

Second-look surgery findings

Among the 27 ears who had second-look surgery, 13 were evaluated by CT scan only, three by MRI only and 11 by both CT scan and MRI. The indication of the second-look surgery was determined by the imaging findings as resumed in Table 1. Recurrent cholesteatoma was noted in 22 cases (81.5%). In the others cases, three ears had fibrous tissue associated with cholesterol granulomas and two ears had only fibrous tissue. According to these findings, CT scan was judged as a poor exam in the diagnosis of recurrent cholesteatoma as it has low specificity (20%) and negative predictive value (NPV) (14.3%) and average sensitivity (68.4%) and positive predictive value (PPV) (76.4%). MRI, on the other hand, proved to be an excellent exam in detecting recurrent cholesteatoma when associating late post-gadolinium T1-weighted and DWI sequences as it reached 100% in sensitivity and NPV. However we noted a significant number of false positives dropping its specificity to 25%. Taken separately, DWI and late post-gadolinium T1 sequences showed both high PPV (83.3% and 71.4%). Nonetheless, with a low NPV (25%), the DWI sequence can't rule out the diagnosis of recurrent cholesteatoma when showing no abnormality.

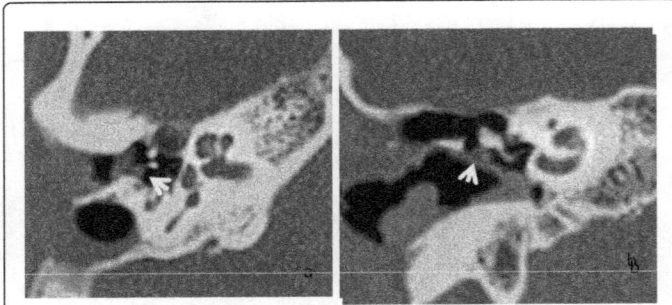

Figure 4: Axial (a) and coronal (b) computed tomography of the right temporal bone showing a mesotympanic pearl-shaped lesion (arrow) of the right middle ear.

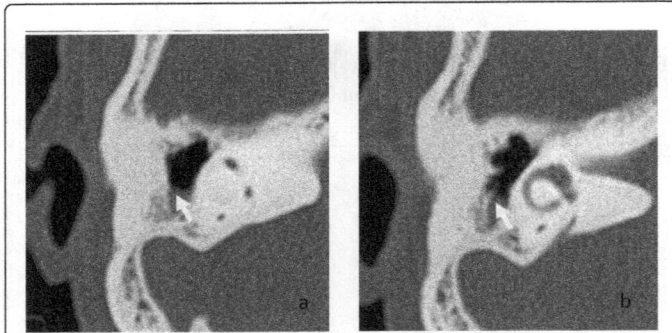

Figure 5: Axial computed tomography of the right temporal bone showing a partial opacification (Arrow) of the middle ear cleft with concave margins.

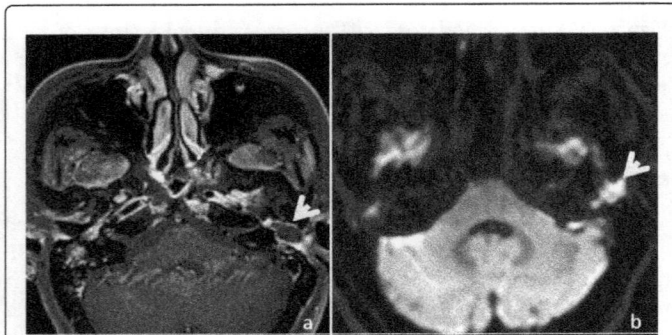

Figure 6: Left temporal bone MRI: Late T1post-Gadolinium axial view (a) and axial DWI view (b) showing a non-enhanced recurrent cholesteatoma (white arrow) with hyperintense signal intensity in DWI.

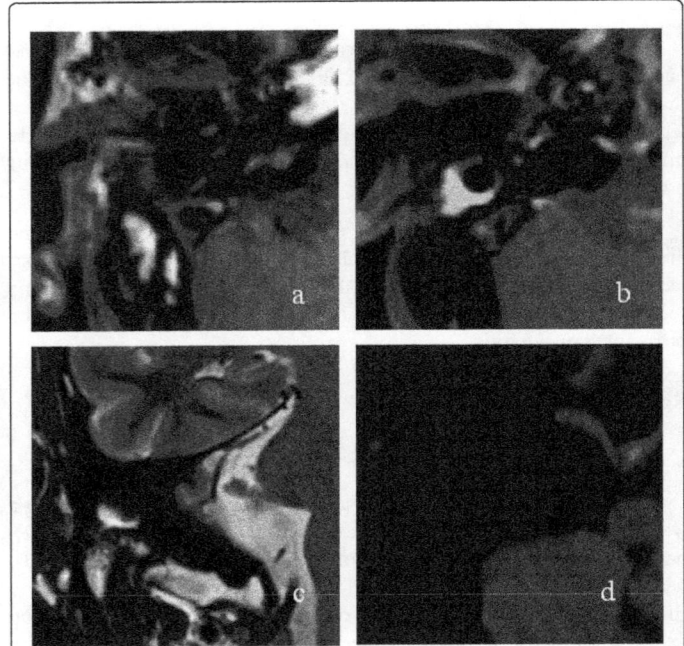

Figure 7: Right temporal bone MRI: T1 pre and post Gadolinium axial views (a,c), T2 coronal view (c) and axial DWI (d) showing a dependent opacity of the middle ear cleft totally enhanced after injection of Gadolinium without hypersignal in DWI.

Discussion

The limits of our study consist in the fact that the 40 ears initially included in the study is a number comparable to those found in other studies when reviewing the literature. However, the number of ears who had both CT scan and MRI (19 ears) was quite low. The fact our study was retrospective made it impossible to have a unique MRI protocol containing all necessary sequences explaining the fact that the DWI sequence wasn't done in all cases due to different MRI machines. The major issues in cholesteatoma surgery are residual and recurrent cholesteatoma. Residual cholesteatoma develops from a vestige of keratinized epithelium left in the middle ear cleft at the first surgery. Its rate varies from 10% to 40% [5] depending on the type and the extent of the cholesteatoma as well as of the operative technique and the surgeon's experience. Recurrent cholesteatoma, on the other hand, is newly appeared cholesteatoma resulting from the recurrence of tympanic membrane retraction or perforation favored by impaired middle ear ventilation. It is rarer than residual cholesteatoma and its rate varies from 10% to 20%b [6]. The known risk factors of recurrent cholesteatoma are the age of patients with a higher risk for children [7], ossicular erosion, the initial extent of cholesteatoma, the lack of the surgeon's experience and the operative technique with higher rates of recurrence with closed techniques [8,9]. Post operative follow-up is recommended at least for 3 years [10] or even for life according to some studies [11]. Patients with recurrent cholesteatoma usually show no symptoms particularly for the residual type. In our study, the most frequent symptom was otorrhea (50% of ears). CT scan is an essential complementary exam in both pre operative and post operative assessment of middle ear cholesteatoma.

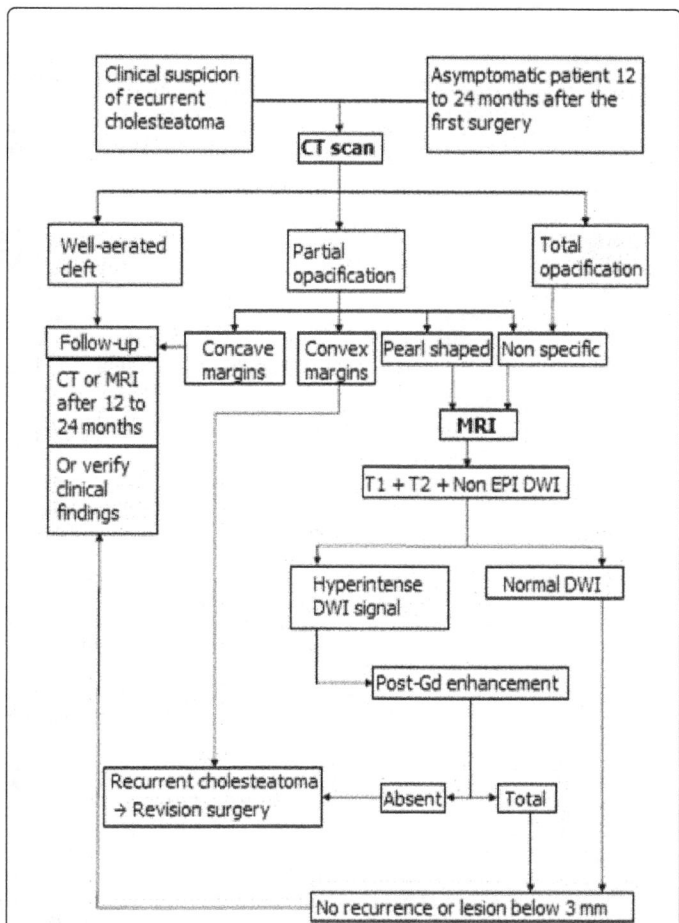

Figure 8: Decisional algorithm of follow-up of patients with middle ear cholesteatoma operated with a closed technique [17,23,27].

Indication	Number of cases	Percentage (%)
Recurrent cholesteatoma on MRI	3	11.1
Partial soft-tissue opacity with convex margins or Pearl-shaped lesion on CT scan+Recurrent cholesteatoma on MRI	6	22.2
Total opacification on CT scan +Recurrent cholesteatoma on MRI	5	18.5
Partial soft-tissue opacity with convex margins or Pearl-shaped lesion on CT scan	11	40.8
Total opacification on CT scan	2	7.4
Total	27	100

Table 1: The indication of the second-look surgery depending on imaging results.

It is recommended to diagnose residual cholesteatoma in asymptomatic patients, in case of confirmed recurrence in the otoscopic exam and in case of unexplained non improvement of hearing loss.CT scan can show a well-aerated cleft almost ruling out recurrent cholesteatoma with an excellent NPV that reached 100% according to Thomassin and al. and Gaillardin et al. [5,12] with no false negatives in both studies. In our study, a low NPV (14.3%) was under estimated by the fact that, as said earlier, a well-aerated cleft is considered safe from recurrent or residual cholesteatoma and thus no second-look surgery is conducted to confirm it. CT scan can also reveal pearl-shaped, highly suggestive of recurrent cholesteatoma particularly when located in the atticus or the retrotympanum [13-15]. CT scan is very effective in detecting these cholesteatoma pearls up to a size of 2 mm. When this type of lesion is shown, the second-look surgery is recommended straight away [6,16]. In our study, pearl-shaped opacification was found in 7 ears with recurrent cholesteatoma confirmed in six cases after second-look surgery. When showing a partial opacification with convex margins, CT scan suspects the recurrence of the cholesteatoma especially when associated with newly appeared bone erosion. This emphasizes the importance of comparing the findings of post operative and pre operative CT scans [14]. In our study, this type of opacification was found in 11 ears, the majority of which (n=8) had an MRI confirming the diagnosis of recurrence in 5 cases which were operated and ruling it out in 3 cases who didn't get to surgery. The second-look surgery revealed recurrent cholesteatoma in 3 ears only. Three patients had surgery based of CT findings only showing recurrence in 2 cases. The principal flaw of CT scan consists on showing either a total or a non specific opacification of the post operative cleft. The reason is that CT scan can't tell the difference between hyperplasic inflammatory mucous, cholesterol granuloma, fibrous tissue and recurrent cholesteatoma all having almost the same density [6,16] .This situation occurs in 20% of cases [14] in CT scans with poor specificity and PPV. In our study, they reached 20% and 76.4% respectively correlating with the results of Geoffray et al. [17] demonstrating that, when showing this kind of opacification, CT scan in unable to confirm of rule out the diagnosis of recurrent cholesteatoma.MRI has emerged as the complementary exam needed to characterize the non specific opacifications shown in CT scans [18]. There is no codified MRI protocol when looking for a recurrent cholesteatoma. However, it should contain T1-weighted sequences pre and post-contrast (the acquisition is made 30 to 45 min after the injection of Gadolinium), T2-weighted sequence and diffusion-weighted imaging with a b-value varying between 800 and 1000 [17,19].

The T1-weighted pre contrast sequence is useful for two reasons. The first is that it is necessary to affirm if there is an enhancement is late contrast sequence [19] and the second is that it can show hyperintense lesions as cholesterol granuloma which can be imperceptible within the enhancement after injection of Gadolinium [15,20]. The principal purpose of the late post-contrast T1-weighted sequence is to differentiate between the absence of enhancement of cholesteatoma and the constant enhancement of fibrous tissues [21]. This enhancement is centripetal [22] and becomes more intense past 45 min [23]. This time limit must be at least 45 min for Lehman et al. [24] and averaged 60 min for Blanco Cabellos et al. [19] and in our study. The major inconveniences of this sequence are the fact that it lengthens the duration of exams [17,21] and depends strongly on the radiologist's experience. It also has frequent false positives lowering its specificity and PPV. These false positives can be due to some material (silastic) used in surgery having the same pearl-shaped and indifference to Gadolinium as cholesteatoma [2]. In 2002, Fitzek and al. were the firsts to use the DWI in temporal bone MRI to detect cholesteatoma and proved that it has diffusion restriction.

Cholesteatoma is hyperintense in DWI not only because of this restriction phenomenon but also due to a T2 shine-through effect. In our study we used the EPI (echo planar imaging) DWI and our results showed lower specificity (50%), PPV (83%) and NPV (25%) than found in literature. The explanation would be the fact that small cholesteatoma pearls can't be diagnosed with this sequence. The minimum size estimated for EPI DWI is 5 mm. Other diffusion imaging techniques were developed in order to have better performances. The TSE DWI technique has a longer duration but lesser susceptibility artifacts and better spatial resolution [17,25,26]. TSE DWI sequence made it possible to detect smaller lesions up to 3 mm equalizing T1 post-contrast sequence though the latter has a better spatial resolution. Some studies showed that TSE DWI has better sensitivity and specificity than T1 post-contrast sequence. De Foer et al. [26] went even further recommending using solely the DWI TSE denying the need for Gadolinium injection by demonstrating that associating both sequences didn't provide significant difference in PPV and NPV in comparison with using TSE DWI only. The newest diffusion technique is the PROPELLER sequence (acronym used by GE heathcare®) manufactured to maximize the signal-to-noise ratio and to minimize artifacts. It has higher performances than the other DWI techniques but has a longer duration (4 to 5 min) with more frequent kinetic artifacts [25]. It can only be acquired in axial plane which limits the exploration of the tegmental area [24]. Some teams decided to give up on late T1 post-contrast sequence and rely only on the DWI technique [26]. Others, including ours, continue with associating both sequences as they give MRI specificity and PPV close to 100% and a NPV averaging 90% [17,23]. This close to perfect NPV is due to the barrier of 3 mm size below which the MRI can't detect cholesteatoma lesions. However, many studies agree that those small lesions grow slowly and consequently they can be diagnosed by another MRI one or two after the first one [17,23,27].The comparison of the results of our study with those of literature enabled us to make a decisional algorithm for the diagnosis of recurrent cholesteatoma for adult patients (Figure 8).

References

1. Bordure P, Bailleul S, Malard O, Wagner R (2009) Otite chronique cholestéatomateuse: Aspects cliniques et thérapeutiques. Encycl Med Chir. Oto-Rhino-Laryngologie 4: 1-16.

2. Khemani S, Singh A, Lingam RK, Kalan A (2011) Imaging of postoperative middle ear cholesteatoma. Clin Radiol 66: 760-767.

3. Migirov L, Tal S, Eyal A, Kronenberg J (2009) MRI, not CT, to rule out recurrent cholesteatoma and avoid unnecessary second-look mastoidectomy. Isr Med Assoc J 11: 144-146.

4. Plouin-Gaudon I, Bossard D, Ayari-Khalfallah S, Froehlich P (2010) Fusion of MRIs and CT scans for surgical treatment of cholesteatoma of the middle ear in children. Arch Otolaryngol Head Neck Surg 136: 878-883.

5. Gaillardin L, Lescanne E, Morinière S, Cottier JP, Robier A (2012) Residual cholesteatoma: Prevalence and location. Follow-up strategy in adults. Eur Ann Otorhinolaryngol Head Neck Dis 129: 136-140.

6. Ayache D, Schmerber S, Lavieille JP, Roger G, Gratacap B (2006) Middle ear cholesteatoma. Ann Otolaryngol Chir Cervicofac 123: 120-137.

7. Preciado DA (2012) Biology of cholesteatoma: Special considerations in pediatric patients. Int J Pediatr Otorhinolaryngol 76: 319-321.

8. Park KT, Song JJ, Moon SJ, Lee JH, Chang SO, et al. (2011) Choice of approach for revision surgery in cases with recurring chronic otitis media with cholesteatoma after the canal wall up procedure. Auris Nasus Larynx 38: 190-195.

9. Tomlin J, Chang D, McCutcheon B, Harris J (2013) Surgical technique and recurrence in cholesteatoma: A meta-analysis. Audiol Neurootol 18: 135-142.

10. Roux A, Bakhos D, Lescanne E, Cottier JP, Robier A (2015) Canal wall reconstruction in cholesteatoma surgeries: Rate of residual. Eur Arch Otorhinolaryngol 272: 2791-2797.

11. Beltaief N, Sellami M, Tababi S, Zainine R, Charfeddine A, et al. (2012) Le cholestéatome de l'oreille moyenne. J Tun ORL 28: 1-6.

12. Thomassin JM, Braccini F (1999) Role of imaging and endoscopy in the follow up and management of cholesteatomas operated by closed technique. Rev Laryngol Otol Rhinol (Bord) 120: 75-81.

13. Ayache D, Williams MT, Lejeune D, Corré A (2005) Usefulness of delayed postcontrast magnetic resonance imaging in the detection of residual cholesteatoma after canal wall-up tympanoplasty. Laryngoscope 115: 607-610.

14. Williams MT, Ayache D (2004) Imaging of the postoperative middle ear. Eur Radiol 14: 482-495.

15. Veillon F, Riehm S, Roedlich MN, Meriot P, Blonde E, et al. (2000) Imaging of middle ear pathology. Semin Roentgenol 35: 2-11.

16. Williams MT, Ayache D (2006) Imaging in adult chronic otitis. J Radiol 87: 1743-1755.

17. Geoffray A, Guesmi M, Nebbia JF, Leloutre B, Bailleux S, et al. (2013) MRI for the diagnosis of recurrent middle ear cholesteatoma in children-can we optimize the technique? Preliminary study. Pediatr Radiol 43: 464-473.

18. Kösling S, Bootz F (2001) CT and MR imaging after middle ear surgery. Eur J Radiol 40: 113-118.

19. Cabellos JAB, Vélez SO, Cáceres IA, Lluch ES, Galobardes J (2011) CT and MRI correlations in patients with suspected cholesteatoma after surgery. Neuroradiol J 24: 367-378.

20. Baráth K, Huber AM, Stämpfli P, Varga Z, Kollias S (2011) Neuroradiology of cholesteatomas. AJNR Am J Neuroradiol 32: 221-229.

21. Venail F, Bonafe A, Poirrier V, Mondain M, Uziel A (2008) Comparison of echo-planar diffusion-weighted imaging and delayed postcontrast T1- weighted MR imaging for the detection of residual cholesteatoma. Am J Neuroradiol 29: 1363-1368.

22. Williams MT, Ayache D, Alberti C, Héran F, Lafitte F, et al. (2003) Detection of postoperative residual cholesteatoma with delayed contrast-enhanced MR imaging: Initial findings. Eur Radiol 13: 169-174.

23. Emonot G, Richard C, Dumollard JM, Veyret C, Martin C (2008) Apport de l'imagerie au diagnostic de cholestéatome residuel. J Fr Oto Rhino Laryngol 94: 366-374.

24. Lehmann P, Saliou G, Brochart C, Page C, Deschepper B, et al. (2008) 3T MR imaging of postoperative recurrent middle ear cholesteatomas: Value of periodically rotated overlapping parallel lines with enhanced reconstruction diffusion-weighted MR imaging. Am J Neuroradiol 30: 423-427.

25. Schwartz KM, Lane JI, Bolster BD Jr, Neff BA (2011) The utility of diffusion-weighted imaging for cholesteatoma evaluation. AJNR Am J Neuroradiol 32: 430-436.

26. De Foer B, Vercruysse JP, Bernaerts A, Meersschaert J, Kenis C, Pouillon M, et al. (2010) Middle ear cholesteatoma: Non–echo-planar diffusion- weighted MR imaging versus delayed gadolinium-enhanced T1-weighted MR imaging. Radiology 255: 866-872.

27. Lincot J, Veillon F, Riehm S, Babay N, Matern JF, et al. (2015) Middle ear cholesteatoma: Compared diagnostic performances of two incremental MRI protocols including non-echo planar diffusion-weighted imaging acquired on 3T and 1.5T scanners. J Neuroradiol 42: 193-201.

30

Sickle Cell Trait, Malaria and Sensorineural Hearing Loss – A Case-Control Study from São Tomé and Príncipe

Cristina Caroça[*1-3], João Pereira de Lima[3], Paula Campelo[2], Elisabete Carolino[4], Helena Caria[5,6], João Paço[1,2] and Susana Nunes Silva[3]

[1]Department of Otolaryngology, NOVA Medical School, Universidade Nova de Lisboa, Campo Mártires da Pátria 130, 1169-056 Lisboa, Portugal

[2]Hospital CUF Infante Santo, 34, 6°, 1350-079 Lisboa, Portugal

[3]Centre for Toxicogenomics and Human Health (ToxOmics), Faculty of Medical Sciences, NOVA Medical School, Universidade Nova de Lisboa, Campo Mártires da Pátria 130, 1169-056 Lisboa, Portugal

[4]Escola Superior de Tecnologia da Saúde de Lisboa, Av. Dom João II Lote 4.69.01, 1990-096 Lisboa

[5]BioISI - Biosystems & Integrative Sciences Institute, Faculty of Science of the University of Lisbon, R. Ernesto de Vasconcelos, 1749-016 Lisboa, Portugal

[6]ESS/IPS, School of Health, Polytechnic Institute of Setúbal, Campus do IPS - Estefanilha, 2910-761 Setúbal, Portugal

*Corresponding author: Cristina Caroça, MD, Department of Otolaryngology, Nova Medical School, Universidade Nova de Lisboa, Campo Mártires da Pátria 130, 1169-056 Lisboa, Portugal, E-mail: cristinacaroca@netcabo.pt

Abstract

Background: Hearing loss is a problem with higher incidence in South Asia, Asia Pacific and sub-Saharan Africa. In these countries there is also associated history of anemia and malaria.

Objective: This study aims to identify a putative role of Beta globin mutation - sickle cell trait and HL in São Tomé and Príncipe population.

Methods: A retrospective case-control study of a convenience sample was collected during Otolaryngologist Humanitarian Missions in São Tomé and Príncipe. Control group includes individuals with normal hearing in both ears, and the case group has participants presenting bilateral or unilateral HL. It was evaluated the potential risk factors and sickle cell trait with HL, as well self-report of malaria infection, consanguinity, familial history of HL. The HbS gene point mutation (Glu6Val) was determined by PCR-RFLP.

Results: Our results showed a statistical significance between HL - oral language and self-report of HL. Taken altogether, our data did not reveal association between sickle cell trait and HL. However, a statistical association between HL and self-report of malaria was found.

Conclusion: No association between sickle cell trait and the high prevalence of HL was found. Self-report of Malaria was found as a risk factor for the development of HL in São Tomé and Príncipe population. The multifactorial profile of HL shall not exclude the relevance of other etiologic factors than Malaria to justify the high prevalence of HL in São Tomé and Príncipe and further investigation must be applied.

Keywords Hearing loss; Sensorineural hearing loss; São tomé and príncipe; Sickle cell trait; Sickle cell disease; Malaria; Hemoglobinopathies

Introduction

More than 360 million people in the World have disabling hearing loss (HL). According to new World Health Organization (WHO) Global Estimates on prevalence of the HL [1,2], there is a higher incidence in South Asia, Asia Pacific and sub-Saharan Africa [1-3]. Sub-Saharan Africa holds 10% of the world's population and two thirds of the world's least developed nations.

More than 1.2 million of the children living in sub-Saharan Africa aged 5 to 14 years old have moderate to severe bilateral HL [3]. The consequences of hearing problems are well known. HL in children can result in developmental delays and lead to significant inability to engage in oral/aural communication.

Anemia has been proposed as an etiologic factor in sensorineural deafness for many years, but there is little supporting evidence [4]. In these African countries there is a high prevalence of anemia and this could be associated with infections, hemoglobinopathies or stunting [5].

Several gene mutations and polymorphisms in the human hosts confer survival advantage and have increased in frequency through natural selection over generations. These include hemoglobinopathies like Sickle Cell Disease (SCD), thalassemias and glucose-6-phosphate dehydrogenase (G6PD) deficiency. Sickle Cell Disease (SCD) refers to a group of symptomatic disorders associated with a specific mutation on the Beta globin (HBB) gene [6]. Sickle hemoglobin (HbS), a structural variant of normal adult hemoglobin, results in the substitution of glutamic acid with valine in the sixth position of β-chain of the hemoglobin (β6Glu-Val) [7]. HbS is the most common pathological hemoglobin variant worldwide [7].

Several studies have suggested that HbS has an effect of protection against Plasmodium falciparum, the etiologic agent of malaria [6], showing that heterozygous people carrying the sickle-cell trait (HbAS) are protected against severe malaria (prevalence of HbAS, in some populations, is above 90%) [6,8].

This mechanism act as natural selection and is co-responsible for the high prevalence of HbS in malaria endemic regions as a result of natural selection over generations [9].

The red cells of individuals with the mutant homozygous gene (HbSS) become sickle shaped in low oxygen tension pressure with reduced oxygen-carrying capacity. The basal turn of the cochlea is particularly sensitive to anoxia, due to the high oxygen consumption rate of the stria vascularis and poor capacity for anaerobic metabolism. In this cases, SNHL start with the loss on the higher frequencies, then the lower frequencies, resulting from the damage at the apical region (low frequencies) and finally loss of the function throughout the entire cochlea [8].

SNHL is one of the several complications of this disease and has been found to occur in 8% of SCD children in Nigeria, 12% in USA, 22% in Jamaica, 36.5% in Kenya and 60% in Ghana [3,8].

In some studies, HbAS in malaria exposure could be also a cause of SNHL [10].

São Tomé and Príncipe it's an archipelago in western equatorial Africa, near Gabon, Equatorial Guinea, Camaroon and Nigeria, with Portuguese as official language [11]. São Tomé and Príncipe was discovered by Portuguese explorers in 1470. The resident population is about 187,000 inhabitants who have a low average age distribution (17-18 years) with low socioeconomic conditions and poor sanitary conditions, as well as a public health infection problem–malaria [12–14].

Since 2011 an otolaryngologist group formed by 2 doctors, 2 nurses and 1 audiologist began humanitarian missions in São Tomé and Príncipe (Project "Health for all"–Instituto Marquês de Valle Flor (IMVF)). Apparently according their clinical registries, this was the first hearing evaluation performed in these islands. Upon the first mission, a high prevalence of SNHL in the population was identified and it was observed upon subsequent missions.

As far as we know this is the first study developed in São Tomé and Príncipe population to evaluate the causes inherent to the high incidence of HL in this population. Such way, this study proposes to answer the question: will it be possible to establish an association between the sickle cell trait (HbAS) and the high incidence of SNHL in São Tomé and Príncipe?

Materials and Methods

Subjects

We present a case-control study, with a convenience sample where the control group include individuals with normal hearing in both ears, and patients with unilateral or bilateral HL compose the case group. The project was submitted and approved by the Medical Ethics Committee of São Tomé and Príncipe and Ethics Research Committee NMS|FCM-UNL.

A total of 316 individuals (136 HL patients and 180 controls with bilateral normal hearing), ranging from 2 to 35 years old, agreed to participate in this study. The limitation to 35 years was chosen to avoid

action of other risk factors of HL, like acoustic trauma, age and the effect of other diseases. We organized into two age groups based on WHO: 1) below 14 years old (2–14 years) as children group and 2) above 15 years old (15–35 years) as adults group. The patients were recruited during consultation provided by the humanitarian missions in São Tomé and Príncipe over a period from February 2012 to May 2014. The controls (normal hearing bilateral) were recruited at consultation at health services, primary schools from São Tomé and local hotel.

All patients signed an informed consent and answered a clinical questionnaire recording risk factors and clinical history. An otolaryngologist observed all. The risk factors included were family history of HL, consanguinity, self-report of malaria infection, pre-natal and perinatal history and history of infections.

All 316 individuals were evaluated regarding their hearing status with Pure Tone Audiogram (PTA) or Auditory Brainstem Response (ABR) depending on collaboration to participate on the audiometric exams.

Audiometric exams were carried out by an audiologist without an audiometric cabin, with earphones-TDH39, in a closed room, with a level of noise measured by iPhone using SchabelDoesIT GbR, Munich, Germany (version 1.0.0), considered acceptable (ANSI S3.1-1999) (R2013). The equipment used was the Madsen Midimate 622 and Vivosonic Integrity V500 audiometer (auditory brainstem response), calibrated according to calibration ISO389 1975/Oslo Recommendation. The Integrity^{TM} V500 system used to collect auditory brainstem is a modular equipment comprised by 4 main components: the computer, the VivoLink (SN: VL0026), the Amplitrode (SN: AJ0270) and the earphones. The earphones used were the ER-3A (ER-3A Left SN:63762 e ER-3A Right SN: 63763) and were calibrated according to ANSI S3.6-1996 and the stimulus used was the CLICK, calibrated in dB equivalent to the sound pressure level (dBpeSPL) according to the procedure IEC 60645-3 for the calibration of short duration stimulus.

Electrophysiological thresholds were translated into the audiometric thresholds for frequencies 2000 Hz and 4000 Hz. No correction factor was applied as is advocated in studies conducted by Jerger and Mauldin [15]; Gorga et al. [16]; van der Drift et al. [17]; Gorga et al. [18] in which establish a strong correlation between the electrophysiological thresholds with the "click" and the audiometric thresholds at 2000 and 4000 Hz.

The hearing loss of each patient was determined based on the better ear and following the WHO classification [19].

Patients with less than 2 years and more than 35 years of age, conductive hearing loss, syndromic hearing loss, obvious environmental causes such as meningitis, cerebral malaria, intra-uterine or neonatal complications, ototoxicity, severe head trauma or developmental delay were excluded.

DNA extraction

Blood samples of all patients and controls were collected into Guthrie cards. Genomic DNA was obtained from each sample using a commercially available kit (QIAamp® DNA micro kit, Qiagen) according to the manufacturer's instructions. All DNA samples were stored at –20°C.

SNP screening

The HbS gene point mutation (Glu6Val) was determined by PCR-RFLP. The primers and PCR conditions for the mutation site of this gene is shown in Table 1. For all of them the nucleotide mutated resulted in either gain or loss of restriction site, which therefore allowed the wild-type (HbAA) and variant alleles to be discriminated by RFLP after appropriate restriction enzyme digestion.

PCR was carried out with 50 ng of DNA in 50 ml reaction volume, containing 1.3x ImmoBuffer, 1.5 mM MgCl$_2$, 0.6 mM dNTP, 1.0 mM of each primer, and 0.75 U of Immolase (Bioline). The amplification started with an initial denaturation step at 95°C for 7 min, cycling parameters were 35 cycles of 95°C for 30 s, specific annealing temperature (60°C) for 30 s, 72°C for 30 s and a final extension at 72°C for 10 min. After amplification, 10 ml of each PCR products were digested with appropriate restriction enzymes (DdeI) for 3 h at 37°C followed by an inactivation step at 65°C for 20 min and electrophoresed in 2% agarose gel with ethidium bromide (0.5 mg/ml) for visualization under ultraviolet light. The expected products for each genotype of the tested gene are shown in Table 1. All the genotype determinations were carried out twice in independent experiments and inconclusive samples were reanalyzed.

Gene	Primers	PCR fragment	Patterns after restriction enzyme digestion
HbAS codon 6 (rs334)	Rv 5'- AGG GTG GGA AAA TAG ACC AA -3'	395 bp	HbAA: 202, 180, 13 bp
	FW 5'- CGG CTG TCA TCA CTT AGA CCT -3'		HbAS: 382, 202,180,13 bp
			HbSS: 382, 13 bp

Table 1: PCR-RFLP conditions for identification of HbAS (rs334) polymorphism.

Statistical Analysis

The Hardy-Weinberg equilibrium of HbS was assessed by Qui-square test, calculated by HW calculator™ - Michael H Court (2005-2008).

Description of the sample was made with descriptive statistics, considering frequency analysis, means and standard deviation (SD).

To study the association between HL and each of the following parameters as district origin, oral language, perception of HL, sex and history of malaria infection, have been used the Qui-squared test.

The association between HbS genotype and the degree of HL of each ear and was analysed with Qui-square test by Monte Carlo Simulation.

To identify risk factors of HL we adopted a Binary Logistic Regression, where HL is a response variable and independent variables were HbS, age groups and self-report of Malaria infection.

All analyses were performed using the IBM, SPSS 20 version.

Results

We evaluated 316 subjects (Table 2) of whom 146 (45.6%) were men and 172 (54.4%) were women, with an age mean of 17.4 ± 9.74 years and a median of 15 years.

	Control-180	Case-136	Case Unil HL	Case Bil HL	p-Value
Age range					0.361
[2-14]	82 (45.6%)	69 (50.7%)	15 (34.1%)	54 (58.7%)	
[15-35]	98 (54.4%)	67 (49.3%)	29 (65.9%)	38 (41.3%)	
Mean Age SD	17.8±9.77	16.9±9.73	20.1±9.29	15.4±9.61	

Sex					0.256
Male:	87 (48.3%)	57 (41.9%)	17 (38.6%)	40 (43.5%)	
Female:	93 (51.7%)	79 (58.1%)	27 (61.4%)	52 (56.5%)	
Oral Language					0.0001
No:	4 (2.2%)	33 (24.3%)	1 (2.3%)	32 (34.8%)	
Yes:	170 (94.5%)	85 (62.5%)	42 (95.4%)	43 (46.7%)	
Indefined:	6 (3.3%)	18 (13.2%)	1 (2.3%)	17 (18.4%)	
Family History Hearing Loss					0.278
No:	140 (77.8%)	115 (84.6%)	40 (90.9%)	75 (81.5%)	
Yes:	34 (18.9%)	20 (14.7%)	4 (9.1%)	16 (17.4%)	
Missing:	6 (3.3%)	1 (0.7%)		1 (1.1%)	
Consanguinity					0.443
No:	171 (95%)	127 (93.4%)	43 (97.7%)	84 (91.3%)	
Yes:	3 (1,7%)	4 (2.9%)	1 (2.3%)	3 (3.3%)	
Missing:	6 (3.3%)	5 (3.7%)		5 (5.4%)	
Malaria					0.07
No:	72 (40%)	41 (30.1%)	11 (25%)	30 (32.6%)	

Yes:	103 (57.2%)	91 (66.9%)	33 (75%)	58 (63.1%)	
Missing	5 (2.8%)	4 (3%)		4 (4.3%)	
Hearing Loss					
Normal:	180 (100%)	44 (32.3%)	44 (100%)		
Mild:		16 (11.8%)		16 (17.4%)	
Moderate:		19 (14%)		19 (20.7%)	
Severe:		17 (12.5%)		17 (18.5%)	
Profound:		40 (29.4%)		40 (43.5%)	
Right Ear					
Normal:	180 (100%)	19 (14%)	19 (43.2%)		
Mild:		26 (19.1%)	13 (29.5%)	13 (14.1%)	
Moderate:		17 (12.5%)	3 (6.8%)	14 (15.2%)	
Severe:		17 (12.5%)	2 (4.5%)	15 (16.3%)	
Profound:		57 (41.9%)	7 (15.9%)	50 (54.3%)	
Left Ear					
Normal:	180 (100%)	25 (18.4%)	25 (56.8%)		
Mild:		18 (13.2%)	8 (18.2%)	10 (10.9%)	
Moderate:		19 (14%)	1 (2.3%)	18 (19.6%)	
Severe:		16 (11.8%)	2 (4.5%)	14 (15.2%)	
Profound:		58 (42.6%)	8 (18.2%)	50 (54.3%)	
Hb					0.743
HbAA:	142 (78.9%)	112 (82.3%)	35 (79.5%)	77 (83.7%)	
HbAS:	35 (19.4%)	22 (16.2%)	9 (20.5%)	13 (14.1%)	
HbSS:	3 (1.7%)	2 (1.5%)	0	2 (2.2%)	
SD – Standard Deviation; HbAA - Wild Type; HbAS - Trait; HbSS - Homozygotic					

Table 2: General characteristics for convenience sample of São Tomé and Príncipe population.

Both groups (case-control) are homogeneous to gender (p=0.256) and age groups (p=0.361).

According to our results, HL is not associated with the district of origin (p=0.058) of each individual.

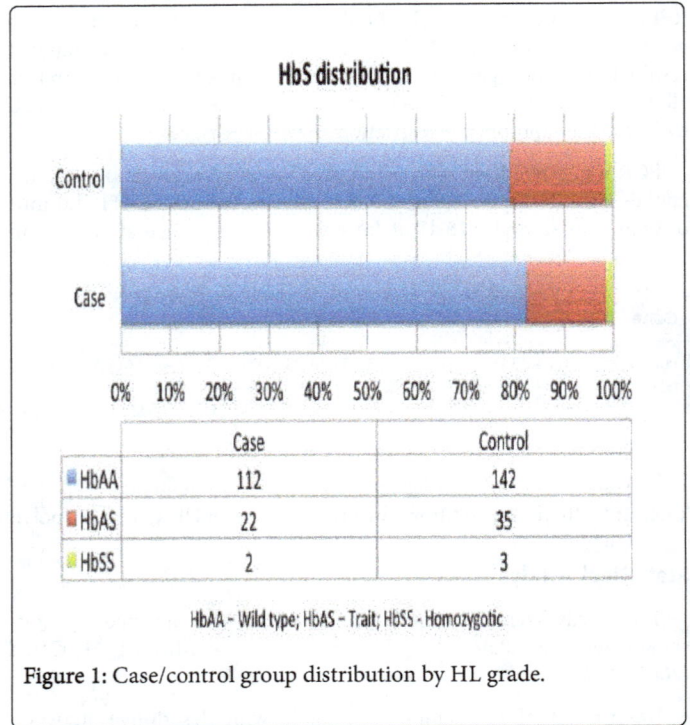

Figure 1: Case/control group distribution by HL grade.

Among the 316 subjects, we found 180 (57.0%) individuals with bilateral normal hearing, 44 (13.9%) unilateral HL (UHL) and 92 (29.1%) with bilateral HL (Figure 1). The individuals with UHL and bilateral HL were included in the case group.

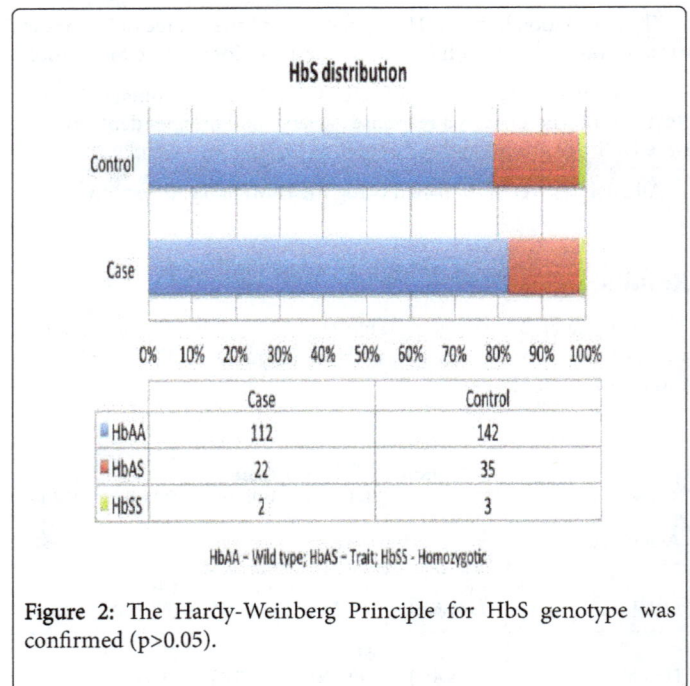

Figure 2: The Hardy-Weinberg Principle for HbS genotype was confirmed (p>0.05).

The Hardy-Weinberg Principle for HbS genotype was confirmed based on the distribution of HbS genotype in control and case group (Figure 2).

When we calculate the media of the tone threshold, we found the left ear (40.02 dB) slight the same than the right (39.85 dB). The audiometric curve in the global sample has a horizontal shape, around mild HL.

The self-reported HL was confirmed by the audiometric evaluation, showing a positive association (p<0.0001) between both parameters. The tendency for self-reported HL was confirmed by the exams (ϕ=0.553; p<0.0001).

Considering oral language for communication, this was absent in 33 (24.3%) of the individuals from case group and in 4 (2.2%) of the control groups these showing a negative association (ϕ=-0.379; p<0.0001) between oral language and HL (p<0.0001). There was a tendency to have oral language in the control group.

A familial history of HL was found to be more prevalent in the control group than in the case group, respectively with 34 controls (18.9%) and 20 patients (14.7%). In the case group, 16 (80%) had bilateral HL and 4 (20%) unilateral HL.

From our sample 3 individuals (1.7%) in the control group and 4 patients (2.9%) in case group confirmed the existence of consanguinity in their families. Thus, no association between HL and consanguinity was performed.

In São Tomé and Principe we did not found any registry about history of malaria infection. At same time, we found that malaria infection is a public health problem and all individuals enrolled recognize malaria infection and can answer about their clinical history regarding this endemic infection. Self-report of malaria infection was more prevalent in the case group with 91 patients reporting a history of malaria (66.9%), being reported by 103 individuals (57.2%) of the control group.

The genotype distribution in our population was shown in Table 2. Concerning our results the HbAS showed no significant predisposition to HL (Table 3).

	Cases n (%)	Controls n (%)	P-value	Crude OR (95% CI)	P-value	Adjusted OR (95% CI)
Age group			0.362		0.07	
[2-14]	69 (45.7%)	82 (54.3%)		Reference		Reference
[15-35]	98 (59.4%)	98 (59.4%)		0.812 [0.520-1.269]		0.633 [0.386-1.038]
Malaria infection			0.071		0.021	
No:	41 (30.1%)	72 (40%)		Reference		Reference
Yes:	91 (66.9%)	103 (57.2%)		1.552 [0.964-2.497]		1.840 [1.097-3.085]
HbS			0.744		0.839	
(HbAA)	112 (82.3%)	142 (78.9%)		Reference		Reference
(HbAS)	22 (16.2%)	35 (19.4%)	0.449	0.797 [0.443-1.435]	0.573	0.842 [0.463-1.530]
(HbSS)	2 (1.5%)	3 (1.7%)	0.855	0.845 [0.139-5.145]	0.832	0.821 [0.133-5.063]

Table 3: Binary logistic regression between HbS and HL without and with risk factors (age group and history of malaria infection), HL: Normal hearing–0–Reference Category is a response variable; independent variables: HbS (0–HbAA wild type, 1- HbAS trait, 2–HbSS homozygotic), age groups (0–[2-14] years, 1–[15-35] years) and history of Malaria infection (0–no, 1–yes).

By applying the model of binary logistic regression the self-report of malaria was identified as a risk factor for HL (Table 3). The history of malaria infection almost doubled the risk of HL (OR=1.840; CI 95% [1.097-3.085]). We also found that, even not statistically significant, the oldest age group presented a decreased risk of HL in 36.7%.

For sickle cell trait we did not verify a significant predisposition to develop HL (OR=0.842; CI95% [0.463-1.530]) as sickle cell disease (OR=0.821; CI95% [0.133-5.063]).

Discussion

The results of this study revealed a prevalence of bilateral SNHL in 92 (29.1%) individuals and unilateral SNHL in 44 (13.9%) of subjects from our convenience sample. The unilateral and bilateral SNHL, accounting for 43% of the total sample, were included in the case study group since the unilateral SNHL also contribute to worse language acquisition and decreased school performance [20].

The horizontal audiologic curve in tonal audiogram was not specific or characteristic to a specific risk factor, meaning that inumerous causes may be responsible for SNHL in São Tomé and Príncipe and not one in particular.

Analysing the risk factors, the history family of HL and consanguinity were excluded from the analysis because they have a small number of cases. They haven't significant association in contrast to what we are expecting, since has been reported the relevance of these factors in HL [21, 22].

The individuals included in this study rarely reported to have consanguineous parents, even knowing that São Tomé and Príncipe are small islands, with high probability of consanguinity.

São Tomé and Príncipe is a population of Sub-Saharan Africa in which several haemoglobinopathies have been identified, including HbSS as the most prevalent [7,23]. It would be expected to obtain an increased prevalence of HbS homozygous (HbSS) and increased HbAS [4,8,10,24] in the São Tomé and Príncipe population. However in our results, HbSS genotype were found only in 16% and 18% for HbAS of the sample.

The HbAS has been reported in many studies as a factor of protection from malaria, reducing its severity [6]. The mechanism that contribute for this protection is the accelerated sickling of parasite-infected HbAS erythrocytes, low growth rates and parasite invasion in HbAS erythrocytes (in low oxygen conditions) and increased phagocytosis of infected HbAS erythrocytes [6]. Recently, had been show that intra-erythrocytic parasite growth is greatly inhibited by HbS polymerization when oxygen levels drop below 5% and, higher parasite-infected sickle erythrocyte phagocytosis by host immune cells has been observed when compared to infected normal erythrocytes [6]. Moreover, HbS erythrocytes infected by P. falciparum lower the surface expression of PfEMP-1, which results in a reduction of cytoadherence and thus protection against severe malaria [6]. This haemoglobin alteration otherwise may lead to thromboembolic events which sought being the source of SNHL [10].

The study model adopted did not confirm this assumption that the HbAS can promote SNHL. In our study we found a significant association between SNHL and a self-report of malaria. Although the patient provides the clinical malaria episode information, we considered their report valid. We must also consider that in the São Tomé Príncipe population exists a strong public awareness of Malaria infection as public health problem and standard procedures and guidelines for infection evaluation are followed, including the collection of thick blood film Plasmodium sp. in the presence of fever and illness.

Our results are supported by others, suggesting also that mild clinical malaria may also be associated with SNHL [25,26].

The malaria infection may trigger the onset of SNHL by pathophysiological processes, thromboembolism and release of inflammatory mediators [26,27]. On the other hand, malaria treatment adopted may be ototoxic. Some studies report reversibility of ototoxicity of some antimalarial [28–32]. In the specific case of children it does not apply [33] especially when is not performed a drug weight adjustment, and children ingest high doses of antimalarial therapy which may induce irreversible ototoxicity [32,33]. Eventually the higher association of the youngest patients of the case group with HL could be supported by the report of children malaria infection in this country during last 14 years [34,35].

The epidemiological profile of Malaria in São Tomé and Príncipe reveals a significant decrease of malaria admissions and deaths over 2006-2007 [34]. Since then, the children were most affected, representing a high proportion relatively to all patients. In 2003 they started some measures to control the disease witch include indoor residual spraying (IRS). In 2004 initiated the intermittent preventive treatment (IPT) with and sulfadoxine and pyrimethamine and changed the antimalarial policy with association of artesunate (AS) and amodiaquine (AQ), as first line treatment, in 2005 implemented the use of insecticide-treated nets (ITN) [34].

Our results support the hypothesis that the sickle cell trait (HbAS) acts as a protective role against malaria and SNHL in São Tomé and Príncipe.

Moreover, although São Tomé and Príncipe region is also affected by other HBB mutations, their prevalence is not relevant [23], justifying no screening for them in our study. There are others haemoglobin diseases, like deficiency of glucose-6-phosphate dehydrogenase, which

ototoxicity is well known when combined with primaquine antimalarial therapy [36,37].

Conclusion

No association between sickle cell trait (HbAS) and the high prevalence of HL was found. However, our study suggests that in this sample, HbAS is preventing HL because is protecting against malaria. Malaria was found as a risk factor for the development of HL in São Tomé and Príncipe population. The multifactorial profile of HL and the horizontal audiologic curve, highly suggests the relevance of other etiologic factors than Malaria to justify the high prevalence of HL in São Tomé and Príncipe and further investigation must be applied.

Acknowledgement

Authors would like to thank to: Democratic Republic of São Tomé and Príncipe, Instituto Marquês de Valle Flôr (IMVF), Instituto Camões, Nova University School – Faculdade de Ciências Médicas de Lisboa, Fundação Calouste Gulbenkian, Mota&Engil, José de Mello Saúde and Audiologists from Hospital CUF Infante Santo (Diogo Ribeiro, Tânia Martins and Vera Lourenço).

This project was part of a PhD for the first author, with a research Grant from Jose de Mello Saúde.

The authors warmly dedicate this study to the memory of their colleague and friend Prof. Jorge Gaspar (1963-2015) who so much contributed with his knowledge and vision to this study.

Funding

Jose de Mello Saúde PhD Grant - to data collection and analysis

Competing Interests

There are no conflicts of interest.

References

1. WHO (2013) Media centre: Millions have hearing loss that can be improved or prevented. WHO Media Cent, pp: 1–2.
2. Olusanya BO, Neumann KJ, Saunders JE (2014) The global burden of disabling hearing impairment: A call to action. Bull World Health Organ 92: 367-373.
3. Tucci D, Merson MH, Wilson BS (2010) A summary of the literature on global hearing impairment: Current status and priorities for action. Otol Neurotol 31: 31-41.
4. Al Okbi MH, Alkindi S, Al Abri RK, Mathew J, Nagwa AA, et al. (2011) Sensorineural hearing loss in sickle cell disease-A prospective study from Oman. Laryngoscope 121: 392-396.
5. Tine RCK, Ndiaye M, Hansson HH, Ndour CT, Faye B, et al. (2012) The association between malaria parasitaemia, erythrocyte polymorphisms, malnutrition and anaemia in children less than 10 years in Senegal: A case control study. BMC Res Notes 5: 565.
6. López C, Saravia C, Gomez A, Hoebeke J, Patarroyo MA (2010) Mechanisms of genetically-based resistance to malaria. Gene 467: 1-12.
7. Piel FB, Patil AP, Howes RE, Nyangiri OA, Gething PW, et al. (2010) Global distribution of the sickle cell gene and geographical confirmation of the malaria hypothesis. Nat Commun 1: 104.
8. Mgbor N, Emodi I (2004) Sensorineural hearing loss in Nigerian children with sickle cell disease. Int J Pediatr Otorhinolaryngol 68: 1413-1416.

9. Driss A, Hibbert JM, Wilson NO, Iqbal SA, Adamkiewicz TV, et al. (2011) Genetic polymorphisms linked to susceptibility to malaria. Malar J 10: 271.

10. García Callejo FJ, Sebastián Gil E, Morant Ventura A, Marco Algarra J (2002) Presentation of 2 cases of sudden deafness in patients with sickle-cell anemia and trait. Acta Otorrinolaringol Esp 53: 371-376.

11. Malheiro JB, Morais JS (2013) São Tomé e Príncipe - Património Arquitetónico, Caleidoscó.

12. Instituto Nacional de Estatística ST e P, Saúde M da, Macro I (2010) São Tomé e Príncipe Inquérito Demográfico e Sanitário, IDS STP 2008-2009.

13. Instituto Nacional de Estatística ST e P (2012) Seminário de divulgação dos dados. In: IV Recens. Geral da Popul. e habitação 2012 (RGPH-2012. Instituto Nacional de estatistica São Tomé e Príncipe 1-100.

14. WHO (2014) Country Profiles. World Health Organization.

15. Jerger J, Mauldin L (1978) Prediction of sensorineural hearing level from the brain stem evoked response. Arch Otolaryngol 104: 456-461.

16. Gorga MP, Worthington DW, Reiland JK, Beauchaine KA, Goldgar DE (1985) Some comparisons between auditory brain stem response thresholds, latencies and the pure-tone audiogram. Ear Hear 6: 105-112.

17. van der Drift JF, Brocaar MP, van Zanten GA (1987) The relation between the pure-tone audiogram and the click auditory brainstem response threshold in cochlear hearing loss. Audiology 26: 1-10.

18. Gorga MP, Johnson TA, Kaminski JK, Beauchaine KL, Garner CA, Neely ST (2006) Using a combination of click- and toneburst-evoked auditory brainstem response measurements to estimate pure-tone thresholds. Ear Hear February 27: 60-74.

19. WHO (2013) Prevention of blindness and deafness-Grades of hearing impairment. In: WHO.

20. Lieu JE, Tye-Murray N, Fu Q (2012) Longitudinal study of children with unilateral hearing loss. Laryngoscope 122: 2088-2095.

21. Driscoll C, Beswick R, Doherty E, D'Silva R, Cross A (2015) The validity of family history as a risk factor in pediatric hearing loss. Int J Pediatr Otorhinolaryngol 79: 654-659.

22. Zakzouk S (2002) Consanguinity and hearing impairment in developing countries: A custom to be discouraged. J Laryngol Otol 116: 811-816.

23. Williams TN, Weatherall DJ (2012) World distribution, population genetics and health burden of the hemoglobinopathies. Cold Spring Harb Perspect Med 2: a011692.

24. Aderibigbe A, Ologe FE, Oyejola BA (2005) Hearing thresholds in sickle cell anemia patients: Emerging new trends? J Natl Med Assoc 97: 1135-1142.

25. Zhao SZ, Mackenzie IJ (2011) Deafness: malaria as a forgotten cause. Ann Trop Paediatr 31: 1-10.

26. Schmutzhard J, Kositz CH, Lackner P, Dietmann A, Fischer M, et al. (2010) Murine malaria is associated with significant hearing impairment. Malar J 9:159.

27. Schmutzhard J, Kositz CH, Lackner P, Pritz C, Glueckert R, et al. (2011) Murine cerebral malaria: Histopathology and ICAM 1 immunohistochemistry of the inner ear. Trop Med Int Health 16: 914-922.

28. Gürkov R, Eshetu T, Miranda IB, Berens-Riha N, Mamo Y, et al. (2008) Ototoxicity of artemether/lumefantrine in the treatment of falciparum malaria: A randomized trial. Malar J 7: 179.

29. Carrara V, Phyo AP, Nwee P, Soe M, Htoo H, et al. (2008) Auditory assessment of patients with acute uncomplicated *Plasmodium falciparum* malaria treated with three-day mefloquine-artesunate on the north-western border of Thailand. Malar J 7:233.

30. Hutagalung R, Htoo H, Nwee P, Arunkamomkiri J, Zwang J, et al. (2006) A case-control auditory evaluation of patients treated with artemether- lumefantrine. Am J Trop Med Hyg 74: 211-214.

31. Roche RJ, Silamut K, Pukrittayakamee S, Looareesuwan S, Molunto P, et al. (1990) Quinine induces reversible high-tone hearing loss. Br J Clin Pharmacol 29: 780-782.

32. Claessen FAP, Van Boxtel CJ, Perenboom RM, Tange RA, Wetsteijn JCFM, Kager PA (1998) Quinine pharmacokinetics: Ototoxic and cardiotoxic effects in healthy Caucasian subjects and in patients with falciparum malaria. Trop Med Int Heal 3: 482–489.

33. Freeland A, Jones J, Mohammed NK (2010) Sensorineural deafness in Tanzanian children-Is ototoxicity a significant cause? A pilot study. Int J Pediatr Otorhinolaryngol 74: 516-519.

34. World Health Organization (2010) Sao Tome and prinicple. Jeune Afr 36: 79.

35. Greenwood BM, Bojang K, Whitty CJ, Targett GA (2005) Malaria. Lancet 365: 1487-1498.

36. Goo YK, Ji SY, Shin H I, Moon JH, Cho SH, et al. (2014) First evaluation of Glucose-6-Phosphate Dehydrogenase (G6PD) deficiency in vivax malaria endemic regions in the Republic of Korea. PLoS One 9: 1-6.

37. Recht J, Ashley E, White N (2014) Safety of 8-aminoquinoline antimalarial medicines. World Health Organization, Switzerland.

31

Simultaneous Fractionated Cisplatin and Radiation Therapy in the Treatment of Advanced Operable Stage III and IV Squamous Cell Carcinoma of the Oral Cavity and Pharynx

Gus J Slotman[*]

Director of Clinical Research, Inspira Health Network, Vineland

[*]**Corresponding author:** Slotman GJ, Director of Clinical Research, Inspira Health Network, 1505 West Sherman Avenue, Suite B, Vineland; E-mail: slotmang@ihn.org

Abstract

Objective: To evaluate simultaneous fractionated cisplatin and radiation therapy in the treatment of advanced operable Stage III and IV squamous cell carcinoma of the oral cavity and pharynx.

Methods: A retrospective chart review of a database with Stage III and IV squamous cell carcinoma of the oral cavity and pharynx patients was conducted. A total of 105 patients with squamous cell carcinoma of the oral cavity and pharynx underwent chemoradiotherapy treatment of two types: CTRT consisted of pre-operative cisplatin, 20 mg/m^2 intravenously for 4 consecutive days during weeks 1, 4, and 7 of radiotherapy; control chemotherapy consisted of several regimens: cisplatin, 75 mg/m^2 intravenously on days 1, 22, and 43 of radiotherapy; carboplatin, 100 mg/m^2 and taxol, 45 mg/m^2 once per week during radiotherapy; or CTRT regimen following surgery. Toxicity to treatment, clinical response, biopsy result, incidence or recurrence, surgery, overall and disease-free survival were measured.

Results: A total of 91 patients underwent CTRT and 14 patients underwent control. Overall, CTRT experienced less high-grade toxicity (14% vs 50%, P<0.05). CTRT had trends of higher clinical complete response (73% vs 57%) and higher incidence of histologic complete response as evidenced by negative biopsy (67% vs 57%). Among patients who had post-treatment surgery, 48% of CTRT surgeries were radical compared to 100% of control surgeries (P=0.07). CTRT had less distant metastasis compared to control (7% vs 50%, P=0.06). Regarding expiratory status, CTRT had less death with disease (56% vs 75%, P=0.33). Kaplan-Meier analysis showed a trend toward increased long-term survival among CTRT compared to control.

Conclusion: Overall, CTRT experienced significantly less toxicity. CTRT showed trends toward higher clinical complete response and histologic complete response compared to control. CTRT also had trends toward less distant metastases and less death with disease compared to control.

Keywords: Squamous cell carcinoma; Head and neck; Cisplatin; Radiotherapy

Introduction

Squamous cell carcinomas of the head and neck (SCCHN) make up approximately 3 percent of all cancer cases in the United States [1]. SCCHN are most common in the oral cavity, pharynx, and larynx. These cancers are curable when detected at an early stage, but most patients present with locally advanced Stage III or IV disease [2]. Traditional treatment for such cancers has involved radical surgery and/or post-operative radiotherapy [3]. More recently, multi-modality therapies have become useful for improving locoregional control and organ preservation, although survival is still poor [2]. Multi-modality therapies involve a combination of surgery, nontraditional radiation therapy, and chemotherapy integration. However, the roles of each technique are not yet standardized.

While no single treatment regimen has been defined as most effective in treating SCCHN, several studies have identified certain multi-modality combinations that produce greater success in terms of organ preservation, survival, locoregional control, and toxicity to treatment. Common multi-modality treatments include docetaxel plus cisplatin followed by fluorouracil infusion for 4 days every 3 weeks; high-dose cisplatin given on days 1, 22, and 43 of radiotherapy; daily low-dose concomitant cisplatin; and a weekly combination of carboplatin and taxol [2,4-6]. These regimens are just a sample of the variety of SCCHN treatments that have been attempted. Many other combinations of radiotherapy and chemotherapy exist. Thus, it is difficult to determine which treatment is best for the patients.

In recent years, investigators have found that concurrent chemotherapy and radiation prior to surgery show synergistic effects in tumor treatment, improving overall disease control and survival [3]. Organ preservation, which is highly valued by most patients, is also improved due to less post-chemoradiotherapy surgery. Several pilot investigations have suggested that low-dose, fractionated cisplatin administered simultaneously with concomitant high-dose radiotherapy may be effective in curing cancer while preserving head and neck function [7-9]. The objective of the present study was to evaluate patients with advanced operable Stage III and IV SCCHN who were treated pre-operatively with 20 mg/m2 IV cisplatin given on 4 consecutive days every 3 weeks during high-dose irradiation therapy (CTRT).

Methods

With the approval of the Inspira Health Network Institutional Review Board, medical records of 91 patients with Stage III and IV squamous cell carcinoma of the oral cavity and/or pharynx who received CTRT were reviewed retrospectively and compared with an unselected control group of 14 patients who underwent other accepted standard, medical and surgical treatment regimens, and received at least part of their care at the Inspira health Network, Vineland, NJ. CTRT chemotherapy consisted of pre-operative cisplatin, 20 mg/m2 intravenously for 4 consecutive days during weeks 1, 4, and 7 of radiotherapy. CTRT patients were included in the outcomes evaluation, on an intent-to-treat basis, if they had at least one course of concomitant chemotherapy during radiation therapy. All control patients completed the cancer treatment regimen prescribed for each. The Southern New Jersey Head and Neck Treatment Network is a group of medical oncologists and radiation oncologists who have treated patients of the senior author (GJS) with CTRT, based on the successes of previously published pilot trials of this regimen and their positive clinical experiences with it. Conversely, control chemotherapy consisted of several regimens: cisplatin, 75 mg/m2 intravenously on days 1, 22, and 43 of radiotherapy; carboplatin, 100 mg/m2 and taxol, 45 mg/m2 once per week during radiotherapy; or CTRT regimen following surgery. The treatment regimens of control patients are described in Table 1, including the drug regimen, surgery, and location of treatment. Both the CTRT and control groups were treated between June 1992 and October 2011. Determination of whether patients received CTRT or control regimens was at the discretion of the treating physician. Due to the retrospective nature of the study, the definition of need for surgery was not controlled. However, all operations at all institutions were performed by trained head and neck surgical oncologists.

Over the course of the study, the radiation therapy technique varied as the technology changed. In the earlier portion of the study, patients were treated with a regimen consisting of single daily fractionation with 6 MV photons and 3D treatment planning followed by a boost, in which they were treated with a hyperfractionated (two fractions/day) regimen with concurrent chemotherapy. In 2006, patients were treated with normal fractionation to a higher total dose, between 70-74 Gy. In the latter part of the treatment study, the patients were treated with a field-within-a-field technique utilizing head and neck IMRT. PTVs were treated between 70-74 Gy. Most treatment regimens were delivered with 6 MV photons with either customized blocks or multi-leaf collimator generated blocks. Verification was performed using port films and later changed to stereoscopic imaging followed by cone beam CT.

The study variables included age, sex, race, vital status, alcohol use, tobacco use, tumor site, tumor grade, clinical stage, surgery, chemoradiotherapy regimen, clinical response, post-CTRT biopsy result, recurrence, and toxicity to treatment. Clinical stage was determined according to the classification of the American Joint Committee on Cancer Staging [10]. Post-chemoradiotherapy biopsy determined whether or not patients whose cancers regressed completely clinically (Clinical Complete Response – CCR) had achieved either a histologically complete response (HCR) or still had residual tumor. Patients with residual disease were recommended for

curative surgery. Toxicity to treatment was determined according to the NCI Common Terminology Criteria for Adverse Events [11].

Statistical analysis was performed using the chi-squared equation for categorical variables. Analysis of variance (ANOVA) was used to compare age. Overall survival and disease-specific survival were analyzed by the Kaplan-Meier logarithmic rank test. Median follow-up was 20 months, with a range of 1 to 128 months. The level of significance was set as $p < 0.05$ (SAS/STAT(R) 9.22 User's Guide).

Patient Characteristics	CTRT (SD)A n=91	CONTROL (SD)B n=14	P Value
Age	59.4 (12.7)	58.1 (9.6)	0.717
Sex (male/female)	70/21	10/4	0.655
Race (white/other)	65/26	11/3	0.578
Alcohol use	54	9	0.729
Tobacco use	71	13	0.196
Tumor site (oral cavity/pharynx)	65/28	11/3	0.502
Tumor stage (III/IV)	18/73	1/13	0.252
Tumor grade (I/II/III)	10/45/13	1/4/5	0.617

A: CTRT treatment consisted of pre-operative cisplatin, 20 mg/m2 intravenously for 4 consecutive days during weeks 1, 4, and 7 of radiotherapy.

B: CONTROL treatment consisted of several regimens: cisplatin, 75 mg/m2 intravenously on days 1, 22, and 43 of radiotherapy; carboplatin, 100 mg/m2 and taxol, 45 mg/m2 once per week during radiotherapy; or CTRT regimen following surgery.

Table 1: Clinical Characteristics of 105 Patients Who Received Treatment for Stage III and IV Squamous Cell Carcinoma of the Oral Cavity and Pharynx Between June 1992 and October.

Results

Patient demographics and tumor characteristics for CTRT and control are displayed in Table 1. Of the 105 patients evaluated in this study, 75 had squamous cell carcinoma of the oral cavity and 30 of the pharynx. No significant differences between CTRT and control regarding age, sex, race, alcohol/tobacco use, tumor site, clinical stage, or tumor grade were found. In the CTRT group, 30 patients (33%) had N0 disease, compared to 5 (36%) patients in the control group. The remaining patients had nodal disease: CTRT had 10 (11%) N1 tumors, 26 (29%) N2 tumors, and 25 (28%) N3 tumors; control had 3 (21%) N1 tumors, 3 (21%) N2 tumors, and 3 (21%) N3 tumors. The CTRT patient group had 80% Stage IV carcinoma (73/91) compared to 93% (13/14) in the control group. Primary CTRT tumors were 1 unknown (1.5%), 1 (1.5%) T1, 19 (21%) T2, and 29 (32%) T3, and 41 (45%) T4. Among control primary tumors there were no unknown or T1, 3 (21%) T2, and 6 (43%) T3, and 5 (36%) T4. No patient in this study had distant metastases at the time of primary treatment. No significant differences were found for tumor stage or TNM.

Toxicity from chemotherapy and radiation therapy is displayed in Table 2. Acute morbidity in CTRT included grade III dehydration, bleeding, and/or hospitalization in 12 (13%) patients and grade IV dehydration in 1 (1%) patient. No CTRT patients had grade V toxicity. In control, morbidity included 5 (33%) patients with grade III toxicity,

1 patient (7%) with grade IV clotting, and 1 (7%) patient with grade V hypoxemia. No toxicity was noted in 38% (35) of CTRT patients and in 0% of control patients (P<0.01). High-grade toxicity (grade 3-5) was significantly increased in control compared to CTRT (50% versus 14%; P<0.05). Three CTRT patients did not complete all cycles of chemotherapy. All control patients completed their prescribed cancer treatment. Although the specific application of radiation therapy evolved during the years in which CTRT patients were treated from daily fractionation to IMRT, toxicity and rates of CCR and HCR did not vary throughout the study.

Toxicity Grade	CTRT n=91	CONTROL n=13A	Total	P Value
No toxicity 0	35 (38%)	0-Jan	35	P<0.01
Low grade toxicity 1	21 (23%)	2 (15%)	23	
2	22 (24%)	4 (31%)	26	P=0.475
High grade toxicity 3	12 (13%)	5 (38%)	17	
4	1 (1%)	1 (8%)	2	P=0.130
5	0	1 (8%)	1	
Total	91	13	104	P<0.05
A: 1 Control patient was unavailable for toxicity determination				

Table 2: Toxicity to chemotherapy/radiation therapy (determined by the NCI common terminology criteria for adverse events).

Response to pre-operative treatment is listed in Table 3. A clinically complete response was seen in 73% (66/91) of CTRT patients versus 57% (8/14) in control (P=0.240). Post-chemoradiotherapy biopsy revealed a histologically complete response in 61 out of 91 CTRT patients (67%) and in 8 out of 14 control patients (57%) (P=0.467).

Treatment Response	CTRT n=91	CONTROL n=14	P Value
Clinical Response			
Clinically Complete Response	66 (73%)	8 (57%)	
Partial Response	25 (27%)	6 (43%)	P=0.240
Biopsy Result			
Histologically Complete Response	61 (68%)	8 (57%)	
Residual Disease	30 (33%)	6 (43%)	P=0.467
Type of Surgery			
Radical Surgery	12 (13%)	4 (29%)	
Neck Dissection Only	11 (12%)	0	P=0.072

Table 3: Response to pre-operative treatment.

Curative cancer surgery results are seen in Table 3. CTRT and control did not differ in the number of patients who required curative

surgery (23/91 versus 4/14; P=0.7913). However, 11 of the CTRT patients had neck dissection only (48% of surgeries) and 12 (52%) had composite resection of the primary tumors with neck dissection and reconstruction. In Control, all 4 (100%) operations were radical composite resections. Thus, organ preservation was achieved in 79/91 (87%) of CTRT, but in only 10/14 (71%) of control patients (P=0.136).

Cancer recurrence and survival data are tabulated in Table 4. Median follow-up time was 20 months, with a range from 1 to 128 months. Recurrences developed in 29 out of 91 (32%) CTRT, and in 6 out of 14 (43%) control (P=0.417). The control group had 14% distant metastases, whereas CTRT had 2% distant metastases (P<0.05). Regarding overall survival, 59 out of 91 CTRT patients are still alive, while 6 out of 14 control patients are alive (65% versus 43%; P=0.115). Overall, 21% of CTRT patients died with disease compared to 50% of control patients (P<0.05).

Figure 1 displays the overall Kaplan-Meier survival for patients with squamous cell carcinoma of the oral cavity and pharynx. With a median follow-up of 20 months, survival overall was 62.79% for CTRT and 50.00% in the control group (P<0.57). Disease-free survival is depicted in Figure 2. For CTRT, disease-free survival was 79.07% for CTRT versus 58.33% in control patients (P<0.16).

Patient Characteristics	CTRT n=91	CONTROL n=14	P Value
Dead			
Died with disease	18 (20%)	6 (43%)	
Died disease-free	8 (9%)	0-Jan	P=0.117
Recurrence			
Local	27 (30%)	4 (29%)	
Distant	2 (2%)	2 (14%)	P=0.064

Table 4: Overall survival, end of life status and recurrence data.

Discussion

The results of this study indicate that the simultaneous administration of low-dose fractionated cisplatin chemotherapy and high-dose irradiation (CTRT) may be an effective primary treatment for patients with advanced operable Stage III and IV SCCHN of the oral cavity and pharynx. Toxicity to treatment was significantly lower with CTRT compared with control and with other standard regimens reported in the literature. Biopsy revealed a trend of more histologic complete responses in CTRT compared to control. No differences were found regarding curative surgery; however, organ preservation was achieved in a higher percentage of CTRT patients. CTRT had fewer distant metastases versus control. Furthermore, patients who underwent CTRT remained disease-free and expired of other causes more frequently than did the control group. Lastly, the Kaplan-Meier survival curves indicate a trend toward better disease-free survival among CTRT patients. Our review of the literature indicates that these treatment effects of CTRT on Stage III and IV SCCHN compared with other cancer protocols have not been reported previously and are significant findings of this study.

While clinical adverse events were common among control patients who underwent other treatment regimens for SCCHN, CTRT toxicity was minimal. Only 13% of CTRT patients suffered grade 3 toxicity, 1 patient had grade 4 toxicity, and no patients experienced grade 5 toxicity. In addition, 38% of CTRT patients completed treatment with no toxicity at all. Previously published clinical trials of concomitant chemoradiotherapy almost universally have reported increased toxicities due to the potency of the drug combinations [3]. In their evaluation of high-dose 100 mg/m2 cisplatin on days 2, 16, and 30 of radiotherapy plus 5-FU, Bourhis et al. observed grade 3 and higher toxicity in 83% of their patients [12]. Unfortunately, these very high rates of toxicity also are common among studies of high-dose cisplatin given every three weeks [4,13]. Alternatively, a study with weekly low-dose cisplatin (30 mg/m^2) during radiotherapy still observed grade 3 to 4 mucositis in 35.2% [14]. In contrast, an early pilot investigation of the regimen that became CTRT (20 mg/m2 cisplatin on day 1 to 4 and 22 to 25 of radiotherapy) reported only 27% grade 3 toxicity and no grade 4 or 5 toxicity, similar to the present results [9]. The results of the present study suggest that chemoradiotherapy protocols in treating SCCHN need to move in the direction of low-dose chemotherapy in fractionated administrations so as to improve patient tolerance of pre-operative treatment without compromising therapeutic effectiveness.

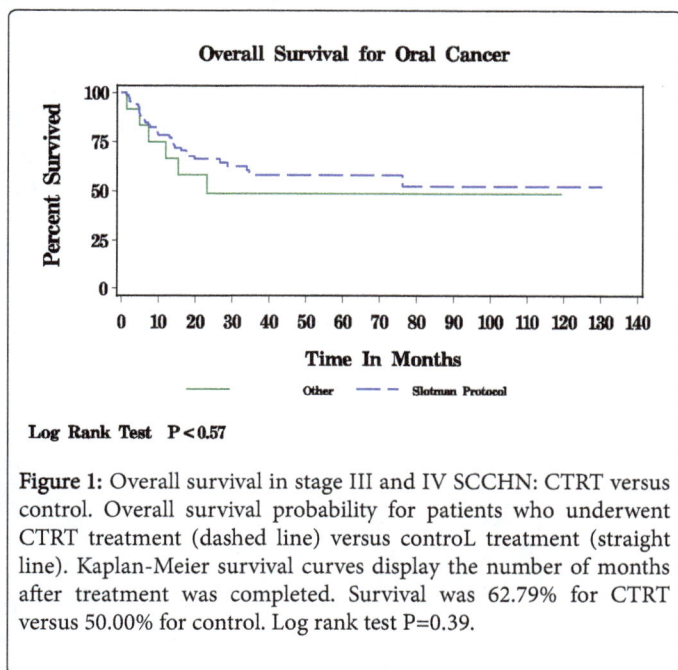

Log Rank Test P < 0.57

Figure 1: Overall survival in stage III and IV SCCHN: CTRT versus control. Overall survival probability for patients who underwent CTRT treatment (dashed line) versus controL treatment (straight line). Kaplan-Meier survival curves display the number of months after treatment was completed. Survival was 62.79% for CTRT versus 50.00% for control. Log rank test P=0.39.

In addition to significantly reducing toxicity, the CTRT chemoradiotherapy combination analyzed in this study resulted in highly effective treatment effects against the cancers. Our complete response rate (CCR) was 73%, and our negative biopsy (as indicated by a histologically complete response (HCR)) was 67%. These outcomes are favorable to those of Paccagnella et al., who treated SCCHN patients with either two cycles of cisplatin 20 mg/m^2, days 1-4, plus 5-FU 800 mg/m^2/day during weeks 1 and 6 of radiotherapy or docetaxel 75 mg/m2 plus cisplatin 80 mg/ M^2, day 1, and 5-FU 800 mg/m^2/day every 3 weeks [15]. The two arms of this study achieved CCR rates of 21.2% and 50%, respectively. Another study tested 100 mg/m^2 cisplatin every 3 weeks plus 5-FU versus the cisplatin regimen plus UFT 200 mg/M^2/d and vinorelbine 25 mg/m2 every 21 days [16]. Again, CCR rates were only 36% and 31%, respectively. Conversely, a pilot CTRT study by Goodman et al. in which patients were treated with cisplatin 20 mg/m2 on days 1 to 4 and 18 to 20 during radiotherapy had an HCR rate of 54% [17]. Consequently, CTRT has significantly better

rates of complete response and negative biopsy than other studies regarding the treatment of SCCHN.

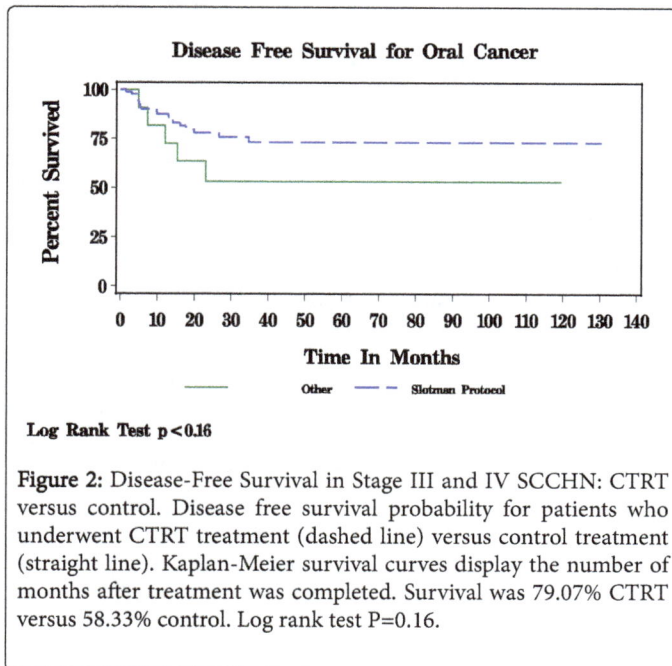

Log Rank Test p < 0.16

Figure 2: Disease-Free Survival in Stage III and IV SCCHN: CTRT versus control. Disease free survival probability for patients who underwent CTRT treatment (dashed line) versus control treatment (straight line). Kaplan-Meier survival curves display the number of months after treatment was completed. Survival was 79.07% CTRT versus 58.33% control. Log rank test P=0.16.

Radical, curative head and neck surgery, with its high complication rates and resulting cosmetic and functional morbidities, has been a major concern in the treatment of SCCHN, particularly in elderly patients. Organ preservation is extremely important to the patient; however, organ function is often compromised when surgery is used to treat SCCHN. Additionally, patients with SCCHN frequently present with unresectable, advanced stage disease at diagnosis [18]. Thus, CTRT was specifically designed to eliminate surgery from the treatment regimen whenever possible. Patients who responded to this treatment not only had a negative biopsy, but also were able to retain full function of their upper aerodigestive tract. Furthermore, only 13% of patients who underwent CTRT required composite resections with complex reconstruction; thus organ preservation was achieved in 87% of CTRT patients. Conversely, a comparison study of two treatments, cisplatin 100 mg/m2 on day 1, 23, and 45 during radiotherapy versus cisplatin 40 mg/m2 weekly for 6 weeks, found that 44.6% and 37% of patients, respectively, required post-treatment surgery [19]. Thus, although CTRT did not differ from control regarding overall surgery, CTRT was more successful in reducing the need for post-treatment surgery when compared to other regimens.

Metastatic disease developed in 2% of the CTRT patients after treatment, while 14% of patients in the control group experienced distant recurrence. The randomized clinical trial reported by Posner et al. documented distant metastasis in 5% of the TPF regimen group and in 9% of the PF group [2]. Thus, the results here indicate that metastatic disease after CTRT distant metastases is comparable to and possibly lower than these published regimens.

The Kaplan-Meier curve for overall survival indicates a disease-free survival for 79% of CTRT patients compared to 58% of control patients at three years post-treatment. Cohen's review of eight prominent chemoradiotherapy studies for advanced stage SSCHN found survival percentages ranging from 17.5% to 55% for three year follow-up periods [3]. In the present investigation, this trend toward increased long-term survival as evidenced by both of the Kaplan-Meier curves for overall survival and disease-free survival suggest that CTRT is comparable with other treatment regimens in terms of survival, and may possibly be more successful. Future studies of CTRT should focus on consistent follow-up with patients for fine to ten years.

There are several limitations in the present study. Of course, a retrospective review is lower on the evidence-based medicine scale than would be a prospective investigation. Incomplete information on individual patients and follow-up data that was not universal restricted analyses, as well. Additionally, the control group was not enrolled by pre-established criteria, and, therefore, varied in the treatments that were applied, resulting in a very heterogeneous array of therapeutic control regimens. Consequently, this study was not a strict two-armed study. Nevertheless, all of the non-CTRT cancer treatments of the control group were currently accepted standard of care for Stage III and IV SCCHN, and thus comprised a reasonably realistic comparison to CTRT. Radiation therapy varied modestly within both patient groups. However, the CTRT chemotherapy regimen was administered consistently. Lastly, the sample sizes were limited by the retrospective nature of the study. F

By comparing the CTRT regimen not only to our control group, but also to other SCCHN regimen publications, the therapeutic benefits of CTRT and their potential for future application are identified. The impressively high CCR and HCR rates achieved in this study while simultaneously reducing toxicity are major improvements to the multi-modality treatment of squamous cell carcinoma of the head and neck. Reduced distant metastases is another positive outcome from CTRT. Lastly, CTRT is comparable in terms of survival with other published regimens, adding effective disease control to minimized adverse treatment effects. Based on the results presented in this paper, we believe that pre-surgery fractionated low-dose cisplatin administered simultaneously with high-dose radiotherapy is a feasible and useful for the management of advance, operable Stage III and Stage IV SCCHN.

References

1. http://www.cancer.org/acs/groups/content/@epidemiologysurveilance/documents/document/acspc-036845.pdf.

2. Posner MR, Hershock DM, Blajman CR, Elizabeth Mickiewicz, Eric Winquist, et al. (2007) Cisplatin and fluoracil alone or with docetaxel in head and neck cancer. NEJM 357: 1705-1715.

3. Cohen EEW, Lingen MW, Vokes EE. (2004) The expanding role of systemic therapy in head and neck cancer J Clin Oncol 22: 1743-1752.

4. Adelstein DJ, Li Y, Adams GL, Wagner H Jr, Kish JA, et al. (2003) An intergroup phase III comparison of standard radiation therapy and two schedules of concurrent chemoradiotherapy in patients with unresectable squamous cell head and neck cancer. J Clin Oncol 21: 92-98.

5. Wolff HA, Overbeck T, Roedel RM, Hermann RM, Herrmann MK, et al. (2009) Toxicity of daily low dose cisplatin in radiochemotherapy for locally advanced head and neck cancer. J Cancer Res Clin Oncol 135: 961-967.

6. Agarwala SS, Cano E, Heron DE, Johnson J, Myers E, et al. (2007) Long-term outcomes with concurrent carboplatin, paclitaxel and radiation therapy for locally advanced, inoperable head and neck cancer. Ann Oncol 18: 1224–1229.

7. Puc MM, Chrzanowski FA, Tran HS, Liu L, Glicksman AS, et al. (2000) Preoperative chemotherapy-sensitized radiation therapy for cervical metastases in head and neck cancer. Arch Otolaryngol Head Neck Surg 126: 337-342.

8. Koness RJ, Glicksman A, Liu L, Coachman N, Landman C, et al. (1997) Recurrence patterns with concurrent platinum-based chemotherapy and accelerated hyperfractionated radiotherapy in stage III and IV head and neck cancer patients. Am J Surg 174: 532-535.

9. Glicksman AS, Wanebo HJ, Slotman G, Li Liu, Christine Landmann, et al. (1997) Concurrent platinum-based chemotherapy and hyperfractionated radiotherapy with late intensification in advanced head and neck cancer. Int J Radiation Oncology Biol Phys 39: 721-729.

10. Greene FL (2002) AJCC Cancer Staging Handbook: From the AJCC Cancer Staging Manual. Springer, New York.

11. National Cancer Institute (2009) Common Terminology Criteria for Adverse Events v4.0. NCI, NIH, DHHS, NIH publication.

12. Bourhis J, Lapeyre M, Tortochaux J, Lusinchi A, Etessami A, et al. (2011) Accelerated radiotherapy and concomitant high dose chemotherapy in non resectable stage IV locally advanced HNSCC: Results of a GORTEC randomized trial Rad Onc 100: 56-61.

13. Castro G, Snitcovsky IML, Gebrim EM, Leitão GM, Nadalin W, et al. (2007) High-dose cisplatin concurrent to conventionally delivered radiotherapy is associated with unacceptable toxicity in unresectable, non-metastatic stage IV head and neck squamous cell carcinoma. Eur Arch Otorhinolaryngol 64: 1475-1482.

14. Rampino M, Ricardi U, Munoz F, Reali A, Barone C, et al. (2011) Concomitant adjuvant chemoradiotherapy with weekly low-dose cisplatin for high-risk squamous cell carcinoma of the head and neck: a phase II prospective trial. Clin Oncol 23: 134-140.

15. Paccagnella A, Ghi MG, Loreggian L, Buffoli A, Koussis H, et al. (2010) Concomitant chemoradiotherapy versus induction docetaxel, cisplatin and 5 fluorouracil (TPF) followed by concomitant chemoradiotherapy in locally advanced head and neck cancer: a phase II randomized study. Ann Oncol 21: 1515-1522.

32

Sublingual Swelling - A Diagnostic Dilemma

Shanmugam VU[1], Vidyachal Ravindra[1*], Ruta Shanmugam[1], Mariappan RG[1], Balaji Swaminathan[1], Prem Nivas[1], Dhanashekaran C[2] and Srinivasan SK[2]

[1]Department of ENT, RMMCH, Annamalai University, Chidambaram, India

[2]Department of Aneasthesia, RMMCH, Annamalai University, Chidambaram, India

*Corresponding author: Vidyachal Ravindra, Post Graduate, Department of ENT, RMMCH, Annamalai University, Chidambaram, India, E-mail: vidyachal3591@gmail.com

Abstract

We report a rare case of sublingual swelling in an 11 month old child which was a diagnostic and surgical challenge. The child presented with a painless, bluish, swelling in the sublingual and submental region with complaints of protrusion of tongue. A pre-operative CT scan was done, but a diagnosis was not truly established. Though it was a case of difficult intubation, surgical excision was done. During surgery Ranula was suspected but histopathological examination revealed it to be Vascular Hamartoma masquerading as a Ranula. Although rare, vascular malformation should be part of differential diagnosis in sublingual and submental swellings.

Keywords Sublingual swelling; Vascular hamartoma; Hemangioma; Lymphangioma

Introduction

Hamartoma is derived from the Greek word hamartia meaning fault or defect and oma denoting tumor. It was coined by Albrecht in 1904 to denote developmental tumor-like malformation [1]. It is defined as a nonneoplastic developmental malformation, comprising of normal mature cells which are native to the anatomic location [1]. Histology shows disorganized architectural pattern with predominance of one of its components. They are common in lung, pancreas, spleen, liver and kidney but very rare in the head and neck region.

It is commonly asymptomatic. But morbidity can arise due to obstruction, infection, infarction, hemorrhage, and rarely due to neoplastic transformation. Deeper masses such as the mass described in this present case, can cause Respiratory and swallowing disturbance. It may occasionally cause life threatening respiratory distress.

Differential diagnostics of neck masses is a challenge. Initially the firm sublingual swelling was assumed to be Pleomorphic Adenoma. But intra-operatively the mass resembled a large Ranula. Post-operative histopathological examination revealed it to be Vascular Hamartoma.

Case Report

We report a rare case of Vascular Hamartoma of the Sublingual Region masquerading as a Ranula. An 11 month old child presented to the ENT OPD with complaints of sublingual swelling of 2 months duration with protrusion of tongue since childhood which was ignored by the parents. Presently, the obstructive nature of the swelling has led to the child to develop difficulty in both respiration and swallowing, which has prompted the parents to come to the hospital. Bimanual palpation revealed a swelling in the floor of the mouth, 3 × 3 cm in size, ovoid in shape, bluish in colour, non-tender and firm in consistency. A provisional differential diagnosis of Ranula, Hemangioma, Lymphangioma, Pleomorphic Adenoma and Congenital Dermoid Cyst was made.

Pre Operative

USG neck

Multi-loculated cystic lesion in Submental Region. Differential Diagnosis-Lymph Cystic Lesion or Plunging Ranula.

CT neck

Hypodense lesion below the mandible in midline displacing the Genioglossus muscle. Extending into the sub-mandibular space. Mylohyoid muscle was pushed down.

The risk of life threatening respiratory distress made surgery necessary. Thus exploration on table with excision was planned under general anesthesia. It was a case of difficult intubation with standby Tracheostomy. Through an external neck incision, swelling was identified on retracting the mylohyoid muscle. Swelling was dissected from its surrounding tissue. Extension into the substance of the tongue was noted. The swelling was removed in toto. Corrugated drain was kept in site. Airway was maintained with Nasopharyngeal airway and Ryle's tube was placed.

Post Operative

Histopathology

Ciliated vascular channels surrounded by fibro-collagenous tissue and skeletal muscle tissue. Final histopathological diagnosis was a Vascular Hamartoma.

Post-operative the child was uneventful and the child was symptomatically better. Nasopharyngeal Airway was removed on the third post-operative day. Ryle's tube was removed on the 6th post-operative day. Residual tongue edema remained. Protrusion of tongue drastically reduced. The floor of mouth swelling resolved and the cervical wound healed normally (Figures 1-4).

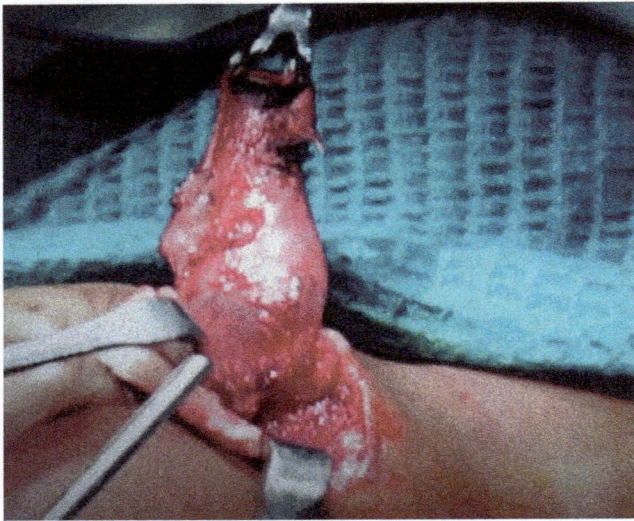

Figure 1: Exposure of the sublingual mass following retraction of Mylohyoid.

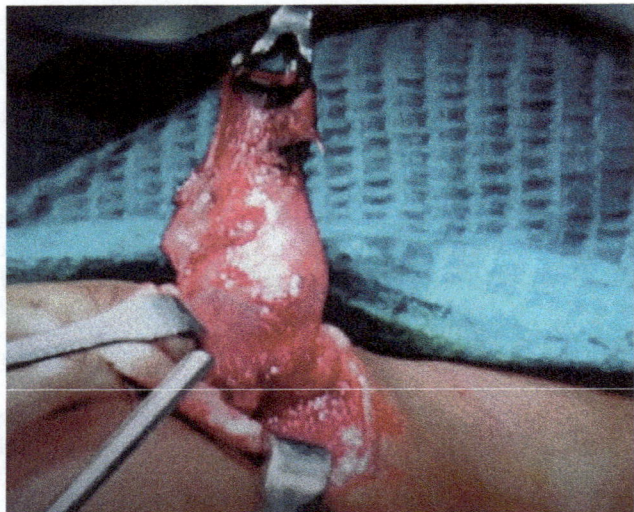

Figure 2: Following dissection of the mass from the surrounding tissue.

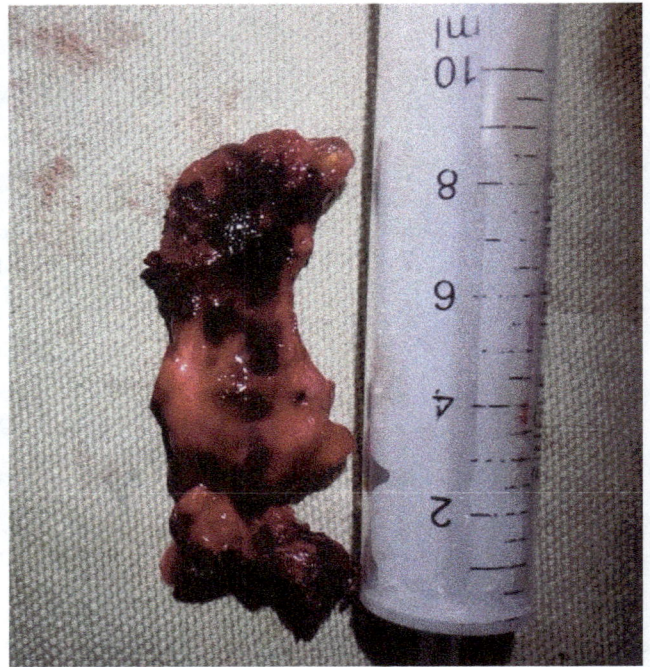

Figure 3: Excised specimen.

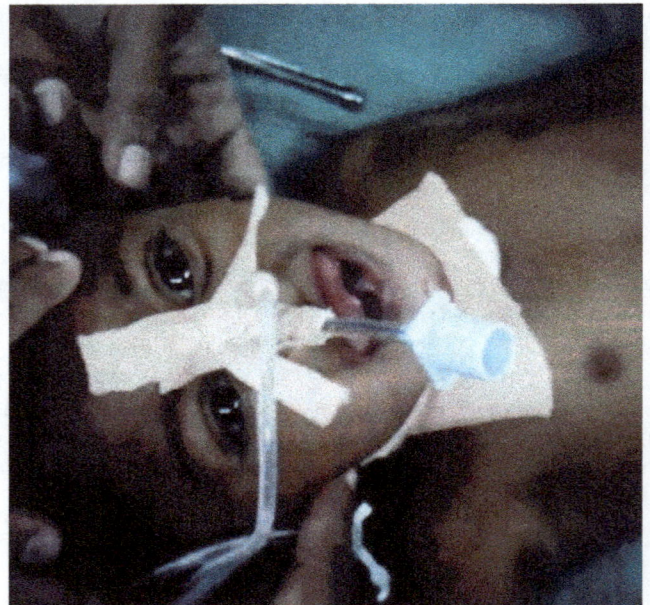

Figure 4: Post-operative picture with nasal airway and Ryle's tube.

Discussion

Vascular Hamartomas are a non-neoplastic abnormality that occurs due to errors in vascular morphogenesis. During organogenesis, abnormalities in the regulating factors can lead to improper proportion and impairment in differentiation [2]. Thus defect in the regulatory pathway of vascular stem cells leads to formation of hamartomatous lesion [2]. They may occur as primary lesion or in association with syndromes such as Sturge-Weber, Klippel-Trenaunary, Proteus Syndrome, Bannayan-Riley-Ruvalcaba Syndrome and Osler-Weber-Rendu Syndrome.

Lymphangioma is a congenital Hamartoma involving the lymphatic system. They are common in the head and neck region but very rare in the oral cavity. They were first described for the first time by Redenbacher in 1828 [3]. In patients less than 20 years of age, they represent 6% of all benign tumors of smooth tissue [3]. Around 50%

are noted at birth and around 90% develop by the age 2 years. Clinically, lymphangiomas of the oral cavity present with a plaque made up of small vesicles with thin walls. These vesicles may be filled with lymph or blood. In the case presented here, these plaques were observed on the lingual surface of the tongue.

Hamartoma are usually exophytic but may rarely present as a flat pigmented lesions. According to a study conducted by Kaplan, though Hamartoma of the oral cavity is very rare, it may occur on the tongue, labial mucosa, buccal mucosa, and median maxillary alveolus.

One of the differential diagnosis that we suspected was a Plunging Ranula. Ranula is a extravasation cyst of the sublingual gland which represents 6% of all oral sialocysts [4]. Plunging Ranula has deep extension beyond the mylohyoid muscle. It can also have massive involvement of the submandibular and parapharyngeal spaces. Its clinical and radiological behavior can be misleadingly similar to other cystic neck masses, particularly the cystic hygroma. But while lymphoid malformations such as Lymphangiomas are present at birth or early childhood, ranulas typically appear in young adults. Both are centered in the submandibular space with a possible continuous extension beneath the free edge of the mylohyoid muscle. Whereas Plunging Ranulas involve only the parapharyngeal and sublingual spaces, lymphangiomas are far more infiltrative, extending further toward the para- and retropharyngeal, carotid, posterior cervical, and visceral spaces and the mediastinum. In case of super-infection or previous surgery the radiological image of the Plunging Ranula can be deceptively similar to lymphangiomas.

In the past, the first line of management of vascular malformations which did not spontaneously involute was radical surgery. One of the disadvantages of radical surgery include injury to muscle and nerves. Furthermore, in toto excision was only possible in about 40% of the cases and these anomalies have a high incidence of recurrence.

Alternative managements like intra-cystic sclero-therapy can lead to disappointing cosmetic and functional result [2]. Presently OK-432 is the preferred intra-lesional sclerosant. It is a lyophilized mixture of low virulent Su Strain of type III group A Streptococcus pyogenes. When administered intra-lesionally it causes inflammation and infiltration with neutrophils and macrophages [5]. In the present case, surgical removal was chosen because of the increasing risk of life threatening respiratory distress and because the possibility of the diagnosis of a Plunging Ranula could not be excluded [6-10].

Conclusion

We report a case of Vascular Hamartoma of the sublingual region masquerading a Plunging Ranula. Although rare, vascular malformation should always be kept in mind in sublingual swellings.

References

1. Patil S, Rao RS, Majumdar B (2015) Hamartomas of the oral cavity. J Int Soc Prev Community Dent 5: 347-353.

2. Kecskes G, Rovo L, Rago P, Katona M, Tornyos S, et al. (2011) Respiratory distress caused by congenital mixed (lymphoid-venous) vascular hamartoma. International Journal of Pediatrics Otorhinolaryngology 6: 229-232.

3. Stănescu L, Georgescu EF, Simionescu C, Georgescu I (2006) Lymphangioma of the oral cavity. Rom J Morphol Embryol 47: 373-377.

4. Mustafa A, Bhokari K, Luqman M, Hameed MS, Kota Z (2013) Plunging ranula: An interesting case report. Open Journal of Stomatology 3:118-121.

5. Athan JJ, Vardhan BG, Muthu MS, Venkatachalapathy, Saraswathy K, et al. (2005) Oral lymphangioma: A case report. J Indian Soc Pedod Prev Dent 23: 185-189.

6. Vohra P, Chandar VV, Patil R, Sharma S (2015) Cavernous hemangioma in the floor of oral cavity masquerading as a ranula. Journal of Indian Academy of Oral Medicine and Radiology 27: 286-90.

7. Arvinder S, Kaur M, Singh S, Chander R, Bhagat S (2013) Giant submental hemangioma: A rare neck mass. Journal of Evolution of Medical and Dental Sciences 2: 9415-9418.

8. Ramdas S, Ramdas A, Ambroise MM, Varghese RG (2015) Submandibular vascular hamartoma with phleboliths mimicking sialolithiasis. Journal of Clinical Sciences 11: 52-4.

9. Kaplan I, Allon I, Shlomi B, Raiser V, Allon DM (2015) A comparative study of oral hamartoma and choristoma. Journal of Interdisciplinary Histopathology 3: 129-134.

10. Corrêa PH, Nunes LC, Johann AC, Aguiar MC, Gomez RS, et al. (2007) Prevalence of oral hemangioma, vascular malformation and varix in a Brazilian population. Braz Oral Res 21: 40-45.

33

Technology Advances in Diagnostics of Vocal Folds Function

Pedersen M*, Akram BH and Agersted AA

The Medical Center Ear, Nose, Throat and Voice Unit, Østergade 18,3 DK 1100 Copenhagen, Denmark

Abstract

There are new aspects in voice research where the patient in the future will benefit from advanced diagnostics. Since a clinical routine with high speed films showed that irregularity of the vocal folds hardly ever was the case, speech therapy for dysfunctions for the vocal fold in many cases was doubted. This was also the case for documentation of irregularity of overtones up to 20.000 Hz with a stable and well documented overtone analyzer. What is next is to bring larynx functions understanding into a position to be part of among others genetic syndrome analysis.

Keywords: Technology advances; Voice; Diagnostics; Treatment

Introduction

The new tools related to high speed films software for clinical use have now been on the market for several years [1]. Combined with electroglottography [2] and kymography, a more nuanced evaluation of the voice is possible. The software includes quantitative measures of the closure of the vocal folds as well as stiffness, a calculation of maximal amplitude versus maximal speed of the vocal folds. Jitter and other measures can also be measured on line on high speed films [3-5]. A new software by the firm Sygyt seems to be clinically feasible to measure overtones exactly and quickly in patients.

Genetic aspects have become in focus as a routine to define the patients' voice related lactose genes [6] and mannose lectin genes [7]. It is not only the vocal folds mucosa which is of interest, but also the whole larynx mucosa. The documentation can till now only be shown in the clinic with the overtone analyzer of the voice (Sygyt Software) before and after treatment. In singers the new aspects are of ectreme importance.

When it comes to treatment - a part from excluding provocations, it seems that the antihistamine fexofenadine is very effective [8] to hinder infections. We know that it hinders swelling and it is an effective prophylaxis in patients with genetic mannose binding lectin, but we need documentation. An aspect for documentation is also to make patients focus on a healthy lifestyle. Other genetics factors should be focused on in the clinical work [9]. It is a problem that in the 1000 multiple genes prospects in Oxford, the voice is not included at all [10], the voice aspects being underrated as a part of verbal communication.

We are focusing on optical coherence tomography [11] as a possible quantitative measure of oedema of the arytenoid region as seen on high speed films in patients with genetic intolerance, allergies and reflux. As in eye diagnostics it is shown to be possible to make economically feasible probes for the larynx at nanometers measurable larynx level [11,12].

Methods of Technical Advances

Analyses are made of a European prize winning female of popular music with high speed films

Software calculations with high speed films (Wolf Ltd.) included

1. Segmentation

2. Kymography

3. Spectral analysis

4. Speed analysis with the formula

$$Stiffness = \frac{max_{tCti}\left(s\left(t\right)\right)}{A_i}$$

Where T_i is the duration of ith cycle in miliseconds (ms), A_i is the dynamic range (max-min) for i^{th} cycle and s(t) is the magnitude of the 1st derivative of considered signal for i^{th} cycle (t C T_i).

Overtones analyses (Sygyt Software, Overtone Analyzer) included

1. Comparison of a normal female voice to a patient voice (non singer)

2. Comparison of a normal female voice to a patient voice (singer).

Results of Technical Advances

With an extremely stable phonovibrogram of a contest winning female singer is presented. Segmentation, kymography, spectral analysis up to 2000 Hz and stiffness analysis (Figures 1-7).

Discussion

It has been discussed if a clinical paradigm shift of understanding larynx functions is underway. There are many new aspects usable online on high speed films, the same is the case with the overtone analyzer where the patients' understanding of what is going on is optimized by comparing on line with a normal male or female voice from the lowest tone to the highest tone, one tone at a time without taking breath in between. The main issue is to document treatment effect of several pharmacological aspects.

The genomic measures bringing voice into the basic genetic communications research for clinical use in the future, is related to our clinical experience with lactose intolerance and mannose binding lectin where patients untreated, are hoarse. They were to be effectively treated

---

*Corresponding author: Pedersen M, The Medical Center Ear, Nose, Throat and Voice Unit, Østergade 18,3 DK 1100 Copenhagen, Denmark; E-mail: m.f.pedersen@dadlnet.dk

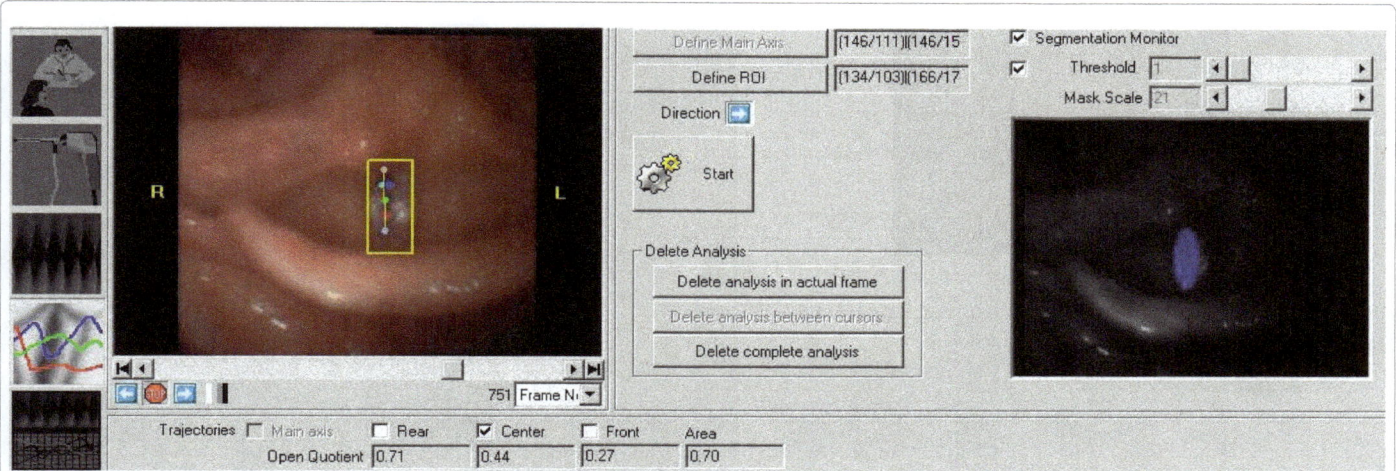

Figure 1: Segmentation of the open quotients are calculated in front – center - rear area - smaller in front between the vocal folds.

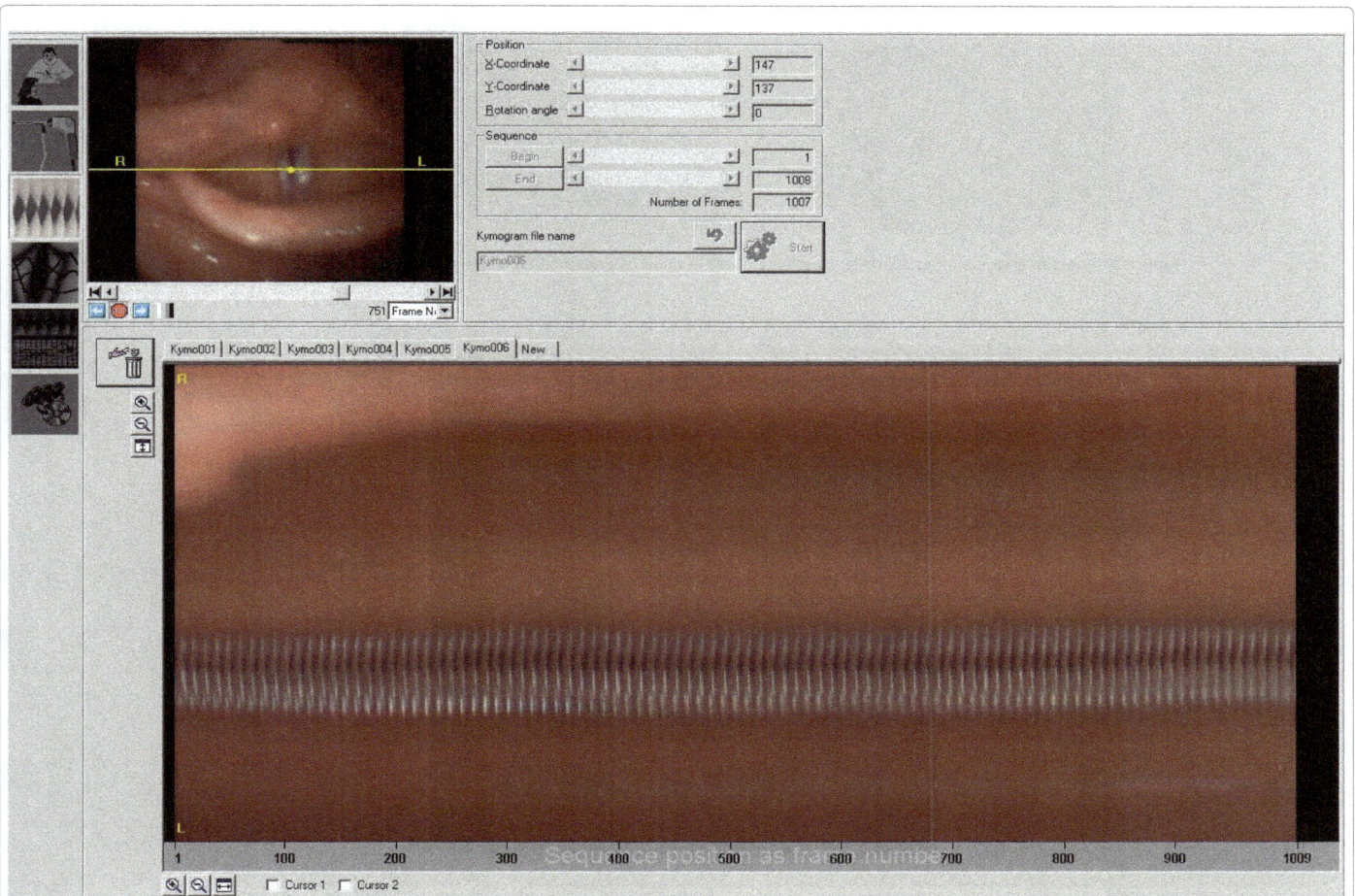

Figure 2: Kymography shows single movements of the vocal folds from above –they are regular.

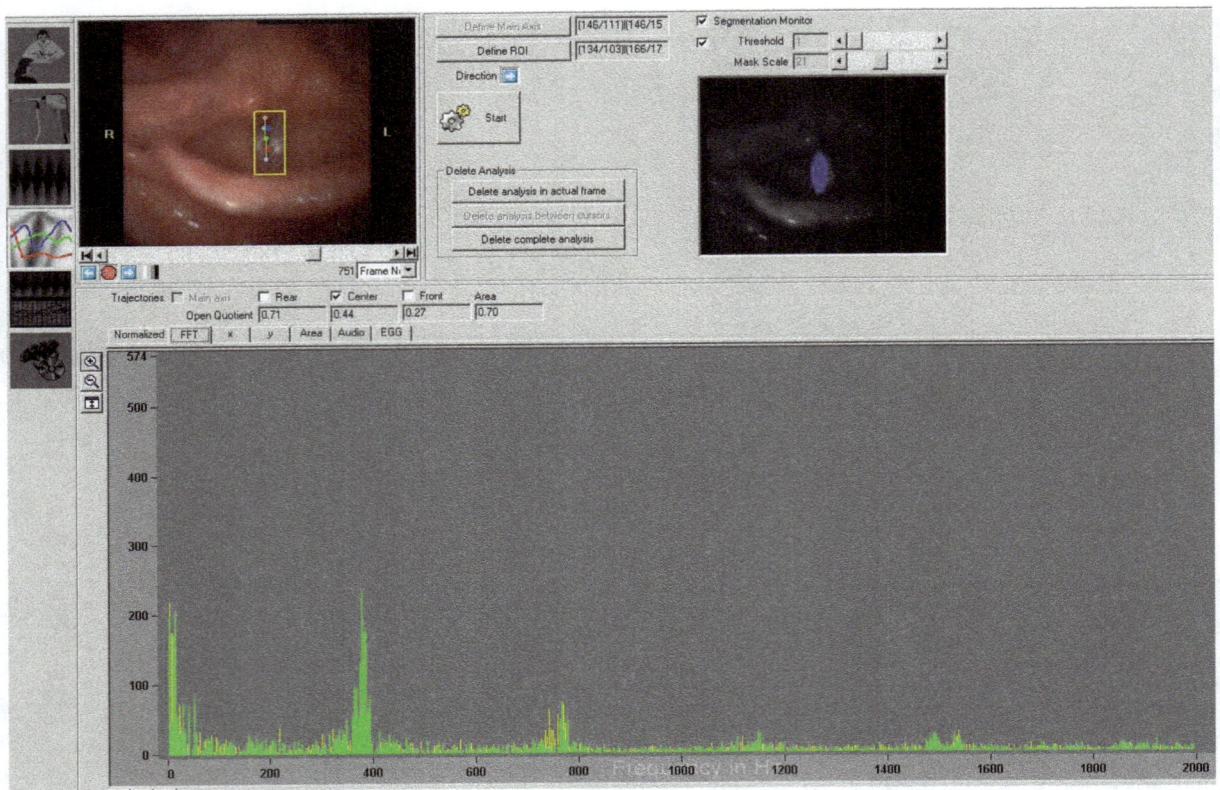

Figure 3: Spectral analysis up to 2000 Hz is extremely well defined as based on high speed films of 4000 pictures per second.

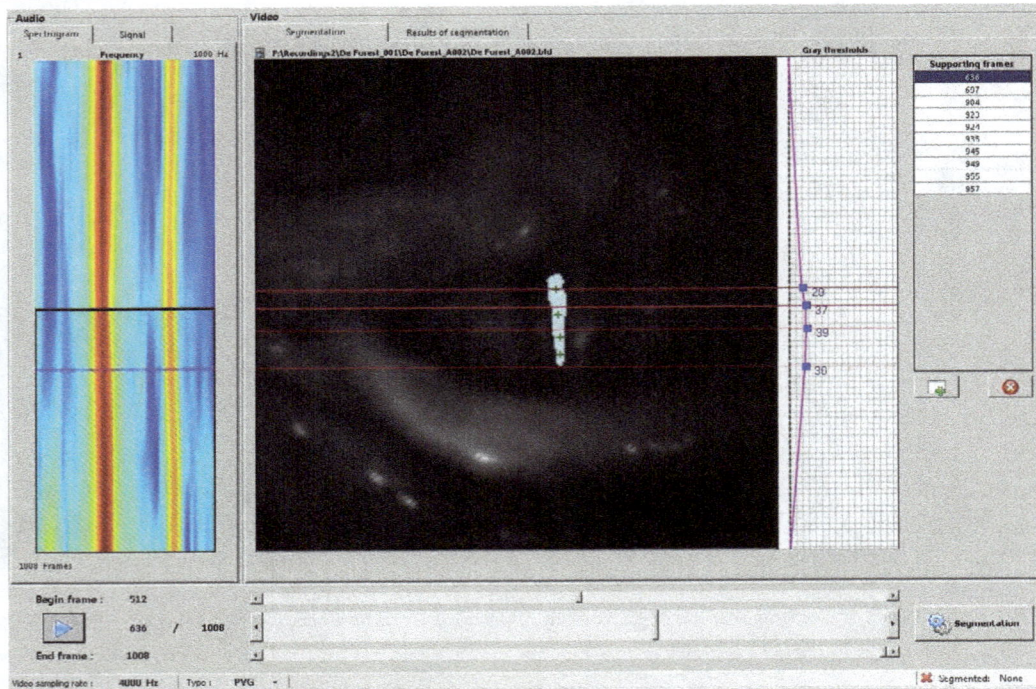

Figure 4: The setup for calculation of measurements of mean stiffness of the Glottal Area Waveform (GAW).

$$Stiffness = \frac{max_{tCti}\left(s(t)\right)}{A_i}$$

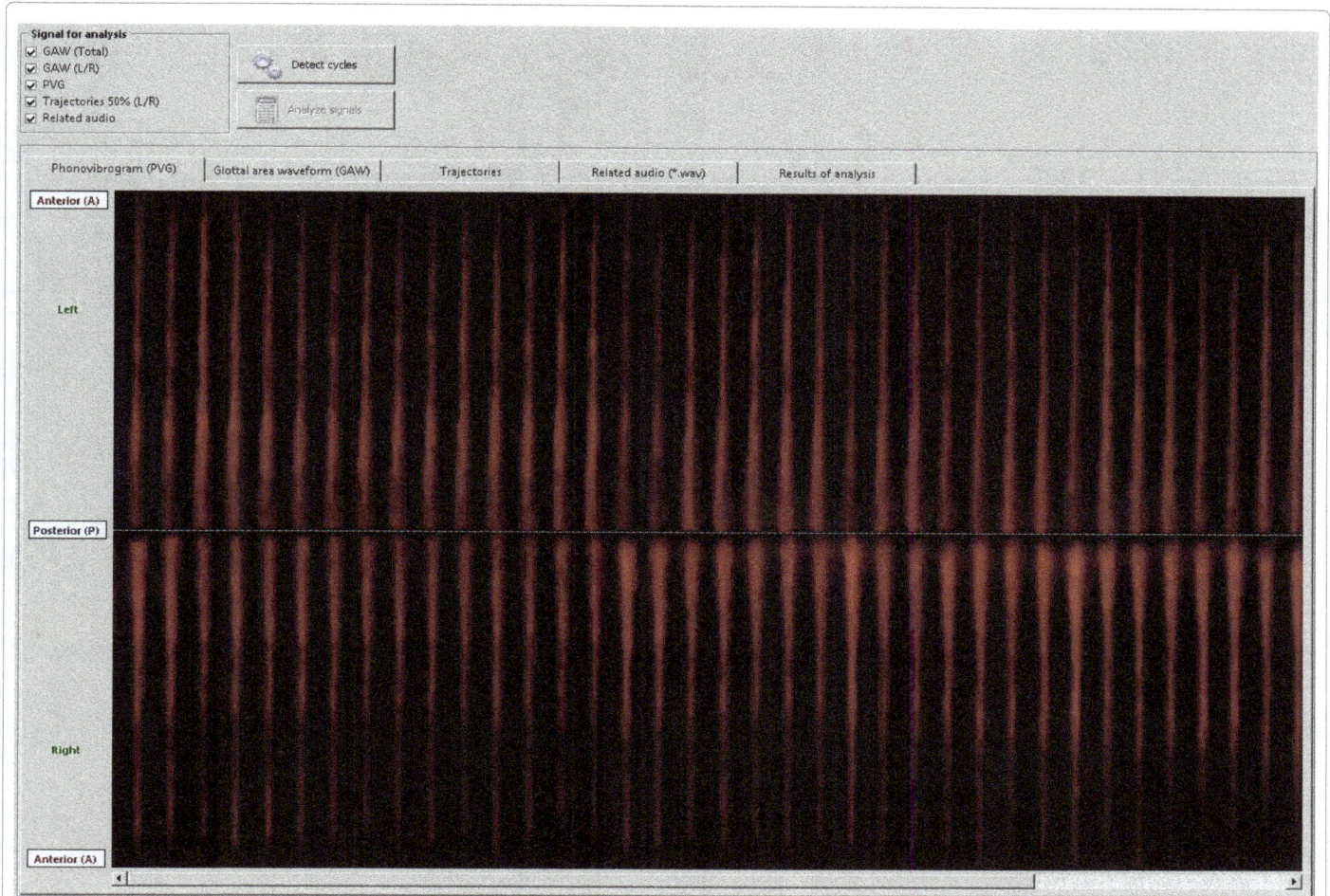

Figure 5: Phonovibrigram of the contest winning female showing the regularity of single movement of the right and left vocal folds. Stiffness analysis: GAW mean 0,38,StD 0,02, min 0,333, max o,413 (average of 30 cycles) GAW right mean 0,391, left 0,483.

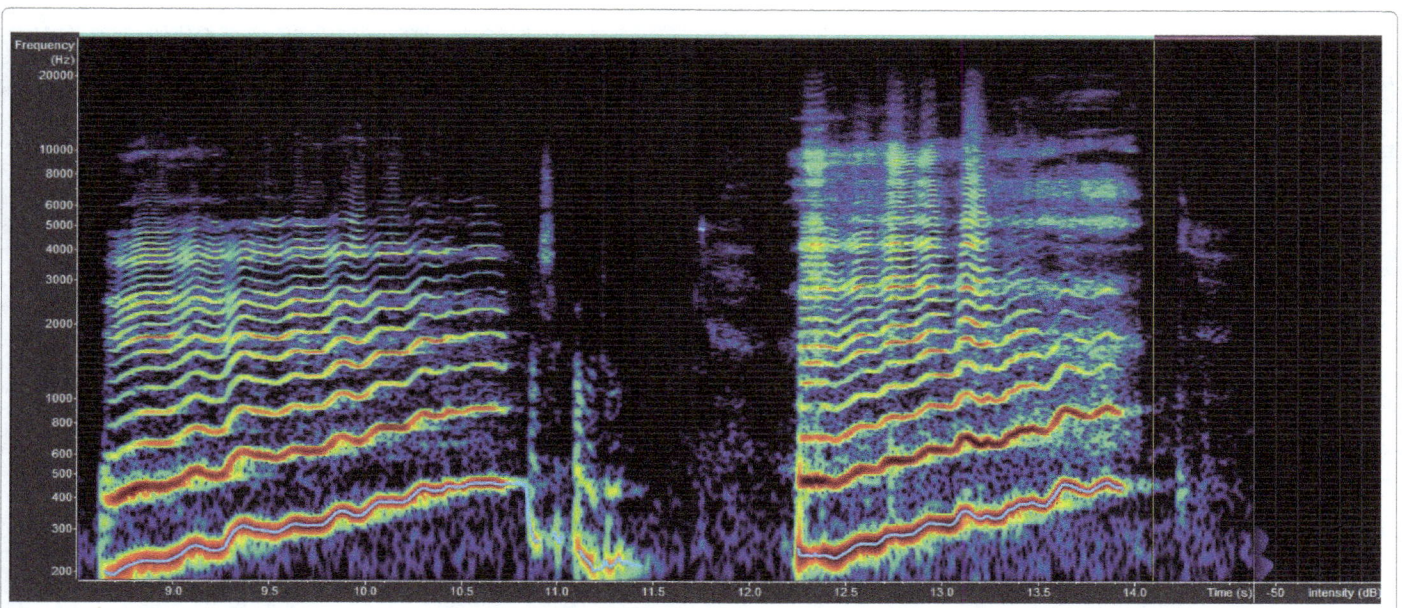

Figure 6: Comparison of a normal female voice (left) to a hoarse female non singer's voice (right), her overtones were less well defined in the upper register (right).

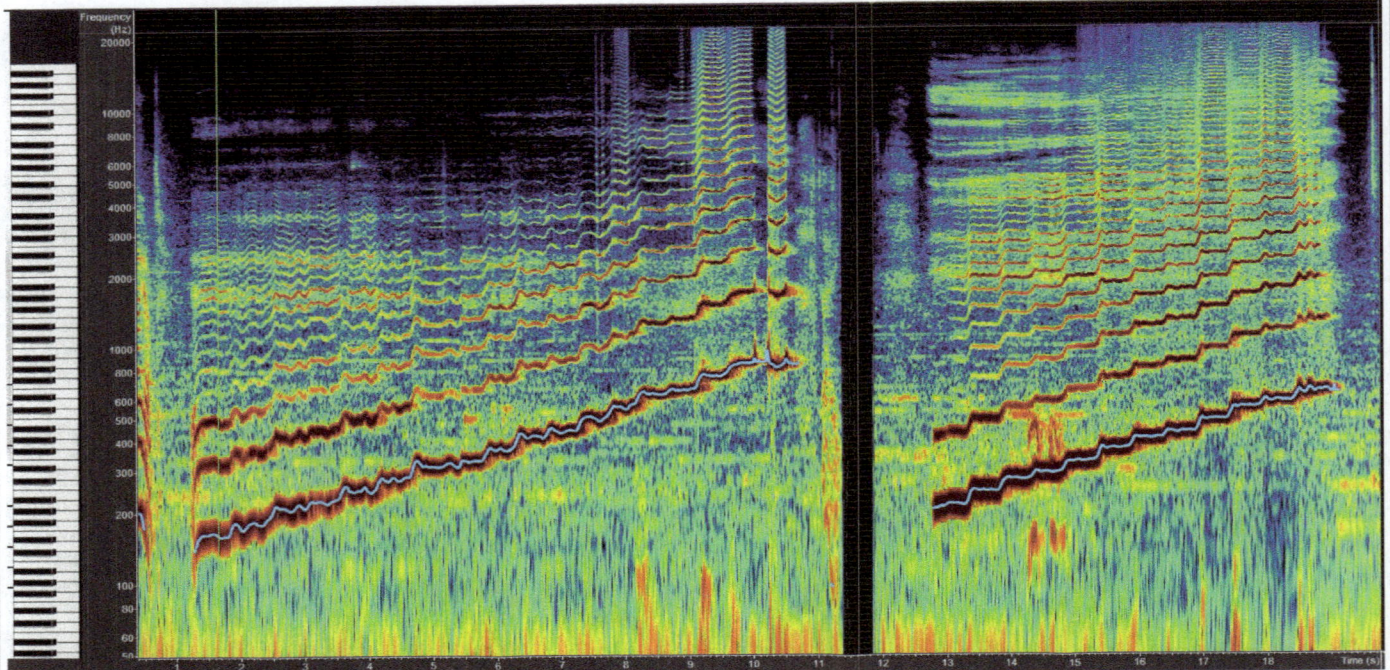

Figure 7: Comparison of a normal female voice (left) to the voice of an acute ill rock singer (right) – the semi tones (first harmonics) in the upper register were weak and she had no semi tones over 600 Hz.

for their hoarseness with lifestyle correction supplemented with the antihistamine fexofenadine as well as local cortisol inhaler in the throat [13,14]. The optical coherence tomography is one of the next steps to document epithelial dysfunctions in the same way as it is done in eye diagnostics and esophageal disorders [12,15].

Conclusion

An approach has been made to present new methods of high speed films and overtone analyses to make refined diagnoses with aspects of treatments of laryngeal disorders including genetics.

References

1. Kunduk M, Doellinger M, McWhorter AJ, Lohscheller J (2010) Assessment of the variability of vocal fold dynamics within and between recordings with high-speed imaging and by phonovibrogram. Laryngoscope 120: 981-987.

2. Pedersen M Fog (1977) Electroglottography compared with synchronized stroboscopy in students of music. The study of sound, Tokyo 18: 423-434.

3. Dollinger M, Berry DA, Huttner B, Bohr C (2011) Assessment of local vocal fold deformation characteristics in an in vitro static tensile test. J Acoust Soc Am 130: 977-985.

4. Banjara H, Mungutwar V, Singh D, Gupta A (2014) Objective and subjective evaluation of larynx in smokers and nonsmokers: a comparative study. Indian J Otolaryngol Head Neck Surg 66: 99-109.

5. Lohscheller J, Svec JG, Dollinger M (2013) Vocal fold vibration amplitude, open quotient, speed quotient and their variability along glottal length: kymographic data from normal subjects. Logoped Phoniatr Vocol 38: 182-192.

6. Zhao J, Fox M, Cong Y, Chu H, Shang Y, et al. (2010) Lactose intolerance in patients with chronic functional diarrhoea: the role of small intestinal bacterial overgrowth. Aliment Pharmacol Ther 31: 892-900.

7. Pedersen M, Eeg M (2012) Does treatment of the laryngeal mucosa reduce dystonic symptoms? A prospective clinical cohort study of mannose binding lectin and other immunological parameters with diagnostic use of phonatory function studies. Eur Arch Otorhinolaryngol 269:1477-1482.

8. Pedersen M (2014) Future aspects of cellular and molecular research in clinical voice treatment. Guest editorial. Advances in Cellular and Molecular Otorhinolaryngology 2: 24442.

9. Pedersen M (2014) Chapter 1.1.18, Genetics, European Manual of Phoniatrics In press.

10. 1000 Genomes Project Consortium, Abecasis GR, Auton A, Brooks LD, DePristo MA, et al. (2012) An integrated map of genetic variation from, 092 human genomes. Nature 491: 56-65.

11. Burns JA (2012) Optical coherence tomography: imaging the larynx. Curr Opin Otolaryngol Head Neck Surg 20: 477-481.

12. Munk MR, Sacu S, Huf W, Sulzbacher F, Mittermuller TJ, et al. (2014) Differential diagnosis of macular edema of different pathophysiologic origins by spectral domain optical coherence tomography. Retina 34: 2218-2232.

13. Pedersen M (2014) Acoustical Voice Measurements did Change after Treatment in Patients with Laryngo-Pharyngeal Reflux: A Prospective Randomized Study including MDVP (Laryngograph Ltd.). Journal of Rhinolaryngo-Otologies 2: 13.

14. Martinucci I, de Bortoli N, Savarino E, Nacci A, Romeo SO, et al. (2013) Optimal treatment of laryngopharyngeal reflux disease. Ther Adv Chronic Dis 4: 287-301.

15. Evans JA, Poneros JM, Bouma BE, Bressner J, Halpern EF, et al. (2006) Optical coherence tomography to identify intramucosal carcinoma and high-grade dysplasia in Barrett's esophagus. Clin Gastroenterol Hepatol 4: 38-43.

34

The Effectiveness of Epinastine Hydrochloride for Pediatric Sleep-Disordered Breathing Related Symptoms Caused By Hyperesthetic Non-Infectious Rhinitis

Hirotaka Hara*, Kazuma Sugahara, Takefumi Mikuriya, Makoto Hashimoto, Shinsaku Tahara and Hiroshi Yamashita

Department of Otolaryngology, Yamaguchi University Graduate School of Medicine, Ube, Japan

Abstract

Objectives: The aims of this study were to prospectively evaluate the effectiveness of oral epinastine hydrochloride in pediatric outpatients with Sleep-Disordered Breathing- (SDB) related symptoms caused by hyperesthetic non-infectious rhinitis, and to assess their Quality of Life (QOL) prior to and following treatment.

Study design: Prospective

Methods: Pediatric outpatients (9 boys and 10 girls; average age, 5.6 years [SD=1.4]), with SDB related symptoms influenced by hyperesthetic non-infectious rhinitis were recruited. The children were all treated with oral epinastine hydrochloride dry syrup for 4 weeks. Before and after the 4-week treatment period, the following data were collected from each participant: otolaryngological findings, obstructive sleep apnea-18 (OSA-18) scores, and evaluation of QOL.

Results: Epinastine hydrochloride significantly improved the swelling of the inferior nasal turbinate mucosa and decreased the quantity of nasal discharge. The initial total mean OSA-18 score was 58.5, whereas the total score reduced to 22.8 after oral epinastine hydrochloride treatment. Significant ($p < 0.01$) differences were found between pre- and post-treatment total OSA-18 scores as well as pre- and post-treatment measurements of domains of sleep disturbance, physical symptoms, and caregiver concerns.

Conclusions: Epinastine hydrochloride therapy may improve nasal findings and QOL in pediatric outpatients with SDB related symptoms caused by hyperesthetic non-infectious rhinitis.

Keywords: Epinastine hydrochloride; Pediatrics; Hyperesthetic non-infectious rhinitis; Allergic rhinitis; Sleep-disordered breathing; OSA-18

Introduction

Sleep-Disordered Breathing (SDB), which includes Obstructive Sleep Apnea (OSA) syndrome and upper airway resistance syndrome, refers to a spectrum of sleep disorders sufficiently intense to cause clinical symptoms.

The exact prevalence of SDB in children is unknown, but the prevalence of OSA is approximately 2% [1]. Studies have shown that the Quality of Life (QOL) of children with OSA syndrome can be affected, and there is now evidence that children with this syndrome may have emotional problems, impaired school performance, hyperactivity, aggressive behavior, or withdrawal behavior [2,3].

The children with nasal and paranasal sinus diseases represented by allergic rhinitis and sinusitis results in nasal breathing disorder and causes sleep disorder breathing easily. Especially in Japan, the prevalence of pediatric allergic rhinitis has been increasing [4]. Polysomnography of children with allergic rhinitis showed that more microarousals compared to control group [5]. Also, the frequency of OSA in children was increased in subjects with positive multi antigen Radio Allegro Sorbent Test (RAST) results compared to those with negative RAST results [6]. Those reports suggested that the relationship between allergic rhinitis and OSA. On the other hand, Arens et al. [7] reported that children with OSA had significantly more opacification of maxillary sinuses, sphenoid sinuses, prominence of inferior nasal turbinate(s), and deviation of the nasal septum and those results suggested the relationship between OSA and paranasal diseases.

A frequent cause of OSA in children is pharyngeal and palatine tonsillar hyperplasia, which causes nasal obstruction and chronic mouth breathing. For this reason, the initial recommended treatment for pediatric OSA is surgical removal of the adenoids and tonsils. However, the frequency of residual mild OSA after adenotonsillectomy is estimated at 45-50% [8-10]. When residual OSA after adenotonsillectomy exists, other approaches are advocated. Rizzi et al. [11] reported that there was a significant correlation (P<0.005) between total nasal resistance and snoring, oral breathing and daytime sleepiness in SDB children. Sullivan et al. [12] reported that the effectiveness of radiofrequency treatment of inferior nasal turbinates against the residual OSA after adenotonsillectomy. Therefore, we hypothesized that the oral anti-allergic drugs for allergic rhinitis would be effective for pediatric SDB caused by hyperesthetic non-infectious rhinitis which includes allergic rhinitis.

The aim of our study was (1) to evaluate the effectiveness of epinastine hydrochloride, a second-generation antihistamine used to treat allergic rhinitis in Japan, for children with symptoms of Sleep-Disordered Breathing (SDB) caused by hyperesthetic non-infectious rhinitis (allergic rhinitis) and (2) to assess, using the questionnaire, the children's QOL prior to and following treatment.

*Corresponding author: Hirotaka Hara, Department of Otolaryngology, Yamaguchi University Graduate School of Medicine, Ube, Yamaguchi, Japan; E-mail: harahiro@yamaguchi-u.ac.jp

Methods

The study protocol was approved by the local Ethics Committee (Yamaguchi Society for allergic disease in otolaryngology, Ube, Japan). The prospective cross-sectional study was conducted between April, 2007 and October, 2007. We studied patients who came to the twenty-four Otolaryngology Outpatient Clinic in Yamaguchi Prefecture, Japan and written informed consents were obtained from all patients. Inclusion criteria were pediatric patients ranged between 3 to 7 years old who presented with both SDB related symptoms during sleep like snore, witnessed apnoeas, frequent arousals, nocturnal sweating, failure to thrive, hyper extended neck, and allergic rhinitis defined as hyperesthetic non-infectious rhinitis by Japanese Guideline for Allergic Rhinitis.

The hyperesthetic non-infectious rhinitis is characterized by hypersensitivity [4]. However, this type of rhinitis is not inflammatory, except for the allergic rhinitis. Therefore, this should reasonably be eliminated from the classification of rhinitis and regarded as a disease similar to allergy or hypersensitivity diseases. However, this was placed into this classification in view of potential clinical convenience.

Exclusion criteria were patients with hypersensitivity against the epinastine hydrochloride, palatine tonsillar hypertrophy, bronchial asthma and/or atopic dermatitis for which treatment was being administered.

All of the children were administered oral epinastine hydrochloride dry syrup (0.05 g/kg, once a day before sleep) for 4 weeks. Before the treatment, complete ear, nose, and throat physical examinations were performed. Sleep studies for diagnose of OSA were not examined.

The QOL of the patients was assessed by asking the patients' caregivers to complete the OSA-18 survey [13] before and 4 weeks after treatment. The OSA-18 survey (Figure 1) consists of 18 items grouped into 5 domains: sleep disturbances (4 items), physical suffering (4 items), emotional distress (3 items), daytime problems (3 items), and caregiver concerns (4 items). The score for each item is 1-7, ranging from "none" to "all of the time." The classification of health-related impact on QOL from the total OSA-18 scores was recommended by Franco et al. [13]. A total score of less than 60 suggests a small impact, whereas scores between 60 and 80 suggest a moderate impact, and scores above 80 suggest a large impact. Wilcoxon rank-sum test were used to evaluate the relationship between patients' QOL, as defined by the OSA-18 scores, and intake of epinastine hydrochloride.

We also conducted a rhinoscopic examination to evaluate the effects of epinastine hydrochloride on inferior nasal turbinate mucosal swelling and nasal discharge before and 4 weeks after treatment. Mucosal swelling and nasal discharge were rated according to the "The Practical Guideline of Management of Allergic Rhinitis criteria" [14]. The extent of inferior nasal turbinate mucosal swelling and nasal discharge was scored (Table 1) before and after epinastine hydrochloride treatment and evaluated with Wilcoxon rank-sum test.

Results

Twenty-one children with hyperesthetic non-infectious rhinitis and sleep-disordered breathing were included in the study. Two subjects did

None of the time	Hardly any of the time	A little of the time	Some of the time	A good bit of the time	Most of the time	All of the time
1	2	3	4	5	6	7

Sleep Disturbance
During the past 4 weeks, how often has your child had...
...loud snoring?
...breath holding spells or pauses at night?
...choking or made gasping sounds while asleep?
...restless sleep or frequent awakenings from sleep?

Physical Symptoms
During the past 4 weeks, how often has your child had...
...mouth breathing because of nasal obstruction?
...frequent colds or upper respiratory infections?
...nasal discharge or a runny nose?
...difficulty in swallowing food?

Emotional Distress
During the past 4 weeks, how often has your child had...
...mood swings or temper tantrums?
...aggressive or hyperactive behavior?
...discipline problems?

Daytime Function
During the past 4 weeks, how often has your child had...
...excessive daytime sleepiness?
...a poor attention span or concentration?
...difficulty getting up in the morning?

Caregiver Concerns
During the past 4 weeks, how often have the problems described above...
...caused you to worry about your child's general health?
...created concern that your child is not getting enough air?
...interfered with your ability to perform daily activities?
...made you frustrated?

MAXIMUM SCORE: 126

Figure 1: OSAS quality of life survey (OSA-18). [8]

Nasal Findings	Score			
	3	2	1	0
Inferior nasal turbinate mucosal swelling	Middle turbinate not seen	Intermediate between (3) and (1)	To centre of middle turbinate	None
Nasal discharge	Filled	Intermediate between (3) and (1)	Small amount adhered to the skin	None

Table 1: Nasal finding score.

Subjects (n = 19)	Mean of pre-treatment scores	Mean of post-treatment scores	Wilcoxon rank-sum test P value
Inferior nasal Turbinate mucosal swelling	2.1 ± 0.40	1.1 ± 0.87	<0.001
Nasal discharge	1.52 ± 0.77	0.74 ± 0.99	0.01

Table 2: Pre and post treatment nasal finding scores.

Domain	Mean of pre-treatment scores	Mean of post-treatment scores	Wilcoxon rank-sum test Pvalue
Sleep disturbances	13.7 ± 9.8	5.0 ± 6.2	0.003
Physical symptoms	14.3 ± 9.9	6.0 ± 7.4	0.006
Emotional distress	10.4 ± 8.6	4.4 ± 5.1	0.015
Daytime problems	8.1 ± 8.4	4.2 ± 6.3	0.12
Caregiver concern	12.1 ± 12.2	3.3 ± 3.9	0.007
Total OSA	58.5 ± 42.1	22.8 ± 24.6	0.003

Table 3: Pre- and post-treatment total and domain OSA-18 scores.

not return the questionnaires after the 4-week treatment; therefore, 19 subjects (9 boys and 10 girls; average age, 5.6 years (SD=1.4)), were evaluated. Epinastine hydrochloride significantly reduced the swelling of the inferior nasal turbinate mucosa and decreased the quantity of nasal discharge. The score for both swelling and nasal discharge significantly decreased after the 4-week treatment ($p<0.001$ and 0.01) (Table 2). Furthermore, the initial total mean OSA-18 score was 58.5; whereas this score reduced to 22.8 after four weeks of oral epinastine hydrochloride treatment. The differences in the total OSA-18 scores, the domains of sleep disturbance, physical symptoms, and caregiver concerns between the start of the study and after 4 weeks of treatment with epinastine hydrochloride were significant (p values=0.003, 0.006, 0.007, and 0.003; Table 3).

Discussion

OSA syndrome is characterized by interactions between nocturnal episodic hypoxemia, hypercapnia, and sleep fragmentation. It is important to emphasize here that delayed treatment of or untreated OSA may result in irreversible morbidity [15]. Gozal et al. reported that in rodent models of OSA oxidative stress and inflammatory processes increase neuronal cell loss in the brain regions responsible for learning, behavior, executive function, and memory [15-18]. Therefore, in addition to OSA symptom severity, the extent of end-organ morbidity may be accounted for by genetic variances in defense mechanisms and injury-related pathways.

The initial recommended treatment for pediatric OSA is surgical removal of the adenoids and tonsils. However, the frequency of residual mild OSA after adenotonsillectomy is estimated at 45-50%, with an additional 20-25% displaying moderate-to-severe OSA after surgery and only 25-35% has no symptoms. When residual OSA after adenotonsillectomy is moderate-to-severe, administration of nasal continuous positive airway pressure (CPAP) is usually recommended [19]. However, the cost–benefit ratio of CPAP in milder cases of residual OSA does not justify its use, and other approaches are advocated.

The effectiveness of nasal steroids against allergic rhinitis has been reported [20-22], but there are few reports concerning the effectiveness of oral anti-allergic drugs for children with allergic rhinitis-induced

SDB. In this study, we evaluated the effect of epinastine hydrochloride on both the improvement in nasal findings, as determined by The Practical Guideline of Management of Allergic Rhinitis criteria [14] and the QOL, which was assessed by the OSA-18 survey. Polysomnography was not performed because it is expensive and difficult to perform due to the small number of sleep technicians in our prefecture.

Epinastine hydrochloride is a second-generation antihistamine used in Japan for allergic rhinitis. Okuda and Okubo reported that in a multicenter, randomized, double-blind, placebo-controlled study in children with perennial allergic rhinitis randomly allocated to receive either epinastine or ketotifen for 2 weeks, the total nasal symptom severity scores were -1.42 for those children treated with epinastine [23]. Okubo and Gotoh also reported that, when used during a nasal provocation test with Japanese cedar pollen allergen, epinastine hydrochloride significantly decreased the number of sneezing attacks and the quantity of nasal discharge for 3 h after drug administration as compared to the placebo [24]. In our study, as in previous reports, epinastine hydrochloride significantly decreased both the swelling of the inferior nasal turbinate mucosa and the quantity of nasal discharge. Both the nasal finding scores for swelling and nasal discharge significantly decreased after the 4-week treatment.

It is well known that the association between SDB and allergic rhinitis appears strongest in children. Epinastine hydrochloride improved swelling of the nasal mucosa and reduced nasal discharge. As a result, nasal obstruction improved and the total mean score of the OSA-18 reduced significantly. The effect of second generation anti-histamine drugs for nasal obstruction is limited, but the nasal cavities of children are narrow and easy to obstruct by a small amount of nasal discharge. Therefore, the epinastine hydrochloride significantly improved the nasal obstruction.

In this study, we used the Japanese translation of the OSA-18. To ensure that the questionnaire had been correctly translated into Japanese, we created an English translation of the Japanese version and verified the accuracy of the translation with the author of the OSA-18. Prior to this study, we also used the Japanese version of the OSA-18 to evaluate the QOL of 5 pediatric SDB patients (age range, 3-7 years; median age, 4.6 years) after adenoidectomy or adenotonsillectomy

[25]. According to the results of the OSA-18, 4 of the children who underwent tonsillectomy or adenotonsillectomy showed improvement in physiological parameters of sleep and in QOL; however, 1 child displayed worsened physiological parameters of sleep after surgery due to re-enlargement of the adenoid, and a decrease in QOL was identified through the OSA-18. Our results demonstrated that the Japanese translation of the OSA-18 must be useful for the evaluation of QOL in SDB children.

Several options have been reported for the medical management of allergic rhinitis-induced OSA in children. Nasal steroids may be beneficial, but they are not recommended for long-term therapy [21]. Nasal steroids may be prescribed temporarily until a referral can be made for treatment. Systemic steroids are occasionally used to decrease upper airway obstruction, such as in patients with infectious mononucleosis (because of anti-inflammatory and lymphocytic effects). One study suggested that systemic steroids failed to affect the size of the tonsils or adenoids, the severity of inflammation as shown on polysomnography, or the symptomatology in patients with OSA [26].

Anti-inflammatory therapy is increasingly being recognized as an alternative to surgery and as an effective intervention in residual mild OSA after adenotonsillectomy. Daily montelukast treatment for 16 weeks was shown to significantly improves adenoid size and polysomnography-recorded, respiratory-related sleep disturbances [27]. While double-blind, placebo-controlled studies have yet to be reported, the use of montelukast for mild SDB before or after adenotonsillectomy is a useful contribution to the currently available therapies for treating SDB in children. A combination of nasal steroids and oral montelukast for 12 weeks has been shown to normalize sleep respiratory parameters in an open-label study conducted in children with residual mild SDB after adenotonsillectomy (Apnea hypopnea index between 1 and 5) [28].

Only a few reports have suggested that effective treatment against nasal congestion of perennial allergic rhinitis improves the quality of sleep. In a study conducted by Santos et al. [29] in a small cohort of subjects (N=31), compared to placebo, the leukotriene receptor antagonist montelukast improved the symptoms of perennial allergic rhinitis and reduced daytime fatigue and daytime somnolence in patients with perennial allergic rhinitis. According to the results of our study, epinastine hydrochloride improved the symptoms of hyperesthetic non-infectious rhinitis and reduced the domains of sleep disturbance of OSA-18. Therefore epinastine hydrochloride is another candidate for alternative therapy for mild OSA.

Our study had several limitations that should be considered. First, we did not administer an allergy test to the children; therefore, object is defined as hyperesthetic non-infectious rhinitis patients. However, judging from frequency, almost all patients were thought to have allergic rhinitis. Further, our study consisted of patients recruited from 24 outpatient clinics in our prefecture; therefore, patient selection was well randomized. Second, any kind of sleep study was not performed. In Japan, due to small numbers of sleep technicians and other social reasons, polysomnography has not been commonly used in children. We are now planning a study in this area with video recording in the near future.

Conclusions

Epinastine hydrochloride therapy demonstrated positive clinical effects on both nasal findings and the QOL of pediatric outpatients with symptoms of SDB caused by allergic rhinitis. Epinastine hydrochloride therapy may be a candidate for anti-inflammatory therapy for allergic rhinitis-induced SDB.

Acknowledgment

We are grateful to the individuals and parents who participated in this study. We would like to thank Hideki Inoue, M.D., Shiro Endo, M.D., Masahiko Ogata, M.D., Yoshihiko Okinaka, M.D., Hiroshi Orita, M.D., Koichiro Kanaya, M.D., Keiko Kanesada, M.D., Yuko Kobayashi, M.D., Hajime Sano, M.D., Shigeko Takemoto, M.D., Kuniyoshi Tanaka, M.D., Tetsuya Tahara, M.D., Yasuhiko Tahara, M.D., Mitsuji Tamura, M.D., Yuko Nagasue, M.D., Keiko Nishikawa, M.D., Masayoshi Nitta, M.D., Takashi Hakuno, M.D., Masaaki Hiyoshi, M.D., Tetsuji Hori, M.D. and Mitsuie Masuda, M.D. for help recruiting subjects.

References

1. Marcus CL (2001) Sleep-disordered breathing in children. Am J RespirCrit Care Med 164: 16-30.

2. Ali NJ, Pitson DJ, Stradling JR (1993) Snoring, sleep disturbance, and behaviour in 4-5 year olds. Arch Dis Child 68: 360-366.

3. Gozal D (1998) Sleep-disordered breathing and school performance in children. Pediatrics 102: 616-620.

4. Okubo K, Kurono Y, Fujieda S, Ogino S, Uchio E, et al. (2011) Japanese guideline for allergic rhinitis. AllergolInt 60: 171-189.

5. Lavie P, Gertner R, Zomer J, Podoshin L (1981) Breathing disorders in sleep associated with 'microarousals' in patients with allergic rhinitis. ActaOtolaryngol 92: 529-533.

6. McColley SA, Carroll JL, Curtis S, Loughlin GM, Sampson HA (1997) High prevalence of allergic sensitization in children with habitual snoring and obstructive sleep apnea. Chest 111: 170-173.

7. Arens R, Sin S, Willen S, Bent J, Parikh SR, et al. (2010) Rhino-sinus involvement in children with obstructive sleep apnea syndrome. PediatrPulmonol 45: 993-998.

8. Mitchell RB, Kelly J (2004) Outcome of adenotonsillectomy for severe obstructive sleep apnea in children. Int J PediatrOtorhinolaryngol 68: 1375-1379.

9. Guilleminault C, Huang YS, Glamann C, Li K, Chan A (2007) Adenotonsillectomy and obstructive sleep apnea in children: a prospective survey. Otolaryngol Head Neck Surg 136: 169-175.

10. Mitchell RB, Kelly J (2007) Outcome of adenotonsillectomy for obstructive sleep apnea in obese and normal-weight children. Otolaryngol Head Neck Surg 137: 43-48.

11. Rizzi M, Onorato J, Andreoli A, Colombo S, Pecis M, et al. (2002) Nasal resistances are useful in identifying children with severe obstructive sleep apnea before polysomnography. Int J PediatrOtorhinolaryngol 65: 7-13.

12. Sullivan S, Li K, Guilleminault C (2008) Nasal obstruction in children with sleep-disordered breathing. Ann Acad Med Singapore 37: 645-648.

13. Franco RA Jr, Rosenfeld RM, Rao M (2000) First place--resident clinical science award 1999. Quality of life for children with obstructive sleep apnea. Otolaryngol Head Neck Surg 123: 9-16.

14. Committee for Practical Guidelines for the management of Allergic Rhinitis (2002) [V. Treatment.] Practical guidelines for management of Allergic rhinitis, 4th edn. Tokyo: Life Science 29-44 (in Japanese).

15. Gozal D, Pope DW Jr (2001) Snoring during early childhood and academic performance at ages thirteen to fourteen years. Pediatrics 107: 1394-1399.

16. Kheirandish L, Gozal D, Pequignot JM, Pequignot J, Row BW (2005) Intermittent hypoxia during development induces long-term alterations in spatial working memory, monoamines, and dendritic branching in rat frontal cortex. Pediatr Res 58: 594-599.

17. Row BW, Liu R, Xu W, Kheirandish L, Gozal D (2003) Intermittent hypoxia is associated with oxidative stress and spatial learning deficits in the rat. Am J RespirCrit Care Med 167: 1548-1553.

18. Xu W, Chi L, Row BW, Xu R, Ke Y, et al. (2004) Increased oxidative stress is associated with chronic intermittent hypoxia-mediated brain cortical neuronal cell apoptosis in a mouse model of sleep apnea. Neuroscience 126: 313-323.

19. Kheirandish-Gozal L, Gozal D (2008) Intranasal budesonide treatment for children with mild obstructive sleep apnea syndrome. Pediatrics 122: e149-155.

20. Nixon GM, Brouillette RT (2002) Obstructive sleep apnea in children: do intranasal corticosteroids help? Am J Respir Med 1: 159-166.

21. Brouillette RT, Manoukian JJ, Ducharme FM, Oudjhane K, Earle LG, et al. (2001) Efficacy of fluticasone nasal spray for pediatric obstructive sleep apnea. J Pediatr 138: 838-844.

22. Demain JG, Goetz DW (1995) Pediatric adenoidal hypertrophy and nasal airway obstruction: reduction with aqueous nasal beclomethasone. Pediatrics 95: 355-364.

23. Okuda M, Okubo K (2003) Double-blind comparative study of Epinastine dry syrup with Ketotifen dry syrup in children with perennial allergic rhinitis. PracticaOto-rhino-laryngologica Suppl114:1-21.

24. Okubo K, Gotoh M (2006) Inhibition of the antigen provoked nasal reaction by second-generation antihistamines in patients with Japanese cedar pollinosis. AllergoInt 55: 261-269.

25. Miyauchi Y, Hara H, Yamashita H (2005) The effect of tonsillectomy or adenotonsillectomy on quality of life in pediatric sleep-disordered breathing patients. Stomato-pharyngol 18:469-475 (in Japanese).

26. Al-Ghamdi SA, Manoukian JJ, Morielli A, Oudjhane K, Ducharme FM, et al. (1997) Do systemic corticosteroids effectively treat obstructive sleep apnea secondary to adenotonsillar hypertrophy? Laryngoscope 107: 1382-1387.

27. Goldbart AD, Goldman JL, Veling MC, Gozal D (2005) Leukotriene modifier therapy for mild sleep-disordered breathing in children. Am J RespirCrit Care Med 172: 364-370.

28. Kheirandish L, Goldbart AD, Gozal D (2006) Intranasal steroids and oral leukotriene modifier therapy in residual sleep-disordered breathing after tonsillectomy and adenoidectomy in children. Pediatrics 117: e61-66.

29. Santos CB, Hanks C, McCann J, Lehman EB, Pratt E, et al. (2008) The role of montelukast on perennial allergic rhinitis and associated sleep disturbances and daytime somnolence. Allergy Asthma Proc 29: 140-145.

35

The Effect of Tonsillectomy on the Salivary Immune Factors

Mohamad A. Bitar*

Department of ENT Surgery, The Children's Hospital at Westmead, Sydney Medical School, University of Sydney, Sydney, Australia

Abstract

Background & objectives: The effect of tonsillectomy on the immune system is a controversial issue. The debate is largely based on contradictory findings in the literature. However, it is unlikely for tonsils to produce a negative systemic effect and it is more logical to think about a local effect that can be transient or long lasting. The aim of this systematic review is to analyze the observed changes in salivary immune factors following tonsillectomy and understand their clinical significance.

Materials & methods: Systematic review of the English literature was performed using Medline, Embase and Cochrane. We used the terms tonsillectomy, adenotonsillectomy, humoral immunity, immune system, saliva in various combination to look for pertinent studies. We excluded duplicate publications, reviews and studies that did not analyze salivary immune factors.

Results: Thirty four manuscripts studied the effect of tonsillectomy on the immune system. Only 9 of them (including 585 patients) looked at the effect on salivary immune factors. All studies analyzed the effect on salivary Immunoglobulin (Ig) A, four of them studied additional factors such as other salivary Ig's, anti-microbial proteins (lactoferrin, peroxidases, lysozyme), anti-viral and anti-bacterial Ig's. One study showed a significant decrease in salivary IgA, another showed a decrease in salivary IgG and a third showed a decrease in salivary IgM, lactoferrin and antimicrobial salivary IgG. Two studies had non-conclusive concerns regarding the observed changes in salivary immune factors, the third study recommended measuring salivary IgA pre and postoperatively. Only 11.1% of the studied patients had on the short term, a significant decrease in SecIgA level that can be attributed to tonsillectomy.

Conclusion: Tonsillectomy does not seem in general to negatively affect the host's salivary immune defenses. The concerns raised are based on a partial apparent down-regulation of the some of the salivary immune components. More longitudinal studies are needed to really understand the clinical effect of any observed change in the salivary immune system.

Introduction

In their critical position at the entrance of the aerodigestive tract, the palatine tonsils play an important role in sampling antigens directly from the epithelial surfaces. The number of bacteria shed into the saliva reaches 100 billion per day in healthy individuals [1]. A healthy environment is maintained in the oral cavity by adequate salivary flow to clear the microbes and by the various local immune factors, in which the tonsils are believed to play an important role [2]. The architecture of the tonsils resembles that of a lymph node in having antigen-presenting cells, T cells, B cells [3]. The palatine tonsils produce antibodies locally and distally through their migrating B cells. They are quite active in the pediatric age group when their size is most prominent knowing that the size is directly proportional to the number of tonsillar B and T cells [4].

Though the tonsils' role in local immunity cannot be underestimated, they are not the only source of salivary immune factors. These factors are synthesized in the salivary glands (e.g. secretory IgA, salivary peroxidase) or originate from both the glands and the blood stream (lysozyme, lactoferrin, and IgM). In addition oral polymorphonuclear leukocytes can release significant amounts of myeloperoxidase, lysozyme, and lactoferrin [2]. On the other hand, there is limited data on the role of tonsils in the immune and non-immune protection of the oropharyngeal area [3].

To better understand the role of tonsils in local oropharyngeal immunity, we underwent a systematic review of the English literature regarding the effect of tonsillectomy on the salivary immune factors.

Methods

A systematic review of the English literature was performed using Medline, Embase and Cochrane. We used the terms tonsillectomy, adenotonsillectomy, humoral immunity, immune system, immunity, saliva to look for pertinent studies. We reviewed the abstract of all articles that studied the effect of tonsillectomy on the immune system. We included in the review only the studies that included salivary immune factors among the studied parameters. We only analyzed the salivary components of the immune system in the reviewed articles. We excluded duplicate publications, reviews and studies that did not include actual measurements of the salivary immune factors (e.g. descriptive studies or those using only questionnaires). We looked at the age of the studied patient, the presence of a control group and or preoperative testing, and the timing of postoperative testing. We attempted to perform a meta-analysis where feasible.

Results

Our search identified 34 manuscripts that studied the effect of

*Corresponding author: Mohamad A. Bitar, Department of ENT Surgery, The Children's Hospital at Westmead, Locked Bag 4001, Westmead, NSW 2560, Australia; E-mail: mbitar-md@hotmail.com

tonsillectomy on the immune system (Figure 1). Of these only 9 (including 585 patients) looked at the effect of tonsillectomy on the salivary immune factors [5-13]. All studies analyzed the effect on salivary Immunoglobulin (Ig) A, four of them studied additional factors such as other salivary Ig's, anti-microbial proteins (lactoferrin, peroxidases, lysozyme), anti-viral and anti-bacterial Ig's (Table 1). One study showed a significant decrease in salivary IgA, another showed a decrease in salivary IgG and a third showed a decrease in salivary IgM, lactoferrin and antimicrobial salivary IgG (Table 2). Two studies had non-conclusive concerns regarding the observed changes in salivary immune factors, the third study recommended measuring salivary IgA pre and postoperatively (Table 1).

As SIgA was the most commonly studied salivary immune factor, it was analyzed by pooling all the results (Table 3). Because there was heterogeneity in the normal reference value for SIgA and some compared postoperative values to controls while others to preoperative values, it was decided to report the values as normal (when normal or above normal) or abnormal (when considered below normal). Only 15.7% of the studied patients had an abnormally low SIgA level. However, in one of the studies that abnormality was present preoperatively which confound the real effect of tonsillectomy. Omitting that study in the analysis will result in having only 11.1% of the patients experiencing a significant decrease in SecIgA level secondary to tonsillectomy.

Discussion

The saliva is a rich medium of microbial and a mixture of anti microbial and immune factors. These factors are supplied via the surrounding blood vessels, the salivary glands and lymphoid tissues. The role of the palatine tonsils in the immune system in general and in the local oropharyngeal immunity in particular has long raised concerns about the immunological sequalae of tonsillectomy. There is no doubt that the tonsils play an important role in the immune defense mechanism of the upper aero-digestive tract.

The tonsils' crypts, which increase the tonsillar surface area up to 300cm^2 are populated by lymphocytes (50-65% B cells, most of which are memory B- cells) forming the lymphoepithelium area. Other cells present include T cells, macrophages, and dendritic cells [4,14]. Unlike lymph nodes, tonsils do not possess afferent lymph vessels; instead antigens are captured directly by epithelial cells known as M cells. M cells capture antigens via endocytosis, translocate them to the basal

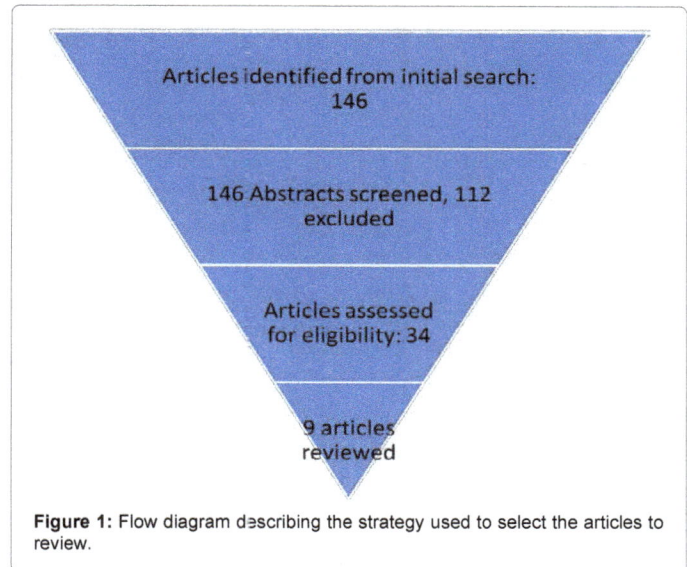

Figure 1: Flow diagram describing the strategy used to select the articles to review.

membrane, then exocytose them intact in intraepithelial spaces [4,15]. This will induce a cascade to activate the primary immune response. This immune reaction is transmitted to the extrafollicular area where T-B lymphocytes interaction generate a long lasting immune response by stimulating differentiation and proliferation of B lymphocytes that move to the lymphoid follicles and act as founder cells in germinal centers [16].

Tonsillar secondary immune response is characterized by a small germinal center reaction and a large extrafollicular plasma cell reaction. Memory B cells in the crypt epithelium play an important role in generating a rapid secondary immune response. In fact, they have a strong antigen presenting ability enabling them to activate memory T helper cells in the crypt epithelium rapidly [4,14,16-18].

Though the main immune role of the tonsils is local, the tonsils are connected to the body immune system through trafficking of immune cells. The naïve T and B cells are transported into the tonsils via the high endothelial venules present in the extrafollicular regions, while plasmablasts migrate from the tonsils via efferent lymphatic vessels that drain in the cervical lymph nodes [4,16]. They then can join the

Authors / Year	Studied immune factors	Conclusion
1) Veltri et al. [5]	Salivary IgA	Tonsillectomy does not modify host's salivary IgA
2) Ostergaard [6]	Salivary IgA, IgG, IgM	No effect of tonsillectomy on salivary IgA level Significant decrease in salivary IgG
3) D'Amelio et al. [7]	Salivary IgA	No negative effect of tonsillectomy on salivary IgA
4) Cantani et al. [8]	Salivary IgA	Recommend measuring salivary IgA level before and after tonsillectomy
5) Lenander-Lumikari et al. [9]	Salivary IgA, IgG, and IgM; salivary anti-microbial proteins lactoferrin, salivary peroxidase, myelo-peroxidase; antibodies against viral antigens and streptococcus mutans	Tonsillectomy does not impair the antimicrobial capacity of human saliva
6) Del Rio-Navarro et al. [10]	Salivary IgA	No negative effect of tonsillectomy on salivary IgA
7) Kirstila et al. [11]	Salivary Ig's (IgA, IgG, and IgM), anti-Streptococcus mutans, anti-viral Ig's, lysozyme, lactoferrin, peroxidases, thiocyanate, hypothiocyanate, agglutinin	Tonsillectomy does not notably impair the saliva-mediated host defence mechanisms. Some concerns were raised regarding some decrease in some immune factors.
8) Jung et al. [12]	Salivary IgA	No significant changes in the local immune system after tonsillectomy
9) Childers et al. [13]	Salivary IgA, Ag-specific salivary IgA in whole and parotid specific saliva	Tonsillectomy does not decrease the salivary IgA level. The increase in parotid saliva specific IgA needs to be explored

Ig, immunoglobulin

Table 1: Reviewed studies and their conclusions.

Study	No	Age (y)	Control	Postop testing (months)	Findings
1) Veltri et al. [5]	17	2-10	Preop levels	1, 3, 9 to 12	**Preop** Normal **Postop** SIgA was not affected
2) Ostergaard [6]	27	6-11	27 Controls Preop levels	30	**Preop:** SIgA significantly lower than controls **Postop:** SIgA increased but level was no significantly different from preop SIgG decreased significantly compared to preop level
3) D'Amelio et al. [7]	274	16-24	726 controls	NS	**Postop:** SIgA levels were non- significantly different
4) Cantani et al. [8]	65	2-11	Preop levels	1	**Preop:** Normal SIgA levels **Postop:** SIgA levels decreased significantly beyond normal.
5) Lenander-Lumikari et al. [9]	53	5-8	Normal children	48	**Postop:** - Higher levels of SIg's, lactoferrin and myeloperoxidase - No difference in anti S mutans IgA and IgG - Higher antibodies level against viruses
6) Del Rio-Navarro et al. [10]	33	3-13	Preop levels	1-4, 5-12, > 12 weeks	**Postop:** SIgA significantly increased
7) Kirstila et al. [11]	25	15-34	Preop levels	1 and 6	**Postop:** At 1month: SIg's levels decreased, but only significantly for IgM. At 6months: - SIgA returned to normal, SIgG increased but SIgM remained low - Non-Ig salivary defense factors remained normal except for lactoferrin -No change in antiviral SIg's except for SIgG against EBV which decreased significantly. -No change of anti Streptococcus mutans SIg's except for SIgG which decreased
8) Jung et al. [12]	66	<4->19	Preop levels 60 controls	1	**Postop:** SIgA decreased to control levels
9) Childers et al. [13]	25	4.4-12.8	25 controls	6-14	**Postop:** - No significant difference in total and specific whole saliva SIgA from controls - Significantly higher levels of specific SIgA in parotid specific saliva

Preop, preoperative; postop, postoperative; SIg, salivary immunoglobulin;

Table 2: Details and results of the reviewed studies.

Study	No	Control	Preop level	Postop level	Time of testing
1) Veltri et al. [5]	17	-	Normal	Normal	Up to 12 months
2) Ostergaard [6]	27	Yes	Abnormal	Abnormal	30
3) D'Amelio et al. [7]	274	Yes	-	Normal	Not specified
4) Cantani et al. [8]	65	-	Normal	Abnormal	1
5) Lenander-Lumikari et al. [9]	53	Yes	-	Normal	48
6) Del Rio-Navarro et al. [10]	33	-	Not specified	Normal	Up to > 12 weeks
7) Kirstila et al. [11]	25	-	Not specified	Normal	Up to 6 months
8) Jung et al. [12]	66	Yes	Not specified	Normal	1
9) Childers et al. [13]	25	Yes	-	Normal	6-14 months

Preop, preoperative; postop, postoperative; SIg, salivary immunoglobulin;

Table 3: Meta-analysis of SIgA levels.

circulation and disseminate to the upper airway mucosa, regional exocrine glands (e.g. lacrimal and salivary glands) and to a lesser extent to the gut mucosa [17].

The effect of tonsillectomy on the systemic immune system is controversial though recent studies showed no significant effect [19-21]. However, it is unclear if tonsillectomy would result in compromising the local immune defenses.

During this review, it was interesting to find that most of the studies that looked at the effect of tonsillectomy on the immune system focused primarily on the systemic humoral and cellular immunity. Only quarter of the published studies dealt with salivary immune factors, especially SIgA; meaning that we need more studies in that field. Though the results of the reviewed studies are reassuring, one should be cautious about considering that this issue has been answered. That is mainly due to the heterogeneity in the way these studies were conducted in terms of

timing of postoperative testing, the presence or absence of controls and sometimes considering the preoperative values as a control reference though it was not always clear if these preoperative values were actually normal compared to control levels.

Despite that, it is reassuring to see that only 2 out of the 9 studies (Cantani et al. [9] and Kirstila et al. [12]) raised some concerns about a negative effect of tonsillectomy on some salivary immune factors with Cantani A et al advising measuring SIgA levels prior and following tonsillectomy [9]. This recommendation can not be adopted without further longitudinal studies in that field to clarify what really happens months to years after tonsillectomy. In fact, Kirstila et al. [12] actually demonstrated a rise in SIgA level 6 months after tonsillectomy following an initial drop at 1 month (similar to Cantani et al. findings). This means that the salivary immune system can compensate for the loss of the tonsillar tissues several months postoperatively.

The most commonly studied salivary immune factor is SIgA which was shown to remain within normal levels in 84.3%. Mind you that in Ostergaard PA study [7], the level of SIgA was already abnormally low preoperatively; which make us doubt that tonsillectomy caused that.

Conclusion

Tonsillectomy does not seem in general to negatively affect the host's salivary immune defenses. The concerns raised are based on a partial apparent down-regulation of the some of the salivary immune components. More longitudinal controlled studies are needed to really understand the clinical effect of any observed change in the salivary immune system.

References

1. Loesche WJ (1988) Ecology of the oral flora in Oral Microbiology and Immunology. MG Newman, R Nisengard eds. Philadephia: WB Saunders Co 351-66.

2. Tenovuo J (1989) Non-immunoglobulin defense factors in human saliva, in Human Saliva: Clinical Chemistry and Microbiology, Vol II, J Tenovuo ed. Boca Raton, FL: CRC Press Inc 55-91.

3. Brandtzaeg P. Immune functions of human nasal mucosa and tonsils in health and disease. In: Bienenstock J, ed. Immunology of the lung and upper respiratory tract. New York: McGraw-Hill,1984: 28–95

4. Nave H, Gebert A, Pabst R (2001) Morphology and immunology of the human palatine tonsil. Anat Embryol (Berl) 204:367-373.

5. Veltri RW, Sprinkle PM, Keller SA, Chicklo JM (1972) Immunoglobulin changes in a pediatric otolaryngic patient sample subsequent to T & A. J Laryngol Otol 86:905-916

6. Ostergaard, PA (1977) IgA levels and carrier rate of pathogenic bacteria in 27 children previously tonsillectomized. Acta pathol. microbiol. scand., C, Immunol 85: 178-186

7. D'Amelio R, Palmisano L, Le Moli S, Seminara R, Aiuti F (1982) Serum and salivary IgA levels in normal subjects: comparison between tonsillectomized and non-tonsillectomized subjects. Int Arch Allergy Appl Immunol 68: 256-259.

8. Cantani A, Bellioni P, Salvinelli F, Businco L (1986) Serum immunoglobulins and secretory IgA deficiency in tonsillectomized children. Ann Allergy 57: 413-416.

9. Lenander-Lumikari M, Tenovuo J, Puhakka HJ (1992) Salivary antimicrobial proteins and mutans streptococci in tonsillectomized children. Pediatr Dent 14: 86-91.

10. Del Rio-Navarro BE, Torres S, Barragan-Tame L (1995) Immunological effects of tonsillectomy/adenectomy in children. Adv Exp Med Biol 371B: 737-739.

11. Kirstila V, Tenovuo J, Ruuskanen O, Suonpaa J, Meurman O, et al. (1996) Longitudinal analysis of human salivary immunoglobulins, nonimmune antimicrobial agents, and microflora after tonsillectomy. Clin Immunol Immunopathol 80: 110-115.

12. Jung KY, Lim HH, Choi G, Choi JO (1996) Age-related changes of IgA immunocytes and serum and salivary IgA after tonsillectomy. Acta Otolaryngol Suppl 523: 115-119.

13. Childers NK, Powell WD, Tong G, Kirk K, Wiatrak B, et al. (2001) Human salivary immunoglobulin and antigen-specific antibody activity after tonsillectomy. Oral Microbiol Immunol 16: 265-269.

14. Brandtzaeg P (2003) Mucosal immunity in infectious disease and allergy. International Congress Series 1257: 11-20.

15. Casselbrant ML (1999) what is wrong in chronic adenoitis/ tonsillitis anatomical considerations. Journal of Pediatric Otorhinolaryngology 49: S133- S135.

16. Van Kempen MJ, Rijkers GT, Van Cauwenberge PB (2000) The immune response in adenoids and tonsils. Int Arch Allergy Immunol 122:8-19

17. Brandtzaeg P, Baekkevold ES, Farstad IN, Jahnsen FL, Johansen FE, et al. (1999) Regional specialization in the mucosal immune system: What happens in the microcompartments? Immunology Today 20: 141-151.

18. Brandtzaeg P (1996) The B-cell development in tonsillar lymphoid follicles. Acta Oto-laryngologica.Supplementum 523: 55-59.

19. Kaygusuz I, Alpay HC, Godekmerdan A (2009) Evaluation of long-term impacts of tonsillectomy on immune functions of children: a follow-up study. Int J Pediatr Otorhinolaryngol. 73: 445-449.

20. Nasrin M, Miah MR, Datta PG (2012) Effect of tonsillectomy on humoral immunity. Bangladesh Med Res Counc Bull 38: 59-61.

21. Santos FP, Weber R, Fortes BC (2013) Short and long term impact of adenotonsillectomy on the immune system. Braz J Otorhinolaryngol 79: 28-34.

36

Treatment of Obstructive Sleep Apnea Syndrome through Orthodontics and Orthognathic Surgery

Omar Shafic Ayub[1], Bruno Ayub[2*], Priscila Vaz Ayub[3], Dirceu Barnabé Ravelli[4], Paulo Domingos Ribeiro[5] and Margareth da Silva Coutinho[6]

[1]Department of Orthodontics and Dentofacial Orthopedics, Dentistry, Federal University of Mato Grosso do Sul - UFMS, Campo Grande, Brazil

[2]University of Franca - UNIFRAN, Franca, Brazil

[3]Orthodontics at the São Paulo State University - UNESP, Araraquara, Brazil

[4]Orthodontics, São Paulo State University - UNESP, Araraquara, Brazil

[5]Department Surgery and Traumatology, Disciplines Sacred Heart University - USC, Bauru, Brazil

[6]Department of Dentistry at the Federal University of Mato Grosso do Sul - UFMS, Campo Grande, Brazil

*Corresponding author: Bruno Ayub, Graduate student in Medicine, University of Franca - UNIFRAN, Franca, Brazil; E-mail: bruno.ayub@hotmail.com

Abstract

Introduction: Obstructive sleep apnea (OSA) results from the presence of abnormal soft and hard tissues in the upper airway, which cause the collapse of the oropharynx in the deeper stages of sleep. Different treatment modalities have been proposed for OSA, aiming to offer a better quality of life for the patients. Orthognathic surgery via maxillary-mandibular advancement (MMA) decreases the collapse of soft and hard tissue structures during sleep and has a high success rate. The facial and occlusal improvement, the enhancement on respiratory function and the less morbid postoperative period are some advantages responsible for the growing acceptance of this technique.

Case report: This case reports a combination of orthodontic treatment and orthognathic surgery via MMA in a 51 year old man with OSA. The initial polysomnography showed an apnea-hypopnea index of 49.2 and arousal index of 21.7. Follow-up polysomnography performed 15 months after surgery revealed significant improvement. The apnea-hypopnea index decreased to 2.9 and the arousal index to 12.3. The patient reported significant improvements in life quality, sleep quality, and nasal breathing capacity, as well as a decrease in daytime sleepiness and snoring. Thus far, the patient has been under postoperative follow-up for 5 years and 6 months, without any complaints of breathing difficulties during the day or night.

Conclusion: The combination of orthodontic and surgical treatment via MMA may be a favorable alternative treatment for improving the respiratory symptoms of patients with OSA and is highly indicated for patients with maxillary-mandibular discrepancies.

Keywords: Obstructive sleep apnea syndrome; Orthognathic surgery; Orthodontics

Introduction

Obstructive sleep apnea (OSA) is a disorder resulting from the presence of abnormal soft and hard tissues in the upper airway, which causes the collapse of the oropharynx in the deeper stages of sleep. OSA is also influenced by the body mass index [1]. The incidence of OSA in the general population is approximately 4%; its incidence peaks between the 4th and 5th decades of life and is 8 to 10 times more common in men than in women [2]. The chronicity of the syndrome causes low blood oxygen level, sleep fragmentation, snoring, fatigue, and hypersomnia. These can lead to work disability and behavioral changes, in addition to cardiorespiratory consequences [3]. Sleep disorders also affect public safety by causing an increase in the number of industrial and automobile accidents [4].

Different treatment modalities for OSA, including surgical or conservative treatment, have been proposed in the literature, seeking to offer a better quality of life for the patients. Continuous positive airway pressure (CPAP) is an immediate, fast, and conservative treatment for OSA; however, treatment adherence is low among patients [5]. The use of intraoral devices (IODs) is another conservative treatment option indicated in patients with mild OSA, with surgical contraindication, or refusing CPAP. However, this treatment may cause occlusal changes and temporomandibular disorders (TMDs), and also have lack of adherence [6]. Surgical techniques such as uvulopalatopharyngoplasty (UPP), hyoid suspension, and partial glossectomy yield limited results, and are mainly performed in cases of mild-to-moderate severity; moreover, they have a high rate of intraoperative and recurrent postoperative complications [7,8].

Orthognathic surgery via maxillary-mandibular advancement (MMA) may be indicated for moderate and severe OSA [9,10] and has 65-100% success rate [9]. Once this technique involves the advancement of both the jaws, permeability of the upper airway increases, decreasing the incidence of airway collapse during sleep. This advancement of hard tissues provide greater stability to the soft tissues of the oropharynx and nasopharynx regions, resolving OSA in 95% of the cases [8]. The preoperative orthodontic treatment that the patients with OSA undergo before MMA enables better surgical stability and better occlusal engagement, ensuring a more predictable treatment over time and aesthetic benefits. A meta-analysis performed by Hsieh et al. [10] showed that MMA produced average reduction rates of 61-92% on the apnea-hypopnea index and 82-92% on the respiratory disturbance index.

This case reports a combination of orthodontic treatment and orthognathic surgery via MMA in a 51 year old man with OSA.

Case Report

A 51 year old male patient, with a history of leukoderma and hypertension, sought dental treatment complaining of "poor sleep, snoring, fatigue, and difficulty in nasal breathing and chewing".

On facial analysis, dolichofacial pattern, non-passive lip seal, increased facial convexity, short chin-neck line, mandibular asymmetry, and nasal apex offset (Figure 1). On intraoral examination, Angle's Class II malocclusion, overjet, severe upper and lower crowding, crossbite maxillary atresia, and deviation from the mean mandibular line (Figure 2).

Radiographic examination revealed skeletal changes matching the patient's facial deformity and severe posterior air space decrease in the nasal and oropharyngeal regions (Figure 3). The initial polysomnographic examination showed an apnea-hypopnea index of 49.2 and arousal index of 21.7. The outlined treatment plan included a combination of an orthodontic approach together with orthognathic surgery.

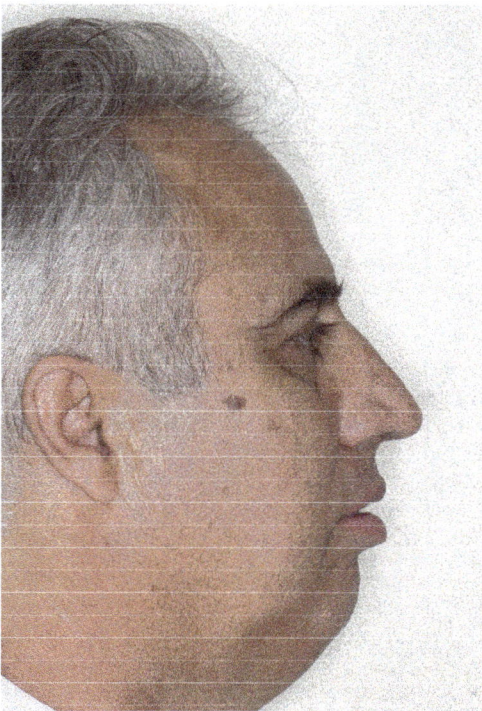

Figure 2: Frontal view of the patient's occlusion.

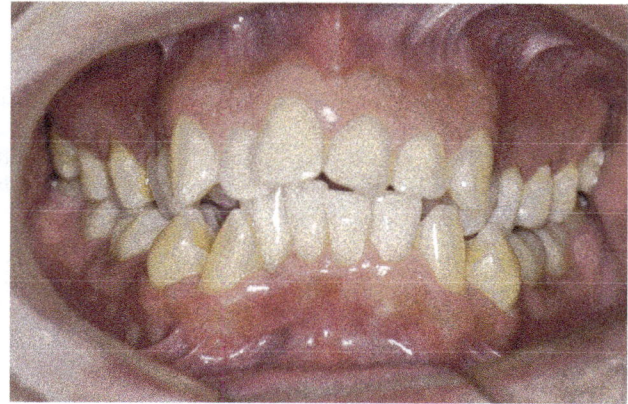

Figure 3: Lateral cephalometric radiograph showing the preoperative reduction of the nasal and oropharyngeal space.

Alignment and leveling of the upper arch was performed using surgically assisted maxillary expansion, without the involvement of the nasal septum. After 5 days, maxillary expansion was initiated using a Haas-type dental-mucus-supported expander appliance. Maxillary expansion was carried out for 40 days postoperatively, until a magnitude of 10.5 mm was achieved. The expander was retained in the upper arch for 6 months and was removed after radiographic confirmation of bone formation in the intermaxillary suture region.

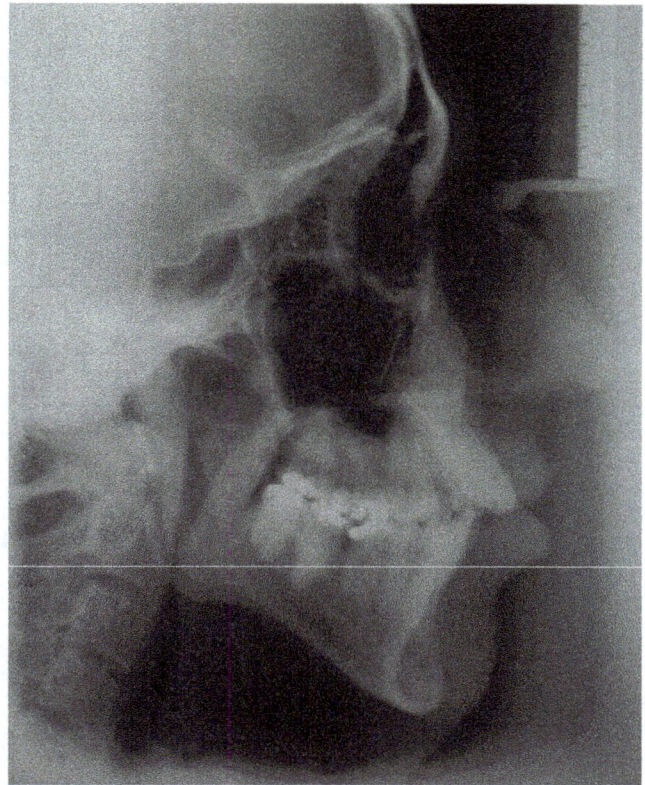

Figure 1: Preoperative lateral profile of the patient.

After the removal of the expander, an acrylic containment apparatus was placed on the palatal concavity throughout the alignment and leveling process of the upper teeth.

The alignment and leveling of the lower arch was performed by extracting a lower first premolar on each side (elements 34 and 44) because of severe crowding in the arch and excessive labial inclination of the lower anterior teeth. Fifteen months after the removal of the expander, we started planning for the bimaxillary orthognathic surgery.

The orthognathic surgery was initiated by performing bilateral sagittal mandibular osteotomies, followed by mandibular advancement of 12 mm on the right side and 14 mm on the left. After surgically guided maxillary-mandibular fixation (MMF) with steel wires, a sagittal internal fixation plate of 2.0 mm thickness with 6 holes was placed on each side of the jaw for clamping and fixation of jaw segments.

Then, a 6 mm advancement mentoplasty was carried out with a decreased vertical height of 1 mm. Subsequently, total bilateral Le Fort I osteotomy (after the mobilization of the maxillary arch), a 10 mm advancement, and 3 mm superior repositioning were performed. During the surgical procedure, the intranasal region was accessed and removed 2/3 of the bilateral inferior turbinates. During the same procedure, a septoplasty in the palatal region of the nasal septum was performed.

The upper osteosynthesis used two 2.0 mm L mini-plates system for canine pillar region and two 1.5 mm L micro-plates system for zygomatic pillar region. Autogenous bone grafts were positioned in the space between the jaw segments. The MMF was removed when the patient was awake and repositioned 12 h after surgery by using intermaxillary elastic bands. The patient remained hospitalized for 36 h after the surgery.

Semi-rigid MMF was used for 24 h in the first 21 days, and the elastic bands were removed 3 times a day only for the main meals. After this period, the patient started postoperative physiotherapy and concluded orthodontic treatment. The orthodontic procedure, including postoperative intercuspation, was completed in 10 months, and the patient reported respiratory and sleep improvements since the early postoperative period (Figure 4).

A follow-up polysomnography performed after 15 months showed significant improvement in OSA. The apnea-hypopnea index had decreased to 2.9 and the arousal index to 12.3. The patient reported a significant improvement in life quality, sleep quality, and nasal breathing capacity, as well as decreased daytime sleepiness and snoring. At 5 years and 6 months after surgery, the patient has no complaints of breathing difficulties at day or night (Figure 5).

Discussion

OSA is characterized by the total cessation of airflow for a period greater than or equal to 10 s [2], and the treatment goal is to reduce the frequency of occurrence of this obstruction. Several clinical symptoms allow the diagnosis of OSA and many of these symptoms could be observed in the current patient. Despite the typical clinical signs, polysomnography is considered the most reliable diagnostic technique to assess the achievement of OSA treatment goals [6].

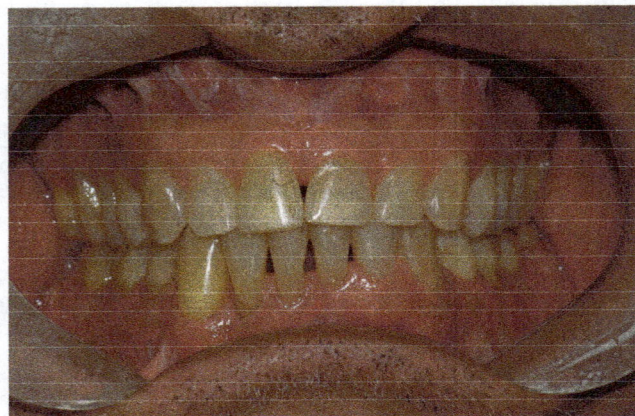

Figure 4: Front aspect of the occlusion after the removal of braces.

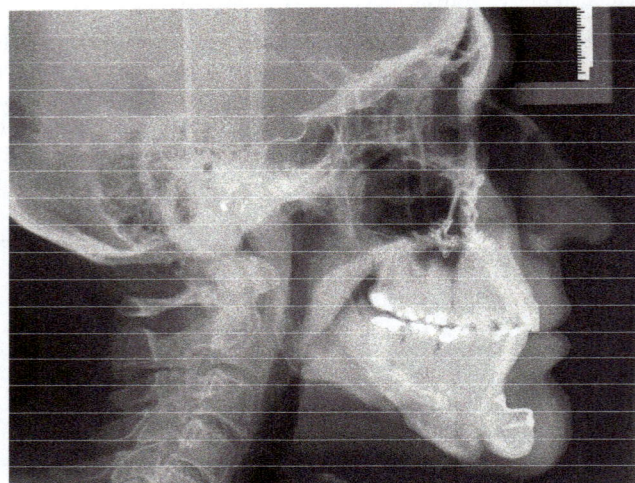

Figure 5: Lateral cephalometric radiograph showing an improved nasal and oropharyngeal space after the removal of braces.

Although various treatment modalities are available for OSA, some have disadvantages. Techniques such as CPAP and IOD depend on patient compliance and their efficacy might be compromised. CPAP has a precise indication and should be used by patients with moderate and severe OSA, as well as those who have no other immediate alternative treatment [5]. The long-term use of IODs has been associated with the appearance of malocclusions and TMDs [6].

Surgical techniques initially proposed for the treatment of OSA, such as UPP, hyoid suspension, and partial glossectomy, aim to manipulate soft tissues. These techniques are associated with postoperative morbidity, which discourages patients from opting these treatments. Postoperative complications and poor long-term effectiveness have sharply reduced the number of such surgical treatments for OSA [5-8].

Orthognathic surgery via MMA was initially first indicated for patients with clinical and cephalometric patter of maxillary-mandibular retrusion. Secondly, after nasal or palatine surgery without significant improvement in OSA [8,10]. In some cases, MMA can provide up to 80% improvement in OSA, as indicated by the apnea-hypopnea post-treatment index (AHI)/disordered breathing index (DBI) [10]. The facial and occlusal improvement, the enhancement on respiratory function and the less morbid postoperative period are some advantages responsible for the growing acceptance of this technique by surgeons and patients.

On this case report, the patient achieved a significant improvement in OSA after surgical treatment, with a decreased apnea-hypopnea index (from 49.2 to 2.9) and arousal index (from 21.7 to 12.3), 15 months after surgery. At 5 years and 6 months after the surgery, the patient is very satisfied with the treatment outcomes and presents a stable occlusion, while reporting aesthetic satisfaction and the absence of any snoring and daytime sleepiness.

Conclusion

The combination of orthodontic and surgical treatment via MMA may be a favorable alternative treatment for improving the respiratory symptoms of patients with OSA and is highly indicated for patients with maxillary-mandibular discrepancies.

References

1. Schendel SA, Broujerdi JA, Jacobson RL (2014) Three-dimensional upper-airway changes with maxillomandibular advancement for obstructive sleep apnea treatment. Am J Orthod Dentofacial Orthop 146: 385-393.
2. Wiegand L, Zwilich CW (1994) Obstructive sleep apnea. St. Louis, Mosby.
3. Eckert DJ, Malhotra A, Jordan AS (2009) Mechanisms of apnea. Prog Cardiovasc Dis 51: 313.
4. Ferrara M, De Gennaro L (2001) How much sleep do we need? Sleep Med 5: 155-179.
5. Weaver TE, Grunstein RR (2008) Adherence to continuous positive airway pressure therapy: The challenge to effective treatment. Proc Am Thorac Soc 5: 173.
6. Dal-Fabbro C, Chaves CM Jr., Bittencourt LRA, Tufik S (2010) Avaliação clínica e polissonográfica do aparelho BRD no tratamento da Síndrome da Apneia Obstrutiva do Sono. Dental Press J Orthod 15: 107-117.
7. Riley RW, Powell NB, Guilleminault C (1993) Obstructive sleep apnea syndrome: A review of 306 consecutively treated surgical patients. Otolaryngol Head Neck Surg 108: 117-125.
8. Ronchi P, Novelli G, Colombo L, Valsecchi S, Oldani A, et al. (2010) Effectiveness of maxillo-mandibular advancement in obstructive sleep apnea patients with and without skeletal anomalies. Int J Oral Maxillofac Surg 39: 541–547.
9. Waite PD, Wooten V, Lachner J, Guyette RF (1989) Maxillomandibular advancement surgery in 23 patients with obstructive sleep apnea syndrome. J Oral Maxillofac Surg 47: 1256–1261.
10. Hsieh YJ, Liao YF (2013) Effects of maxillomandibular advancement on the upper airway and surrounding structures in patients with obstructive sleep apnoea: A systematic review. Br J Oral Maxillofac Surg 51: 834-840.

37

Auditory Cortical Temporal Processing Abilities in Young Adults

Aseel Almeqbel[1*] and Catherine McMahon[2]

[1]Department of Hearing and Speech Sciences, Faculty of Allied Health Sciences, Health Sciences Center, Kuwait University, Kuwait

[2]Linguistics Department, Faculty of Human Sciences, Macquarie University, The HEARing Cooperative Research Centre (CRC), Sydney, Australia

*Corresponding author: Aseel Almeqbel, Department of Hearing and Speech Sciences, Faculty of Allied Health Sciences, Health Sciences Center, Kuwait University, P.O. Box 31470, 90805, Sulaibikat, Kuwait; E-mail: aseel.m@hsc.edu.kw

Abstract

Purpose: To evaluate whether cortical encoding of temporal processing ability, using the N1 peak of the cortical auditory evoked potential, could be measured in normally hearing young adults using three paradigms: voice-onset-time, speech-in-noise and amplitude-modulated broadband noise.

Research design: Cortical auditory evoked potentials (CAEPs) were elicited using: (1) naturally produced stop consonant-vowel (CV) syllables /da/-/ta/ and /ba/-/pa/; (2) speech-in-noise stimuli using the speech sound /da/ with varying signal-to-noise ratios (SNRs); and (3) 16 Hz amplitude-modulated (AM) BBN presented in two conditions: (i) alone (representing a temporally modulated stimulus) and (ii) following an unmodulated BBN (representing a temporal change in the stimulus) using four modulation depths; (4) Behavioural tests of temporal modulation transfer function (TMTF) and speech perception using CNC word list were carried out. All stimuli were presented at 65 Db SPL in the sound field.

Study sample: Participants were adults (12 Females and 8 Males) aged 1830 years with normal hearing.

Results: Results showed: (1) a significant means difference in N1 latency ($p<0.05$) between /da/ vs. /ta/ and /ba/ vs. /pa/; (2) significant N1 latency prolongation with decreasing signal-to-noise ratios for the speech sound /da/; and (3) the N1 latency did not significantly change for different modulations depths when measured for the AMBBN alone or when following a BBN.

Conclusion: Changes in the N1 latency provide a measure of temporal changes in a stimulus for VOT and speech-in-noise. N1 latency could be used as an objective measure of temporal processing ability in individuals with temporal processing disorder who are difficult to assess by behavioural response.

Keywords: Temporal processing; Auditory; Evoked potentials; Adults

Introduction

Auditory temporal processing ability can be defined as the perception of sound or change in a sound within a defined time [1]. Some have argued that the auditory temporal processing is an essential component of most auditory processing capacity, which can be seen at several levels, ranging from neuronal sensitivity to the effects of stimulus onset time, to cortical processing of auditory information such as speech stimuli [1]. A number of studies have shown further that a sustained disruption to auditory temporal processing in newborns and young children can disrupt the perception of speech stimuli, which can lead to poor phonological processing, and in turn to poor reading and language development [2-4]. In particular, this type of causal relationship has been proposed in cases of auditory processing disorder, dyslexia and specific language impairment (SLI) [1,4,5]. Therefore it is important to identify a temporal processing deficit early to minimize subsequent potential impacts on speech, language and reading development. One of the main limitations in identifying such deficits in infants and young children is that these individuals are unable to provide reliable behavioural responses to measures that

assess temporal processing. On the other hand, cortical auditory evoked potential (CAEPs) are now emerging as an instrument that can be used to evaluate temporal changes in sound stimuli [6,7], and are considered to represent the perception of temporal differences.

Research has shown that in normal-hearing individuals the auditory cortical area plays a predominant role in encoding temporal acoustic elements of the speech signal such as voice-onset-time (VOT) [8], speech signals in noise [9] and amplitude modulations [10], all of which are crucial to speech and language processing. When identifying words or sentences, human listeners make use of a temporal cue such as VOT to distinguish between stop consonants that differ in timing of onset. In particular, VOT is represented in the primary and secondary auditory cortical area by synchronized activity that is time-locked to consonant release and voicing onset [11]. VOT corresponds to the duration of the delay between the release of the stop consonant and the start of voicing and this feature is related to the timing cues for VOT perception [11,12]. Voiced syllable-initial stop consonants in English (such as /ba/-/da/) have a short time interval between the release of the consonant and the onset of voicing compared with voiceless stop consonants (e.g., /pa/-/ta/). Studies using synthesized speech tokens with onset times of 0–80 ms representing the continuum between /da/ and /ta/ have demonstrated that a delay of 0–30 ms was identified as the voiced /da/, while stimuli with VOT of 50–80 ms were consistently identified as voiceless /ta/ [13]. Because the 40 ms stimulus was identified as either sound nearly half of the time, it appears that in a normal auditory system the human listener is required to resolve sounds with at least a 20 ms accuracy to differentiate between voiced and voiceless stop consonants.

The ability of the hearing system to detect and resolve a speech signal embedded in competing background noise is critical for successful communication in difficult listening environment. Numerous factors contribute to the capability to hear a signal in the presence of competing noise, including reduced audibility as well as the way in which signals in noise are encoded through the central and peripheral auditory system. In particular, the cortical auditory system has been involved in discriminating stimuli in background noise; that is, the cortical neurons respond primarily to the stimulus onset but do not fire to continuous static background noise [14,15], which suggests that they must resolve timing differences of milliseconds. In other words, the auditory nerve fibres discharge continuously to the masker so that the signal response is a modulation of the firing rate produced by the masker. In cortical neurons, however, there is no steady discharge to the masker, so that the dynamic range of the neurons are available to encode the onset of the signal [14,15]. Thus, cortical neurons are more effective at encoding the signal-to-noise ratio rather than changes in signal intensity per se [16].

Amplitude modulations within speech (as represented by the speech envelope) are important temporal cues for identifying linguistic contrast [17] and conveying sufficient information for its intelligibility. Temporal smearing of these modulations will affect its intelligibility and therefore speech perception [18]. Psychoacoustic studies have demonstrated that the slow rate of modulation frequencies of 4–16 Hz are both necessary and almost sufficient for correct speech identification in quiet and in noise [18,19]. For example, Drullman et al. [19] investigated the effect of temporal smearing on sentence intelligibility and phoneme recognition. They demonstrated that perceiving only modulations above 16 Hz yields almost the same speech perception threshold for sentences in noise; however, for modulations lower than 16 Hz, sentence intelligibility in quiet is heavily affected. In particular, stop consonant speech sounds are affected more than vowels due to their short duration [19]. It seems that to perceive these modulation frequencies within speech requires a high level of temporal resolution in both frequency and time for adequate perception and intelligibility.

Psychoacoustic testing of temporal processing ability, such as voice-onset-time, speech-in-noise and amplitude modulation detection as a function of modulation frequency, have been used behaviourally to evaluate populations with temporal processing deficits such as auditory neuropathy spectrum disorder (ANSD) [7,20-26] and dyslexia [27-30]. These studies reveal abnormal temporal processing ability in a high proportion of individuals with ANSD and dyslexia, which is assumed to underpin the poor speech perception, language and reading skills measured in these populations. Given the difficulties in testing younger populations behaviourally, objective measures of temporal processing using the CAEP would be an advantage in ensuring early detection and remediation.

The CAEP reflects synchronized electroencephalography (EEG) activity in response to sound stimuli and has been found to maintain high temporal resolution [31,32]. The waveform morphology of the CAEP can be defined in terms of amplitude and latency. These voltage changes over time are presumed to result from post-synaptic potentials within the brain, and are influenced by the amount of recruited neurons, synchrony of the neural response and extent of neuronal activation [33]. The CAEP waveforms are made up of several components, including the P1-N1-P2 complex, which reflects synchronous neural activity of structures in the thalamo-cortical portion of the auditory system in response to stimulus onset and other acoustic changes of a continued stimulus [34,35]. That is, the P1-N1-P2 complex could reflect a change from silence to sound (onset response), sound to silence (offset response), or amplitude or frequency modulations of a sustained tone [36]. Alternatively, it may occur in response to changes in ongoing, more complex, sounds such as speech [37-39]. Martin and Boothroyd [38] first coined the phrase "Acoustic Change Complex" (ACC) to describe the cortical response evoked by a change in stimulus, including changes of spectral envelope alone or of periodicity alone with no change in amplitude, or amplitude alone in the absence of changes of spectral envelope or periodicity [40].

Human electrophysiological studies using CAEPs have demonstrated that the auditory N1 latency is sensitive to temporal cues of the acoustic stimuli rather than intensity cues [7,41,42]. Onishi and Davis [41] demonstrated that the latency of N1 in young adults with normal hearing was shortest with fast stimulus rise times and lengthened as rise times were extended. In contrast, when rise time was held constant, changing stimulus intensity had little influence on N1 latency. Two other studies have supported this finding: Michalewski et al. [7] demonstrated that N1 latency in normally hearing young adults was constant over different intensity levels (50–100 dB SPL) and Rapin et al. [42] showed that N1 latency over different intensity levels (30–70 dB SPL) of pure tones was stable.

Data from single neurones in the primary auditory cortex of anaesthetised cats have demonstrated that it is the SNR rather than the absolute level of the sound that is an essential factor affecting the latency of the evoked potentials [14]. Specifically, Phillips and Farmer [14] showed that when the level of noise was increased, the level of tone also had to be increased by the same amount to maintain an equivalent response from a given cortical neuron; these responses are typically transient and time-locked to signal onset. This finding indicates that latency of the evoked potentials is more sensitive in detecting timing cues of the acoustic signal in the presence of noise rather than the intensity cues of that signal. Previous studies have demonstrated the sensitivity of the N1 latency of the CAEP to temporally different stimuli in normally hearing and in temporally disordered populations. Kaplan-Neeman et al. [43] and Whiting et al. [36] measured changes in the N1 latency to speech-in-noise paradigms using different SNRs in young adults with normal hearing, showing that the latency increases with increasing noise levels. Whiting et al. [36], for instance, increased a broadband noise from 50 to 80 dB SPL in 10 dB steps, while recording cortical evoked responses to speech tokens (/da/ and /ba/) presented at 65 and 80 dB SPL. As the noise level increased, N1 latencies increased systematically. In terms of SNR (20 dB to -5 dB), a systematic N1 latency delay was observed; that is, N1 latencies increased as SNR decreased. In other study, Kaplan-Neeman et al. [43] recorded CAEPs in a /da/-/ga/ discrimination paradigm with varying background noise levels (15 dB to -6 dB). The authors observed a systematic increase in N1 latency as the SNRs decreased for both stimuli. Both studies applied an oddball paradigm to evoke the discriminatory P3 cortical response when individuals perceive a target stimulus.

In a temporally disordered population such as those with ANSD, Michalewski et al. [7] measured the passively evoked N1-P1-N2 cortical response to 1 kHz tones and compared this with the response measured in adults with normal hearing. They showed that the N1 latency was prolonged in ANSD and that this prolongation correlated significantly with psychoacoustic testing of gap detection and speech perception. Their findings emphasize the role of the neural synchrony and the degree of auditory nerve responses to the latency N1 component of the CAEP, suggesting that N1 latency may provide a reliable objective testing of auditory temporal processing.

Few studies showed the effect of modulating temporal characteristics of a stimulus on the CAEP. Because of the clinical applicability of this procedure to children with disrupted temporal cues, and the importance of early detection and remediation, this study aimed to develop and evaluate temporal acuity from the auditory cortex by modulating the temporal cues of sound stimuli. In particular, these are changes to voice-onset-time, speech-in-noise ratios and amplitude modulation depths.

Methods

Participants

Twenty young adult participants with normal hearing (8 males, 12 females) aged 18–30 years (mean 25.2, SD 2.2) were recruited. Participants were divided into two groups (A and B) of 10 participants each. Group A participated in voice-onset-time and speech-in-noise testing and group B participated in amplitude- modulation of broadband noise testing to reduce the possibility of participants becoming fatigued by the long test time.

All had pure-tone air conduction thresholds ≤ 15 dB HL at octave frequencies from 250 Hz to 8 kHz with normal tympanograms, no history of hearing or speech problems and noise exposure, and no reported previous history of reading or learning problems. All participants included in this study had speech perception scores ≥ 96% using CNC word lists (open-set-speech perception) and normal temporal processing, evaluated using a Temporal Modulation Transfer Function (TMTF) test, the averaged mean was -19 dB (± 1.48 dB).

Procedure

Air and bone conduction pure-tone thresholds were determined using a calibrated clinical audiometer (AC33 Interacoustics two channels) using a modified version of the Hughson and Westlake procedure [44]. Tympanometry used a calibrated immittance meter (GSI-Tymp star V2, calibrated as per ANSI, 1987). Tympanograms were obtained for a 226 Hz probe tone. A Consonant-Nucleus-Consonant (CNC) word test was used to assess open-set speech perception ability.

Temporal modulation transfer function (TMTF)

To develop the stimuli for the TMTF test, two sounds were generated: un-modulated broadband noise (BBN) and amplitude modulated BBN, of 500 ms duration with a rise/fall (ramp) of 20 ms. The stimuli were generated using a 16-bit digital to analog converter with a sampling frequency of 44.1 kHz and low pass filtered with a cut off frequency of 20 kHz. The modulated BBN stimuli were derived by multiplying the BBN by a dc-shifted sine wave. Modulation depth of the AMBBN (fm 16 Hz) stimuli was controlled by varying the amplitude of the modulating sine wave [27,45].

Amplitude modulation detection threshold at low modulation rate (fm 16 Hz) was obtained using an adaptive two down one up, forced choice procedure (2I-2AFC) that estimates modulation depth necessary for 70.7% correct detection [46]. The participants' task was to identify the interval containing the modulation. No feedback was given after each trial. The step size and thresholds of modulation were based on the modulation depth in decibels (20 log m, where m refers to depth of modulation). The step size of modulation was initially 4 dB and reduced to 2 dB after two reversals. The mean of the last three reversals in a block of 14 were taken as threshold. The poorest detection threshold that could be measured was 0 dB, and corresponded to an AM of one (100% modulation depth); the more negative the value of 20 log m, the better the detection threshold. The Stimuli were played in a computer (a PC Toshiba); the participant received the output of the stimuli that were calibrated using Bruel and Kjaer SLM type 2250, microphone number 419 presented at 65 dB SPL sound field.

Voice-onset-time (VOT)

The main aim of this test was to determine the perceptual distinction between voiced and voiceless stop consonant-vowel-syllables electrophysiologically. Four naturally produced stop consonant-vowel-syllables /da/-/ta/ and /ba/-/pa/ were recorded by an Australian female speaker. These speech stimuli were selected to allow comparison between the current study and the numerous studies in which these stimuli have been used [13,39,47-51]. The speech stimuli used in those previous studies, however, were synthesized, whereas the speech stimuli used in the current study were naturally recorded, resulting in differences between the formant frequencies and the voicing time (see Table 1). In addition, it has been recommended that naturally recorded speech be used for evoked potential research, since the aim is to apply results to speech perception in everyday life [52].

Stimulus stop CV	VOT (ms)	Formant frequency (Hz)
/da/	0,03	F0: 180.7
		F1: 816.1
		F2: 1465.8
ta/	0,95	F0: 182.0
		F1: 801.3
		F2: 1300.9
/ba/	0,06	F0: 174.8
		F1: 797.6
		F2: 1199.8
/pa/	0,67	F0: 189.0
		F1: 785.1
		F2: 1143.6

Table 1: Details of the stimuli, stimulus type, VOT and formant frequency.

Speech stimuli were recorded using an AKG C535 condenser microphone connected to a Mackie sound mixer, with the microphone positioned 150 mm in front and at 45 degrees to the speaker's mouth. The mixer output was connected via an M-Audio Delta 66 USB sound device to a Windows computer running Cool Edit audio recording software and captured at 44.1 KHz 16 bit wave format. All speech stimuli were collected in a single session to maintain consistency of voice quality.

After selection and recording, speech stimuli were modified using Cool Edit 2000 software. All speech stimuli of 200 ms duration were ramped with 20 ms rise and fall time to prevent any audible click arising from the rapid onset or offset of the waveform.

The inter-stimulus interval (ISI), calculated from the onset of the preceding stimulus to the onset of the next stimulus was 1207 ms, as it has been shown that a slower stimulation rate results in more robust CAEP waveforms in immature auditory nervous systems [53].

Speech-in-noise

The main aim of the speech-in-noise test (varying SNRs) was to determine the effect of signal-to-noise ratio (SNR) on the CAEP, specifically the N1 latency, in an effort to further our understanding of how noise affects responses to the temporal cues of the speech signal. We developed varying signal-to-noise ratios with the speech stimulus /da/ to measure this ability. The speech stimulus /da/ was naturally recorded by an Australian female speaker using an AKG C535 condenser microphone connected to a Mackie sound mixer, with the microphone positioned 150 mm in front and at 45 degrees to the speaker's mouth. The mixer output was connected via an M-Audio Delta 66 USB sound device to a Windows computer running Cool Edit audio recording software and captured at 44.1 KHz 16 bit wave format. A speech stimulus was of 60 ms duration and ramped with a 20 ms rise and fall time to prevent any audible click arising from the rapid onset or offset of the waveform.

After a speech stimulus was selected and recorded, the broadband noise of 600 ms was generated using Praat software, which changed the signal-to-noise ratio using Matlab software with respect to the 65 dB SPL /da/ sound and then combined them to create a /da/ embedded in different noise levels. Noise levels were 45, 55, 60, 65, 70, 75 and 85 dB SPL. These noise levels were chosen to create seven signal-to-noise ratios (SNRs) (Quiet (+20 dB), +10 dB, +5 dB, 0 dB, -5 dB, -10 dB, -20 dB). The inter-stimulus interval (ISI), calculated from the onset of the preceding stimulus to the onset of the next stimulus was 1667 ms.

Amplitude modulation (AM) of broadband noise

The main aim of this test was to measure the change in the N1 latency of the cortical response to an amplitude-modulated signal. Two stimuli were used: (i) a 300 ms amplitude-modulated broadband noise to determine whether the cortical response was sensitive to temporal changes in a single stimulus and (ii) a 600 ms un-modulated broadband noise followed by a 300 ms amplitude modulated broadband noise to determine whether the cortical response was sensitive to a temporally different stimulus. The modulation frequency was 16 Hz, and all stimuli had a 20 ms rise and fall time. The stimuli were generated using a 16-bit digital-to-analog converter with a sampling frequency of 44.1 kHz and low pass filtered with a cutoff frequency of 20 kHz. The depth of the modulation was controlled by varying the amplitude of the modulating sine wave. The inter-stimulus interval (ISI), calculated from the onset of the preceding stimulus to the onset of the next stimulus was 1307 ms for the first condition and 1907 ms for the second condition.

Stimulus presentation

All stimuli used in these procedures were presented at 65 dB SPL (as measured at the participant's head), which approximates normal conversational level. It was confirmed with each participant that this level was at a loud but comfortable listening level. Presentation was via a loudspeaker speaker placed 1 m from the participant's seat at 0 azimuth.

Set-up

Participants sat on a comfortable chair in a quiet room at Electrophysiology Clinic and watched a DVD of their own choice. The volume was silenced and subtitles were activated to ensure that participants would be engaged with the movie and pay no attention to the stimuli. All participants were instructed to be relaxed, pay no attention to the sounds being presented and not to fall asleep.

Data acquisition

A NeuroScan and 32-channel NuAmps evoked potential system was used for evoked potential recording. All sounds were presented using Neuroscan STIM 2 stimulus presentation system.

Recording

Evoked potentials were recorded in continuous mode (gain 500, filter 0.1–100 Hz) and converted using analog-to-digital sampling rate of 1000 Hz using scan (version 4.3) via gold electrodes placed at C3, C4, Cz with reference electrode A2 on the right mastoid bone and ground on the contralateral ear on the mastoid bone.

Adults participated in two 2 h recording sessions, including the electrode application and CAEP recording. None of the participants showed signs of fatigue during the testing. All sound levels were calibrated using Bruel and Kjaer SLM type 2250, microphone number 419.

Off-line data analysis

EEG files with a -100 to 500 ms time window were obtained from the continuous file. Any responses on scalp electrodes exceeding $\pm$ 50 μV were rejected. Prior to averaging, EEG files were baseline corrected using a pre-stimulus period (-100 ms). Averaging was digitally band pass filtered offline from 1 to 30 Hz (zeroshift, 12 dB/octave) in order to enhance detection of the CAEP components and smooth the waves for the final figures. For each participant, the individual grand average waveform was computed, visually identified and subjected to suitable statistical analyses using SPSS (version 18) to investigate the aims of the current study. The smaller groups of participants necessitated the use of non-parametric analysis.

Results

/da/ vs. / ta/

The Wilcoxon Signed-Rank test was performed to compare the mean N1 latency of the stop CV voiced /da/ vs. voiceless /ta/. Also referred to as the Wilcoxon matched pairs signed rank test, this is the non-parametric alternative to the repeated measures t-test. Results show a significant mean difference in N1 latency between the two conditions (Z=-2.814, p<0.05).

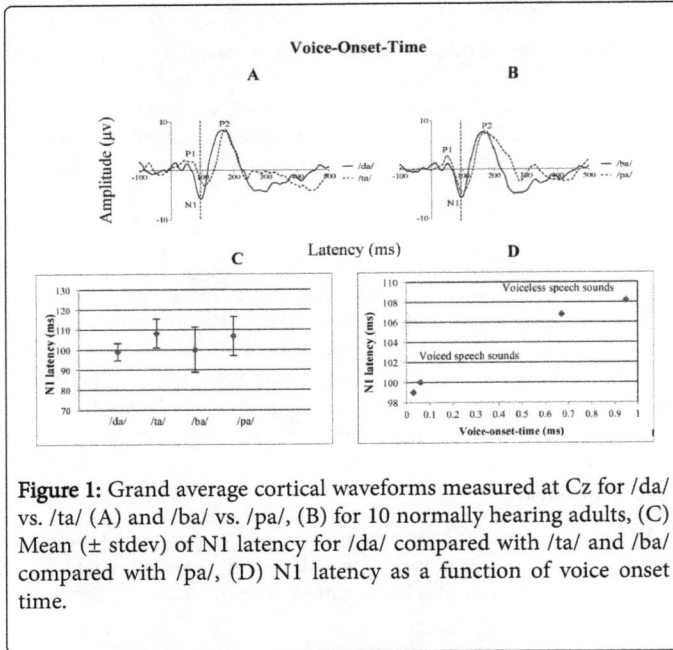

Figure 1: Grand average cortical waveforms measured at Cz for /da/ vs. /ta/ (A) and /ba/ vs. /pa/, (B) for 10 normally hearing adults, (C) Mean (± stdev) of N1 latency for /da/ compared with /ta/ and /ba/ compared with /pa/, (D) N1 latency as a function of voice onset time.

There was an early N1 latency for the stop CV voiced /da/ and later N1 latency for the stop CV voiceless /ta/ as shown in Figure 1A. For example, the mean N1 latency for /da/ was 99 ms (± 4.36 ms) and the mean N1 latency for /ta/ was 108 ms (± 7.20 ms) as shown in Figure 1C.

/ba/ vs. /pa/

The Wilcoxon Signed-Rank test performed to compare the mean N1 latency of the stop CV voiced /ba/ vs. the stop CV voiceless /pa/ showed a significant mean difference between /ba/ vs. /pa/ (Z=-2.809, p<0.05). There was an early latency for N1 for the stop CV voiced /ba/ and later N1 latency for the stop CV voiceless /pa/ as shown in Figure 1B. For example, the mean N1 latency for /ba/ was 100 ms (± 11.21 ms) and the mean N1 latency for /pa/ was 106 ms (± 9.72 ms) as shown in Figure 1C.

Speech-in-noise

The Friedman Test (the non-parametric alternative to the one-way repeated measures analysis of variance) was performed to compare the mean N1 latencies of all SNR conditions. Results indicated a statistically significant difference in N1 latency of the CAEP across the SNR conditions (Chi square [5]=36.037, p<0.05) as shown in Figures 2A and 2B. Inspection of the mean values showed an increase in N1 latency of the CAEP from signal-to-noise levels of +20 dB 96.0 ms (± 5.41 ms), +10 dB 102.6 ms (± 8.85 ms), +5 dB 118.3 ms (± 13.17 ms), 0 dB 123.5 ms (± 15.27 ms), -5 dB 129.1 ms (± 15.80 ms) and -10 dB 145.3 ms (± 18.72 ms). No observable response was measured at -20 dB for all participants.

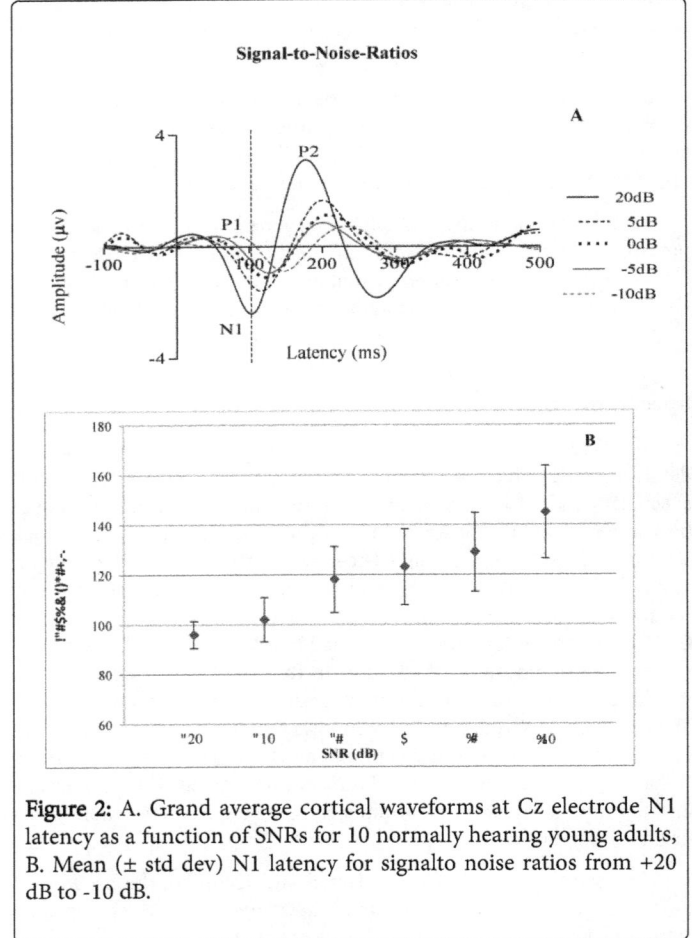

Figure 2: A. Grand average cortical waveforms at Cz electrode N1 latency as a function of SNRs for 10 normally hearing young adults, B. Mean (± std dev) N1 latency for signal to noise ratios from +20 dB to -10 dB.

Amplitude-modulation (AM) of broadband noise

The aim of this test was to objectively assess the sensitivity of normal-hearing listeners to amplitude-modulation (AM) of broadband noise, important for speech intelligibility [28]. Two conditions were evaluated to measure the temporal processing ability of normally hearing adults: (i) 300 ms AM-BBN and (ii) 300 ms AM-BBN following a 600 ms BBN. The Friedman Test was performed to compare the mean N1 latency of all modulation depths. Results indicated no statistically significant difference in N1 latency of the CAEP across the five modulation depths for the AM-BBN stimulus alone (100%, 75%, 50%, 25%, 0% AM) (Chi square [4]=6.85, p>0.05) as shown in Figure 3A, although slight non-significant and non-systematic differences in N1 latency were observed. Similarly, for the responses measured to the AM-BBN following a BBN, results indicated no statistically significant difference in N1 latency of the CAEP across the modulation depth levels (100%, 70%, 50%, 25%, 0%AM) (Chi square [4]=4.161, p>0.05). In this test condition, when the unmodulated BBN was followed by AM-BBN with 0% amplitude-modulation depth, there was no identifiable N1 component for all participants in the study, as shown in Figure 3B.

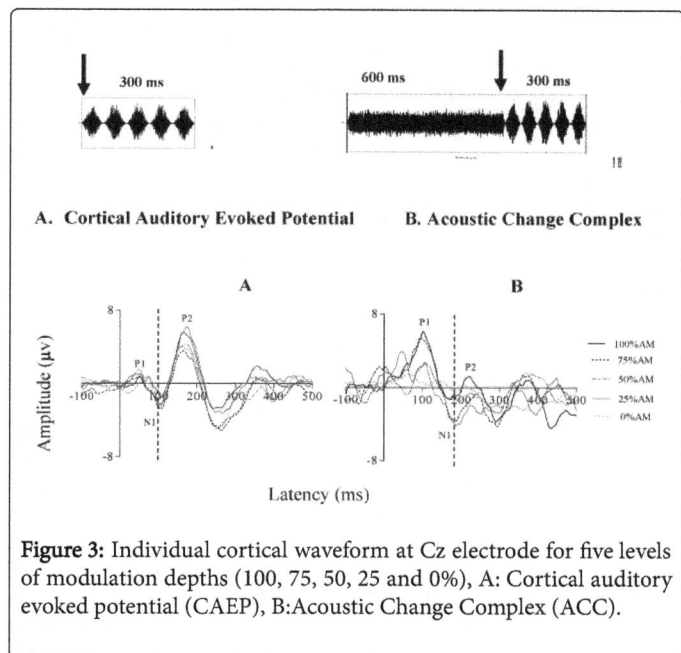

Figure 3: Individual cortical waveform at Cz electrode for five levels of modulation depths (100, 75, 50, 25 and 0%), A: Cortical auditory evoked potential (CAEP), B:Acoustic Change Complex (ACC).

Further analysis was carried out using a Wilcoxon Signed-Rank Test to compare the difference between two conditions (300 ms AM-BBN versus 300 ms AM-BBN following a 600 ms BBN) tested at each depth separately. Results show a statistically significant difference in N1 latency between the two conditions at 100% (Z=-2.706, p<0.05), at 75% (Z=-2.708, p<0.05), at 50% (Z=-2.705, p<0.05) and at 25% (Z=-2.707, p<0.05).

Discussion

The aim of this study was to develop and evaluate three electrophysiological measures of temporal processing in normally hearing adults with normal temporal processing abilities measured using TMTF. As previous studies had shown that the N1 latency of the CAEP was more sensitive to the neural timing of the acoustic stimuli than other CAEP components, changes in its latency formed the basis of the study. Overall, we observed a systematic difference in N1 latency for changes in voice-onset time and signal-to-noise ratios but not for the amplitude-modulated BBN presented alone or following an unmodulated BBN. Despite this pattern of results, significant differences of the N1 latency were measured for the AM-BBN alone compared with the same signal following a BBN when tested at each depth separately.

Voice-onset-time

The main finding from the VOT temporal measure was that the latency of N1 cortical responses for the stop voiced CVs /da/ and /ba/ was earlier than for the stop voiceless CVs /ta/ and /pa/ suggesting that normally hearing adults coded the voiced and voiceless stop CV syllables differently. A possible reason for the early latency for the stop voiced CVs /da/ and /ba/ and later latency for the stop voiceless /ta/ and /pa/ is that the voiced and voiceless stop CVs are encoded differently at the cortical level in normal-hearing listeners because of the neural timing differences (temporal spacing) between the two speech stimuli [8]. In the human auditory cortex these temporal cues are represented by the synchronized responses of neuronal populations

timed-locked to the onset of the acoustic stimulus [11,47,54]. That is, the CAEP has time-locked components with latencies that are determined by the temporal cues of these speech stimuli.

Our results are consistent with previous studies that have found an early CAEP latency for stimuli with shorter VOT, such as /da/ and /ba/, and later CAEP latency for stimuli with longer VOT, such as /ta/ and /pa/ [13]. In addition, our results support those of previous studies that have proposed N1 latency is sensitive to the neural timing of the acoustic stimuli and can be used as an objective test to evaluate perceptual dysfunction in a disordered population with poor temporal processing ability.

The temporal cue of sounds such as VOT is important for speech perception. For example, a voiced stop consonant in word-initial position such as in /da/ is distinguished from its voiceless counterpart /ta/ by temporal cues. That is, the distinction between these two syllables is the interval between consonant release and the onset of voicing.

Psychoacoustical studies have established the importance of VOTs as a temporal cue for the perceptual discrimination of voiced from voiceless speech sounds. The perception of voicing onset depends mainly on voice-onset-time and the short formant transition from consonant to vowel [55]. Individuals with temporal processing deficits, such as those with ANSD, have been found to have poor perception of voicing onset of stop consonant-vowel syllables. For example, Narne and Vanaja [24] found that individuals with ANSD have speech perceptual errors involving stop consonants (e.g., /d/-/t/) which are distinguished by voice-onset-time, thus perceiving the voiced sound /d/ as voiceless /t/ [24]. VOTs are short acoustic events that have been shown to be important in differentiating stop consonants [56], and the poor perception of voicing onset in individuals with ANSD may reflect their difficulty in detecting the duration of these short acoustic events due to temporal processing disruption [57]. Interestingly, children with language and reading difficulties and associated temporal processing problems also often exhibit impairment in speech sound discrimination, especially VOT contrast [58].

We have shown electrophysiologically in this study that the VOT of stop CV syllables induced a temporal cortical response that systematically varied in N1 latency in a manner related to the time at which stimulus voicing began (see Figure 1D). The implication of these results is important in measuring these four CV syllables /da/, /ta/ and /ba/, /pa/ that differ in voicing onset electrophysiologically using the CAEP in infants and young children who are suspected to have temporal processing disorders. This type of assessment may perhaps assist in early identification and intervention of temporal processing disruption.

Speech-in-noise

There was a clear effect of SNRs on N1 latency in this study, to the extent that, as the noise level increased, the latency of N1 was significantly prolonged. These results suggest a delay in the cortical neurons to detect the onset of the speech stimulus /da/ with increasing noise level in normally hearing adult participants. With the most difficult listening condition, -20 dB SNR, there was no identifiable N1 waveform for any participant. This finding highlights the possibility that in situations at -20 dB SNR in normal communication, speech intelligibility will be significantly deteriorated in normally hearing adult listeners.

Individuals with ANSD typically complain of an impaired ability to understand speech especially in the presence of background noise [23,59]. The auditory processes that contribute to the speech perceptual deficit in background noise appear to be related to the abnormal temporal processing function in ANSD [26,57]. Cunningham et al. [59] have shown that some individuals with ANSD in their study who have speech perception scores of 90% in quiet had their speech perception scores reduced to 40% when tested at 10 dB SNR and their speech perception scores showed a further marked drop down to 5% at 0 dB SNR. Kraus et al. [20] presented a case study with ANSD, with normal hearing thresholds and speech perception of 100% scores in quiet; however, in the presence of background noise at +3 dB SNR the speech perception scores were 10%. Furthermore, many studies have shown that children diagnosed with language-based learning disabilities, such as dyslexia and specific language impairment, exhibit distortion of the timing of cortical responses when acoustic signals are presented in noise [60,61].

The implication of these results is important for a population with SNR problems, such as ANSD, and for those with temporal processing deficit. Further studies examining speech signal-to-noise encoding in these populations are necessary to understand how listening is impaired by changing temporal information at the level of the cortex. This research may assist in early identification of and intervention for temporal processing disruption in infants, young children and those adults whose auditory temporal processing abilities may be difficult to assess by behavioural measures.

Amplitude-modulated broadband noise

This study of young normally hearing adults found that the N1 peak of the CAEP could be elicited to different modulation depths (100%, 75%, 50%, 25% and 0%). This finding reflects the ability of cortical neurons to detect overall amplitude changes (temporal) within the acoustic signal objectively, even the smallest changes, such as 25% AM. That is, the temporal modulation information within the acoustic stimuli was represented by the N1 component at the level of the auditory cortex. These small changes within the acoustic stimuli are important for speech intelligibility, since human speech consists of time varying signals and the information contained in the dynamic temporal structure is crucial for speech identification and communication. Individuals s with poor temporal processing ability have particular difficulty in detecting these small changes in the amplitude of the acoustic signal [22,26,57]. This difficulty consequently affects their speech intelligibility, which is further worsened in the presence of background noise.

Although the results reported here indicate a slight shift in N1 latency when the modulation depths changed in both conditions, this effect was not significant. In the first condition (AM-BBN 300 ms), we assume that the reason behind our not observing significant changes in N1 latency in response to changes in amplitude modulation depths was that the CAEP waveform is dominated by the onset and thus reflects characteristics of the stimulus onset time [11,47,54]. That is, the onset time for all modulation depths (non-stimuli) was 0 ms but the amplitude depths varied; therefore, the cortical neurons were less sensitive to the modulation depths in this condition, and so we were unable to observe significant changes in N1 latency.

For the second condition, un-modulated BBN (600 ms) + AM (300 ms), we assume that the reason for not observing systematic and significant changes in N1 latency in response to varying amplitude modulation depths was that the first N1 latency corresponds to the onset of the un-modulated BBN (600 ms), which is a change from silence to sound (an onset response). Furthermore, the second N1 latency corresponds to the onset of the changing from the un-modulated BBN to AMBBN, which is part of the ongoing stimuli "acoustic changes complex" (ACC), and so the second part reflects the acoustic changes in the stimuli [40]. The ACC has been reliably recorded in our participants and our data confirm that it is possible to detect N1 latency in response to modulation depths of ongoing stimuli. Even though it is possible to detect N1 latency of the ACC responses to AM-BBN part, the response is considerably smaller than that observed to the un-modulated BBN (600 ms). We assume here that the cortical regions activated by the two stimuli (un-modulated + modulated AM-BBN) are not entirely separated, but overlap. In the overlapping region, the "line-busy effect" hypothesis of Stevens and Davis [61] would explain the reduction in overall amplitude of the AMBBN (ACC), because the cortical neurons were already activated (firing) by the un-modulated BBN (onset response) and interfere with synchronous responses to AMBBN (ACC). This overlap would result in an overall decrease in the numbers of cortical neurons that respond synchronously to the AM-BBN [63-82]. Therefore fewer cortical neurons firing to the second part ACC of the ongoing stimuli would evoke smaller responses of the N1 component, which is significantly smaller than that for onset responses of un-modulated BBN. Consequently, we would not observe any significant effect in N1 latency in response to the modulation depths for the ACC.

A second possibility is that the cortical neurons activated by the two stimuli (un-modulated BBN + AM-BBN) are separate; that is, the ACC is a response to a "new sound" which occurred because of the gap between the two stimuli. The ACC in that case is an onset response rather than an ongoing AM-BBN sound, and perhaps there are different populations of cortical neurons firing to that "new sound".

This N1 latency of acoustic change complex and the behavioural detection of the AM-BBN we obtained can indicate presence or absence of the person's sensitivity of the AM-BBN detection ability of the ongoing stimuli. Although we did not observe any significant effect on N1 latency, further study of N1 amplitude and other CAEP components, such as P1 and P2 and N2 components, might elucidate whether different generators could be activated in response to the amplitude modulated signal. Clearly, however, much additional work will be needed to establish the clinical utility of this measure.

Conclusion

The results from the present study suggest that N1 latency can be used as an objective testing of temporal processing ability in participants with a temporal processing disruption who are particularly challenged by the presence of background noise and who are difficult to assess by behavioural response. However, further work needs to be done with a larger population with normal hearing and with a temporally disordered population to clinically validate these tests. The present study represents the first publication of normative data for adults responding to one of our electrophysiological temporal processing measures (AM-BBN). However, as this the first time we have measured the AM paradigm and the aim was to investigate whether N1 latency could be elicited in response to different AM depths in young adults, further investigation is necessary to understand the relation between N1 amplitude and AM.

References

1. Musiek F (2003) Temporal processing: The basics. Hearing Journal 56: 52.

2. Farmer M, Klein R (1995) The evidence for a temporal processing deficit linked to dyslexia: A review. Psychonomic Bulletin & Review 2: 460-493.

3. Tallal P, Miller SL, Bedi G, Byma G, Wang X, et al. (1996) Language comprehension in language-learning impaired children improved with acoustically modified speech. Science 271: 81-84.

4. Wright BA, Lombardino LJ, King WM, Puranik CS, Leonard CM, et al. (1997) Deficits in auditory temporal and spectral resolution in language-impaired children. Nature 387: 176-178.

5. Tallal P, Miller S, Fitch RH (1993) Neurobiological basis of speech: A case for the preeminence of temporal processing. Annals of the New York Academy of Sciences 682: 27-47.

6. Michalewski HJ, Starr A, Zeng FG, Dimitrijevic A (2009) N100 cortical potentials accompanying disrupted auditory nerve activity in auditory neuropathy (AN): Effects of signal intensity and continuous noise. Clinical Neurophysiology 120: 1352-1363.

7. Michalewski HJ, Starr A, Nguyen T, Kong Y, Zeng F, et al. (2005) Auditory temporal processing in normal-hearing individuals and patients with auditory neuropathy. Clinical Neurophysiology 116: 669-680.

8. Roman S, Canevet G, Lorenzi C, Triglia J, Liegeois-Chauvel C (2003) Voice onset time encoding in patients with left and right cochlear implants. Neuroreport 15: 601-605.

9. Warrier C, Johnson K, Hayes E, Nicol T, Kraus N (2004) Learning impaired children exhibit timing deficits and training-related improvements in auditory cortical responses to speech in noise. Experimental Brain Research 157: 431-441

10. Giraud AL, Lorenzi C, Ashburner J, Wable J, Johnsrude I, et al. (2000) Representation of the temporal envelope of sounds in the human brain. J Neurophysiol 84: 1588-1598.

11. Steinschneider M, Volvov I, Noh M, Garell C, Howard M (1999) Temporal encoding of the voice onset time phonetic parameter by field potentials recorded directly from human auditory cortex. Journal of Neurophysiology 82: 2346-2357.

12. Lisker L, Abramson A (1964) A cross-language study of voicing in initial stops: Acoustical measurements. Word 20: 384-422.

13. Sharma A, Dorman MF (1999) Cortical auditory evoked potential correlates of categorical perception of voice-onset time. J Acoust Soc Am 106: 1078-1083.

14. Phillips DP, Farmer ME (1990) Acquired word deafness, and the temporal grain of sound representation in the primary auditory cortex. Behavioural Brain Research 40: 85-94.

15. Phillips DP, Hall SE (1986) Spike-rate intensity functions of cat cortical neurons studied with combined tone-noise stimuli. J Acoust Soc Am 80: 177-187.

16. Billings CJ, Tremblay KL, Stecker C, Tolin W (2009) Human evoked cortical activity to signal-to-noise ratio and absolute signal level. Hear Res 254: 15-24.

17. Rosen S (1992) Temporal information in speech: Acoustic, auditory and linguistic aspects. Philosophical Transactions: Biological Sciences 336: 367-373.

18. Houtgast T, Steeneken HJ (1985) A review of the MTF concept in room acoustics and its use for estimating speech intelligibility in auditoria. Journal of the Acoustical Society of America 77: 1069-1077.

19. Drullman R, Festen JM, Plomp R (1994) Effect of temporal envelope smearing on speech reception. J Acoust Soc Am 95: 1053-1064.

20. Kraus N, Bradlow AR, Cheatham MA, Cunningham J, King CD, et al. (2000) Consequences of neural asynchrony: A case of auditory neuropathy. J Assoc Res Otolaryngol 1: 33-45.

21. Kumar AU, Jayaram M (2005) Auditory processing in individuals with auditory neuropathy. Behav Brain Funct 1: 21.

22. Rance G, McKay C, Grayden D (2004) Perceptual characterization of children with auditory neuropathy. Ear Hear 25: 34-46.

23. Rance G, Barker E, Mok M, Dowell R, Rincon A, et al. (2007) Speech perception in noise for children with auditory neuropathy/dys-synchrony type hearing loss. Ear Hear 28: 351-360.

24. Narne VK, Vanaja CS (2008) Effect of envelope enhancement on speech perception in individuals with auditory neuropathy. Ear Hear 29: 45-53.

25. Narne VK, Vanaja C (2008) Speech identification and cortical potentials in individuals with auditory neuropathy. Behav Brain Funct 4: 15.

26. Zeng FG, Oba S, Garde S, Sininger Y, Starr A (1999) Temporal and speech processing deficits in auditory neuropathy Neuroreport 10: 3429-3435.

27. Lorenzi C, Dumont A, Füllgrabe C (2000) Use of temporal envelope cues by children with developmental dyslexia. Journal of Speech Language and Hearing Research 43: 1367-1379.

28. Menell P, McAnally K, Stein J (1999) Psychophysical sensitivity and physiological response to amplitude modulation in adult dyslexic listeners. Journal of Speech, Language, and Hearing Research 42: 797-803.

29. Rocheron I, Lorenzi C, Füllgrabe C, Dumont A (2002) Temporal envelope perception in dyslexic children. Neuroreport 13: 1683-1687.

30. Witton C, Talcott JB, Hansen PC, Richardson AJ, Griffiths TD, et al. (1998) Sensitivity to dynamic auditory and visual stimuli predicts nonword reading ability in both dyslexic and normal readers. Current Biology 8: 1791-1797.

31. Hall III, WJ (1990) Handbook of audiotry eveoked responses. Massachusetts: Allyn and Bacon.

32. Van Wassenhove V, Grant KW, Poeppel D (2003) Electrophysiology of auditory-visual speech integration. Auditory Visual Speech Processing. St. Jorioz, France.

33. Eggermont J (2007) Electric and magnetic fields of synchronous neural activity. In: Burkard RM, Don M, Eggermont J (eds.) Auditory evoked potentials, Philadephia: Lippincott Williams & Wilkins.

34. Näätänen R, Picton T (1987) The N1 wave of the Human electric and magnetic responses to sound: A review and an analysis of the component structure. Psychophysiology 24: 375-425.

35. Wolpaw JR, Penry JK (1975) A temporal component of the auditory evoked response. Electroencephalogr Clin Neurophysiol 39: 609-620.

36. Whiting KA, Martin BA, Stapells DR (1998) The effects of broadband noise masking on cortical event-related potentials to speech sounds /ba/ and /da/. Ear Hear 19: 218-231.

37. Kaukoranta E, Hari R, Lounasmaa OV (1987) Responses of the human auditory cortex to vowel onset after fricative consonants. Exp Brain Res 69: 19-23.

38. Martin BA, Boothroyd A (1999) Cortical, auditory, event-related potentials in response to periodic and aperiodic stimuli with the same spectral envelope. Ear Hear 20: 33-44.

39. Tremblay KL, Piskosz M, Souza P (2003) Effects of age and age-related hearing loss on the neural representation of speech cues. Clin Neurophysiol 114: 1332-1343.

40. Martin BA, Boothroyd A (2000) Cortical, auditory, evoked potentials in response to changes of spectrum and amplitude. J Acoust Soc Am 107: 2155-2161.

41. Onishi S, Davis H (1968) Effects of duration and rise time of tone bursts on evoked V potentials. J Acoust Soc Am 44: 582-591.

42. Rapin I, Schimmel H, Tourk LM, Krasnegor NA, Pollak C (1966) Evoked responses to clicks and tones of varying intensity in waking adults. Electroencephalogr Clin Neurophysiol 21: 335-344.

43. Kaplan-Neeman R, Kishon-Rabin L, Henkin Y, Muchnik C (2006) Identification of syllables in noise: electrophysiological and behavioral correlates. J Acoust Soc Am 120: 926-933.

44. Cahart R, Jerger J (1959) Preferred method for clinical determination of pure tone thresholds. Journal of Speech and Hearing Disorders 24: 330-345.

45. Viemeister NF (1979) Temporal modulation transfer functions based upon modulation thresholds. J Acoust Soc Am 66: 1364-1380.

46. Levitt H (1971) Transformed up-down methods in psychoacoustics. J Acoust Soc Am 49: Suppl 2: 467+.

47. Giraud K, Demonet J, Habib M, Chauvel P, Liegeois-Chauvel C (2005) Auditory evoked potential patterns to voiced and voiceless speech sounds in adult developmental dyslexics with persistent deficits. Cerebral Cortex 15: 1524-1534.

48. Sharma A, Dorman MF, Spahr AJ (2002) A sensitive period for the development of the central auditory system in children with cochlear implants: Implications for age of implantation. Ear Hear 23: 532-539.

49. Sharma A, Kraus N, McGee T, Nicol T (1997) Developmental changes in P1 and N1 central auditory responses elicited by consonant-vowel syllables. Clinical Neuropathysiolgy 104: 540-545.

50. Sharma A, Marsh CM, Dorman MF (2000) Relationship between N1 evoked potential morphology and the perception of voicing. J Acoust Soc Am 108: 3030-3035.

51. Sharma A, Dorman M, Kral A (2005) The influence of a sensitive period on central auditory development in children with unilateral and bilateral cochlear implants. Hearing Research 203: 134-143.

52. Picton TW, Alain C, Otten L, Ritter W, Achim A (2000) Mismatch negativity: Different water in the same river. Audiol Neurootol 5: 111-139.

53. Gilley PM, Sharma A, Dorman M, Martin K (2005) Developmental changes in refractoriness of the cortical auditory evoked potential. Clinical Neuropysiology 116: 648-657.

54. Eggermont JJ (2001) Between sound and perception: Reviewing the search for a neural code. Hear Res 157: 1-42.

55. Summerfield Q, Haggard M (1977) On the dissociation of spectral and temporal cues to the voicing distinction in initial stop consonants. J Acoust Soc Am 62: 435-448.

56. Pickett J (1999) The acoustics of speech communication. MA: Allyn & Bacon.

57. Zeng FG, Kong YY, Michalewski HJ, Starr A (2005) Perceptual consequences of disrupted auditory nerve activity. J Neurophysiol 93: 3050-3063.

58. Hornickel J, Skoe E, Nicol T, Zecker S, Kraus N (2009) Subcortical differentiation of stop consonants relates to reading and speech-in-noise perception. Proc Natl Acad Sci U S A 106: 13022-13027.

59. Cunningham J, Nicol T, Zecker S, Bradlow A, Kraus N (2001) Neurobiologic responses to speech in noise in children with learning problems: Deficits and strategies for improvement. Clinical Neurophysiology 112: 758-767.

60. Wible B, Nicol T, Kraus N (2002) Abnormal neural encoding of repeated speech stimuli in noise in children with learning problems. Clin Neurophysiol 113: 485-494.

61. Stevens S, Davis H (1938) Hearing: Its psychology and physiology. New York: Wiley.

62. Miller MI, Barta PE, Sachs MB (1987) Strategies for the representation of a tone in background noise in the temporal aspects of the discharge patterns of auditory-nerve fibers. J Acoust Soc Am 81: 665-679.

63. Phillips DP (1990) Neural representation of sound amplitude in the auditory cortex: effects of noise masking. Behav Brain Res 37: 197-214.

64. Schneider BA, Hamstra SJ (1999) Gap detection thresholds as a function of tonal duration for younger and older listeners. J Acoust Soc Am 106: 371-380.

65. Zeng FG, Liu S (2006) Speech perception in individuals with auditory neuropathy. J Speech Lang Hear Res 49: 367-380.

66. Bacon SP, Viemeister NF (1985) Temporal modulation transfer functions in normal-hearing and hearing-impaired listeners. Audiology 24: 117-134.

67. Barnet AB (1975) Auditory evoked potentials during sleep in normal children from ten days to three years of age. Electroencephalogr Clin Neurophysiol 39: 29-41.

68. Berlin CI, Bordelon J, Hurley A (1997) Autoimmune inner ear disease: Basic science and audiological issues. In: Berlin CI (eds.) Neurotransmission and Hearing Loss: Basic Science, Diagnosis and Management pp: 137-146.

69. Berlin CI, Bordelon J, St John P, Wilensky D, Hurley A, et al. (1998) Reversing click polarity may uncover auditory neuropathy in infants. Ear Hear 19: 37-47.

70. Berlin C, Hood L, Cecola P (1993) Dose type I afferent neuron dysfunction reveal itself through lack of efferent suppression? Hearing Research 65: 40-54.

71. Berlin C, Hood L, Goforth-Barter L, Bordelon J (1999) Clinical application of auditory efferent studies. In: Berlin CI (eds) The efferent auditory system: Basic sciences and clinical applications. Singular Publishing Group, San Diego.

72. Berlin C, Hood L, Hurley A, Wen H (1994) Contralateral suppression of otoacoustic emissions: An index of the function of the medial olivocochlear system. Archives of Otolaryngology – Head and Neck Surgery 110: 3-21.

73. Berlin C, Hood L, Hurley A, Wen H (1996) Hearing aids: Only for hearing impaired patients with abnormal otoacoustic emissions. In: Berlin C (eds) Hair cells and hearing aids. Singular Publishing Group, San Diego.

74. Berlin C, Hood L, Morlet T, Rose K, Brashears S (2003) Auditory neuropathy/dys-synchrony: Diagnosis and management. Mental Retardation and Developmental Disabilities Research Reviews 9: 225-231.

75. Berlin C, Hood L, Rose K (2001) On renaming auditory neuropathy as auditory dys-synchrony. Audiology Today 13: 15-22.

76. Berlin CI, Morlet T, Hood LJ (2003) Auditory neuropathy/dyssynchrony: its diagnosis and management. Pediatr Clin North Am 50: 331-340, vii- viii.

77. Billings CJ, Tremblay KL, Souza PE, Binns MA (2007) Effects of hearing aid amplification and stimulus intensity on cortical auditory evoked potentials. Audiology and Neuro-Otology 12: 234-246.

78. Bishop DV (1997) Uncommon understanding: Development and disorders of language comprehension in children. Hove: Psychology press.

79. Bishop DV, Carlyon R, Deeks J, Bishop S (1999) Auditory temporal processing impairment: Neither necessary nor sufficient for causing language impairment in children. Journal of Speech, Language, and Hearing Research 42: 1295-1310.

80. Bradlow AR, Kraus N, Hayes E (2003) Speaking clearly for children with learning disabilities: Sentence perception in noise. Journal of Speech Language and Hearing Research 46: 80-97.

81. Drullman R, Festen JM, Plomp R (1994) Effect of reducing slow temporal modulations on speech reception. J Acoust Soc Am 95: 2670-2680.

82. Mason JC, De Michele A, Stevens C, Ruth RA, Hashisaki GT (2003) Cochlear implantation in patients with auditory neuropathy of varied etiologies. Laryngoscope 113: 45-49.

38

A Simple Minimally Invasive Technique to Reduce the Size of Pneumatized Middle Turbinate (Concha Bullosa)

Zeyad Mandour, Remon Kalza and Samy Elwany[*]

Department of Otolaryngology, Alexandria Medical School, Alexandria, Egypt

[*]**Corresponding author:** Samy Elwany, MD, FACS, Department of Otolaryngology, Alexandria Medical School, Alexandria, Egypt, E-mail: samy.elwany@alexmed.edu.eg

Abstract

Pneumatized middle turbinate, concha bullosa, is a common anatomic variant. In the vast majority of cases it is asymptomatic. In some patients it may cause contact headache or secondary sinusitis. It may also hamper access to the middle meatus during endoscopic sinus surgery. In this paper we describe a simple minimally invasive turbinoplasty technique to reduce the size of concha bullosa. The technique was used in 42 patients. The patients were followed up for 12-18 months. The turbinates retained their reduced size and stability at the end of the follow up period. Also, we did not observe any mucocele formation or adhesions between the turbinates and the surrounding structures. The technique is best used when the air cells within the turbinates are large. Resective techniques, on the other hand, may be used when enlargement of the turbinates is due to hypertrophy of its tissues rather than the presence of air cells.

Keywords: Concha; Bullosa; Middle turbinate, Turbinoplasty

Introduction

Pneumatization of the middle turbinate is a common anatomic variant, which has been named "Concha Bullosa" by Zuckerkandl in 1893. Three types of middle turbinate pneumatization: lamellar, bulbous and extensive, have been described based on the site and extent of pneumatisation [1]. The reported incidence of concha bullosa varies between 14-53% in various studies [2]. In the vast majority of cases concha bullosa is asymptomatic. However, Excessive enlargement of the middle turbinate can result in contact headache [3] and narrowing of the drainage pathway of the anterior group of paranasal sinuses. It may also impair intraoperative endoscopic access to the osteomeatal complex.

Several techniques have been described for management of concha bullosa including some technically challenging turbinoplasty procedures [4]. We describe, herein, a simple non-technically demanding procedure to reduce the size of symptomatic pneumatized middle turbinates.

Materials and Methods

The procedure was performed on Forty-two patients (26 males and 16 females), with CT evidence of pneumatized middle turbinate, during the period from January 2012 and December 2014. The indications for surgery were chronic rhinosinusitis, contact headache, or as an initial step to provide access to the osteomeatal complex during endoscopic nasal surgery. Patients with allergic rhinitis and those who had previous surgeries were excluded from the study. Twenty patients had extensive type of pneumatization (combined lamellar and bulbous), 18 patients had bulbous type, and 4 patients had lamellar type. All patients completed a validated outcomes instrument (SNOT-22) [5] before surgery and at the end of the follow

up period. IRB approval was obtained from the Committee of Medical Ethics and Research.

The patients received the routine postoperative care of nasal procedures The patients were followed up postoperatively on weekly basis for one month, monthly for 3 months, and then every 3 months for at least 12-18 months.

Surgical technique

The procedure was performed under general anesthesia. Seven patients, however, requested local anesthesia.

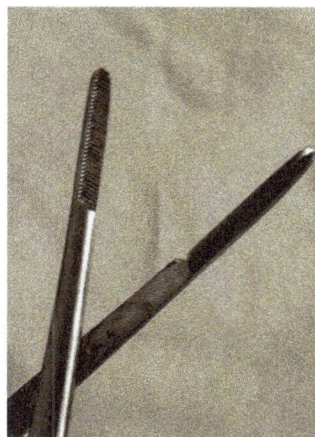

Figure 1: The instrument used for crushing the pneumatized turbinate. Note the large crushing surface of the blade.

The enlarged pneumatized portion of the middle turbinate was gently crushed between the blades of Kressner turbinate crushing

Variable	Preoperative score	Postoperative Score	Significance (p)
SNOT-22	58 (5)	21 (2)	0.01*

Table 1: SNOT-22 Quality of life score–Mean/SD, *Mann-Whitney U Test. Level of significance p<0.05.

Discussion

Pneumatized middle turbinates sometimes encroach upon the middle meatus, narrow the osteomeatal complex, hinder intraoperative endoscopic access to the middle meatus, and hamper postoperative control of the postoperative bed.

Excision of the lateral lamella of the concha bullosa, which is a commonly performed procedure, is associated with reported postoperative adhesions in 15% of patients especially if the procedure was combined with surgery of the paranasal sinuses [3]. In an attempt to decrease the rate of postoperative adhesions and improve the postoperative outcomes, several authors described more technically demanding procedures that were associated with a smaller incidence of postoperative adhesions.

None of our patients developed mucocele within the crushed turbinate. Mucocele is believed to develop secondary to osteal obstruction. In approximately 55% of cases the concha bullosa represents an extension of anterior ethmoid pneumatization and its ostium thus opens in the middle meatus. Posterior ethmoid air cells account for pneumatization of the remaining 45% which therefore drain into the superior meatus [6]. The ostium of the conchal cell is always present in the highest level of the cavity of the concha bullosa regardless the size and location of the conchal cell [5] This, apparently, shielded the ostium from traumatic injury during the crushing procedure.

In our series the turbinates retained their reduced postoperative size. We believe that crushing of the conchal walls results in micro-fractures that, upon healing, result into permanent remodeling of the turbinate to its new size and shape.

Excessive surgical manipulation of the concha bullosa in the form of dissection of its mucosa or bony lamella can potentially destabilize the middle turbinate. The described technique does not entail undue manipulations of the middle turbinate and was not associated with destabilization of the middle turbinate in any of our cases.

Conclusion

Our technique is a simple procedure that can result in predictable outcomes. The technique is not associated with the risk of destabilization of the middle turbinate, and does not increase the risk for mucocele formation within the middle turbinate. It also reduces the risk of postoperative adhesions. The technique is best used when the air cells within the turbinates are large. Resective techniques, on the other hand, may be used when enlargement of the turbinates is due to hypertrophy of its tissues rather than the presence of air cells.

References

1. HatipoÄŸlu HG, Cetin MA, YÃ¼ksel E (2005) Concha bullosa types: Their relationship with sinusitis, ostiomeatal and frontal recess disease. Diagn Interv Radiol 11: 145-149.

2. Stallman JS, Lobo JN, Som PM (2004) The incidence of concha bullosa and its relationship to nasal septal deviation and paranasal sinus disease. AJNR Am J Neuroradiol 25: 1613-1618.

3. Shihada R, Luntz M (2012) A concha bullosa mucopyocele manifesting as migraine headaches: A case report and literature review. Ear Nose Throat J 91: E16-18.

4. Har-el G, Slavit DH (1996) Turbinoplasty for concha bullosa: A non-synechiae-forming alternative to middle turbinectomy. Rhinology 34: 54-56.

5. Marambaia PP, Lima MG, Santos KP, Gomes Ade M, de Sousa MM, et al. (2013) Evaluation of the quality of life of patients with chronic rhinosinusitis by means of the SNOT-22 questionnaire. Braz J Otorhinolaryngol 79: 54-58.

6. DoÄŸru H, DÃ¶ner F, Uygur K, Gedikli O, Cetin M (1999) Pneumatized inferior turbinate. Am J Otolaryngol 20: 139-141.

39

A Twelve Months Follow-Up: Influence of Origin and Duration of Hearing-Loss on Tnrts after Cochlear Implantation

Florian Christov[*], Patrick Munder, Laura Berg, Judith Arnolds, Heike Bagus, Stephan Lang, Diana Arweiler-Harbeck

Uniklinik Essen, HNO, Essen, Germany

[*]**Corresponding author:** Florian Christov, Uniklinik Essen, HNO, Essen, Germany; E-mail: florian.christov@uk-essen.de

Abstract

Introduction: People with profound sensorineural hearing loss benefit from cochlear implantation. Nevertheless there are discrepancies as far as signal processing and hearing results are concerned. The large variety of patients in terms of age, cause and duration of deafness is one explanation. Neural response telemetry (tNRT) gives information about the function of the hearing nerve and the device. Previous studies couldn`t exactly show evident correlations between NRTs and cause or length of hearing-loss. Aim of the present study was the re-evaluation of tNRTs in a 12 months follow-up as a function of duration and reason of deafness.

Patients and methods: 168 patients (82 female, 86 male) implanted at the department between 2008 and 2013 with an implant of Cochlear® were included into the study. 71 patients received a CI512 and 52 patients a CI24RE device, while 45 patients were supplied with the slim straight electrode array CI422. tNRTs were measured at each of the 22 electrodes intraoperatively, after 6 and after 12 months.

Results: tNRT-values showed a reduction of tNRT-values over parts of the monitored period. Patients with Menière`s disease showed slightly higher values but the differences regarding the cause of deafness weren`t significant. Implant recipients with a mean time of hearing loss or a mean time of hearing aid supply showed a tendency of lower tNRTs. However the results weren't significant.

Conclusion: Within the first six months after CI implantation tNRTs decreased significantly. Patients with Menière's disease showed decent higher tNRTs. Patients with a period of deafness longer than two years presented lower tNRT thresholds. Participants with a mean time hearing aid supply prior CI surgery also provided a trend towards lower tNRTs. The impact of tNRTs on residual hearing in dependence of different shaped electrode arrays as well as the effect on speech perception should be focused in upcoming studies.

Keywords: Cochlea implant; NRT; ECAP; Hearing loss; Electrode; Deafness; Hearing aid

Introduction

People with severe to profound sensorineural hearing loss benefit from cochlear implantation [1,2] Nevertheless there are meanderings with regard to diverse age groups: Younger patients tend to have better hearing results than the older ones [3,4]. The large variety of patients in terms of cause and duration of deafness could be another explanation for the different hearing outcomes. The predictability of hearing success after cochlear implantation at a certain point of time is one of the most often discussed questions. As a matter of course the patient asks for the likeliness of a good hearing result after surgery. Electric compound action potentials (ECAPs) are an objective indicator for the nerve- and device- function and are determined for each of the 22 electrodes on both the slim straight (CI 422) and the precurved (CI24 RE and CI 512) arrays. Having been utilized for more than 20 years now, the importance for the clinical use is still in focus of applied research and application feasibilities in further development [5,6].

ECAPs are potentials from the hearing nerve after stimulation from a CI-electrode and correspond to wave I of the ABR. The stimulation occurs at one electrode and the answering potential gets recorded at the after next electrode. Thus stimulation artefacts can be avoided. A logical theory is that lower values are expected to result in better hearing abilities, because the nerve-reaction already occurs at a minor stimulation level. Intra- and postoperative measurements of ECAPs and determination of the threshold level are very important for a successful supply with cochlear implants and are already part of the daily routine [7]. Intraoperative ECAPs confirm the CI- function and record the hearing nerves answer to direct stimulation. Postoperative ECAPs are additionally important for the very first CI - fitting process as well as in the following controls [7].

ECAPs can be measured by using the NRT-System (Neural Response Telemetry). They are detected visually by marking the first potential that appears after the lowest stimulation level (vNRT). The more common method is to measure several potentials at different stimulation levels and calculate a regression value (tNRT) [8]. However there are even more options to obtain NRTs: In the fitting process of the cochlear implant MAPs (mapping) can be used to optimize the patient`s hearing result: A T-Level (behavioral threshold) demonstrates the threshold at which a sound can be recognized and a C-Level (comfort level) distinguishes a comfortable volume [8]. Though it is not recommended to use NRTs for programming only [9]. It is known that NRTs decrease after surgery [10] and even in case of intraoperative absence NRTs can appear and/or increase with a latency of some months [11]. Literature provides contrary opinions to what extent there is an effect of the patient's age [3,4,12]. Previous studies couldn't exactly show evident correlations between NRTs and cause or length of hearing-loss either [2,13]. King et al. analyzed for 21 patients that NRT-thresholds and the slope of the NRT growth function are predictors for the C-Level in patients with a hearing loss less than 20 years [14]. Nevertheless for a larger collective there is no comprehensive knowledge about other parameters influencing NRT values. A further question is if there is a change of these factors in the course of time. Aim of the present study was the evaluation of tNRTs of 168 individuals in a 12 months follow-up as a function of duration and reason of deafness.

Patients and Methods

168 patients (82 female, 86 male) implanted at the department between 2008 and 2013 with an implant of Cochlear® were included into the study. 123 were supplied with a perimodiolar electrode-array: 71 patients with a CI512 and 52 patients with a CI24RE. 45 patients received the slim straight CI422. Electrode insertion was performed 44 times via the round window and 124 times via cochleostomy. A retrospective analysis of tNRTs during operation as well as 6 and 12 months after surgery was performed. Patients with incomplete data set of tNRTs were excluded.

After inserting the electrode array into the cochlear NRTs were determined in an open operative site at each of the 22 electrodes automatically by a program of the company. Every electrode shows specific amplitudes after stimulating the nerve with different intensity levels. By detecting the regression value of above-threshold potentials at each electrode the tNRTs are obtained. A profile of the cochlear implant is shown in a chart and gives information of the tNRTs of each electrode (in CL=current level).

Quantity and mean-scores were calculated for all 22 electrodes and both different array-types. The analysis of variance and the Wilcoxon-Test were determined using SPSS-22. Significant results were set for p<0.05. The comprehensive experience of performing more than 1000 cochlear implants at the clinic showed a useful cut for good results at a tNRT<164 CL. This study was performed in accordance with the Declaration of Helsinki and was approved by the local ethics committee.

Results

In all age cohorts tNRTs were reproducible intra- and postoperatively. An analysis of all tNRT-values over all patients and each electrode at three points of time revealed a reduction of tNRT-values over the monitored period. The mean value of the tNRTs improved after 6 months significantly (p=0.000) from 174.14 to 156.38 and despite a slightly following not significant increase (p=0.403) the value remained at this lower standard after 12 months (157.79). Figure 1 shows the mean tNRTs of all patients and electrodes at three points of time.

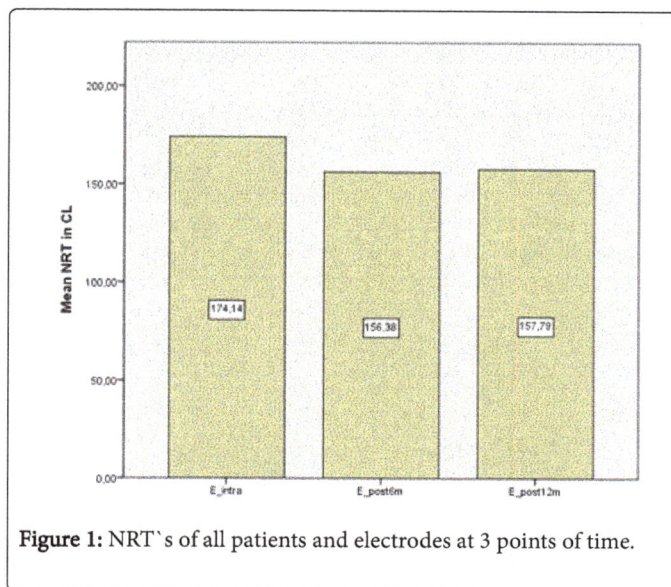

Figure 1: NRT's of all patients and electrodes at 3 points of time.

Origin of hearing loss

Taking into account the eight main causes of deafness, the largest three groups included the patients with unknown (n=92), genetic (n=44) and post-inflammatory (n=18) reasons of deafness. The genetic group can be subdivided into Connexin26 associated hearing loss (n=5) and other genetic (n=39) reasons. Menières disease (n=5), posttraumatic (n=3) and toxic (n=4) causes were less frequently (Figure 2). In the analysis of variance (ANOVA) of slim straight electrodes the differences between the groups weren't significant intraoperatively (p=0.806) or after 6 (p=0.757) and 12 (p=0.480) months. Perimodiolar electrodes didn't show significant results either (p=0.935 and p=0.756 and p=0.453). For statistically reasons the minor cluster of autoimmune (n=1) and otosclerotic (n=1) patients had to be excluded for this calculation.

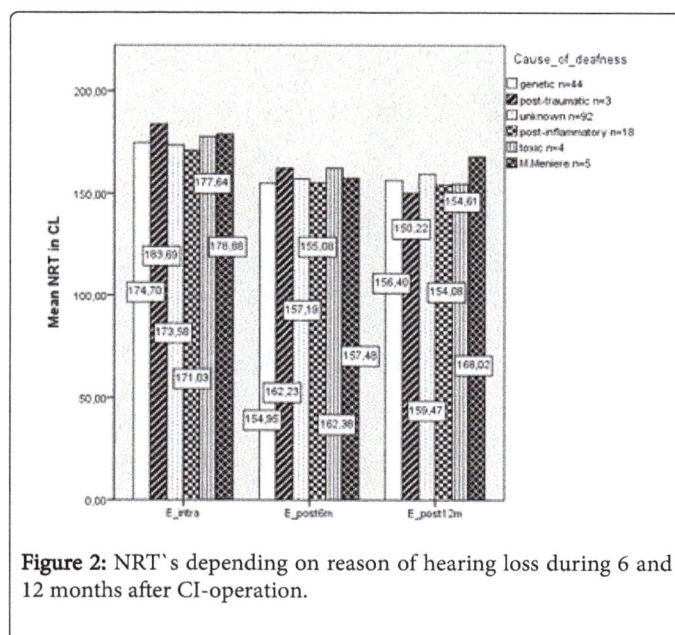

Figure 2: NRT's depending on reason of hearing loss during 6 and 12 months after CI-operation.

Duration of hearing loss

The patients were divided into four groups regarding the time of hearing loss before cochlear implantation (<1 year (n=41), 1-2 years (n=18), 2-6 years (n=37), >6 years (n=72)). The analysis of variance for slim straight electrodes didn`t show significant differences intraoperatively (p=0.555), after 6 (p=0.514) and after 12 months (0.281). Similar results were obtained for the precurved models (p=0.293 und p=0.168 und p=0.195). In the 12 months control decent tendencies of slightly higher tNRT-values were seen in patients with a hearing loss for less than 2 years (Figure 3).

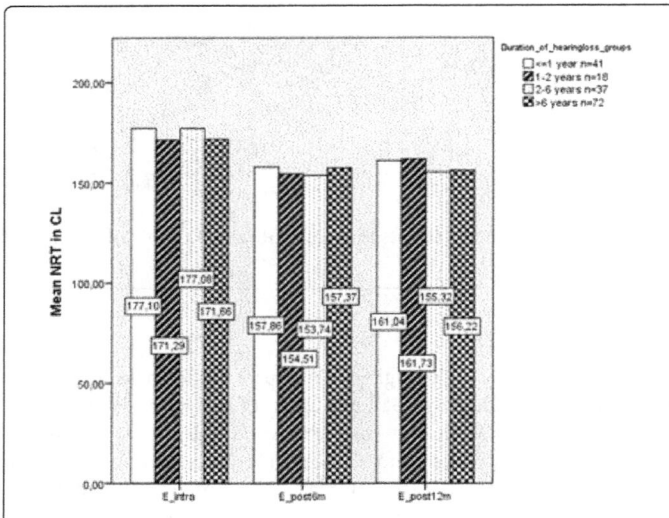

Figure 3: NRT`s depending on duration of deafness during, 6 and 12 months after CI implantation.

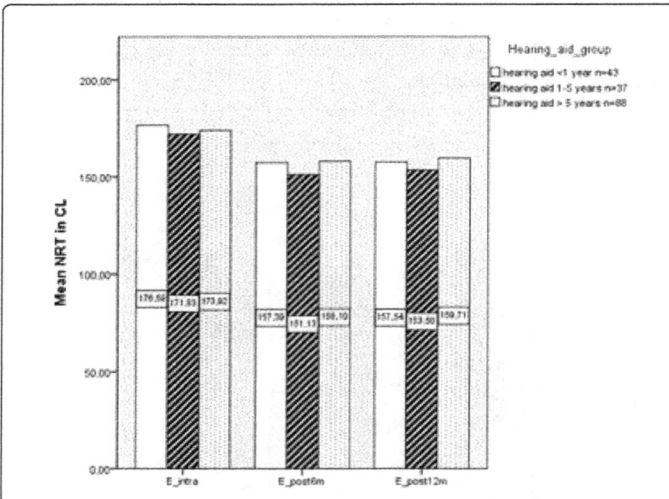

Figure 4: NRT`s depending on duration of hearing aid supply prior CI during, 6 and 12 months after CI implantation.

43 CI users had been supplied with a hearing aid for less than one year. While another 37 patients wore a hearing aid 1 to 5 years in advance, 88 participants used a device longer than 5 years prior to CI implantation (Figure 4). The cluster of patients utilizing a hearing aid 1-5 years prior to CI implantation showed slightly lower tNRT values

than the others. However there were no significant results intraoperatively (p=0.548), after 6 (p=0.142) and after 12 months (p=0.197) either.

Discussion

Electric compound action potentials (ECAPs) are an indicator for the hearing nerve- and the device- performance in and after CI implantation [7]. A logical theory is that lower values are expected to result in better hearing outcome as the nerve's reaction occurs to a lower stimulation level. In the course of observed time there are changes of the tNRTs depending on different factors. Mittmann et al. for example discussed the influence of the electrode array's position inside the cochlea by using a NRT-ratio and proved a high correlation to the results of a radiological control [15]. The impact of further parameters and the possibility of exerting influence on ECAP performance are discussed separately in the following:

NRT in the course of time

Contour advanced electrode arrays are known to result in lower thresholds compared to the slim straight types [10]. However in the present investigation both showed similar characteristics regarding different items: A significant drop of tNRTs could be revealed after 6 months. Chen et al. though showed a significant decrease of tNRTs already after 24 h caused by an almost immediate restoration of neuronal sensitivity and interaction between matrix and electrodes [16]. It is possible that the CI-users of the investigated cohort would have shown the same phenomenon if they were reevaluated at an earlier point of time after implantation than after 6 months. Experience shows that tNRTs as well as the impedances are lower in closed operative settings than determined in an open operative site. Chen et al. didn`t specify the exact measuring circumstances. That might be an explanation for the origin of the rapid NRT-decrease. In contrast Tanamati et al. claimed in their study, that during the first year no significant changes to ECAPs could be found [17]. Brown et al. supported this thesis and assumed only small changes in the development of ECAPs over a 5 to 6 years observation [18]. However, the present results are not in contrast to these observations, as it could be demonstrated as well, that tNRT values kept stable after the initial drop.

Origin of hearing loss

With regard to the cause of deafness significant correlations to tNRT thresholds couldn't be shown. The same conclusion was drawn by Kutscher et al. [13] who didn`t see a correlation between the recovery function and etiology of hearing loss. Anyhow the results of the present survey clarified that the cluster of patients with Ménière's disease at all three points of time had higher NRTs than the two largest groups (genetic and unknown origin). Nevertheless the outcome was statistically not significant. The difference was most obvious 1 year after implantation. McRackan et al. also claimed that the hearing outcome of Ménière's disease patients is worse than in the general CI population [19]. Assuming that lower ECAPs are associated with better hearing results, the thesis of McRackan and co-workers can be supported. However cochlear implantation is still the best option to treat profound hearing-loss in patients with Mèniere`s disease [20]. Miyagawa et al. focused on the genetic causes of deafness and claimed that patients with certain gene mutations show relatively good results. [21] Kraaijenga et al. showed that otosclerosis and meningitis are negative predictors for the hearing outcome [22].

Duration of hearing loss

Nehmè et al. negated an influence of the duration of hearing loss on the ECAP outcome [23]. Their cohort was mainly made up of congenitally deafened patients. The period of deafness corresponded to the age at CI operation and the age at implantation didn't affect the NRTs. These results were in agreement with the current study which didn't figure out significant differences concerning the length of deafness either. However it could be clarified that 12 months after surgery there was a tendency of lower tNRT thresholds in patients with a duration of hearing loss longer than two years before implantation. These results can be explained with a presumably lighter hearing loss than after a rapid profound deafness (which normally gets implanted earlier) and more various cohorts in the present study. Nehmè et al. investigated only 34 mainly congenitally deafened patients [23], while in the current study 168 CI users with congenital and acquired hearing loss were included. Zeh et al. added, that even in the period of rehabilitation of cochlea implantation there were no differences with regard to the duration of deafness [2].

Kutscher et al. proclaimed there is no correlation between nerve recovery function and time of hearing aid use prior to CI [13]. Lazard et al. supports the thesis that the hearing aid use has a significant influence on the outcome of the hearing performance [24]. In spite there weren't significant results in the recent study either decent lower tNRTs for patients who utilized a device 1-5 years before operation could be shown. It can be assumed, that patients with a mean time hearing aid provision have better residual hearing conditions and may more often suffer from a slowly progressive hearing loss. The interest for a cochlear implant develops stealthy in the course of time and this issue is accompanied with lower tNRTs. An explanation for the poorer outcome of the short-term supply (less than one year) could be a rapid more severe hearing loss, that couldn't be treated satisfactorily with conventional hearing aids. The need for cochlear implantation comes straight away and a more profound hearing loss might have been the reason for higher tNRTs. In contrast, if patients have been suffering from profound hearing loss for many years without benefitting from the hearing device for a long time, a degeneration of the hearing nerve might already have occurred. This phenomenon is also reflected in higher tNRT thresholds. An explanation for Kutscher et al.'s contrary thesis [13] might be the smaller collective (n=50). Furthermore only Nucleus24 devices were included, while in the present study CI 422, CI 512 and CI 24 RE were analyzed. A detailed investigation on this issue is the main emphasis of further upcoming publications.

Conclusion

Within the first six months after CI implantation tNRTs decreased significantly and remained stable in the following course of time. Despite of a small number of patients with Ménière's disease, this group showed decent higher tNRTs than CI users with other reasons of hearing loss. Patients with a period of deafness longer than two years presented lower tNRT thresholds. Participants with a mean time hearing aid supply prior CI surgery also provided a trend towards lower tNRTs. The impact of tNRTs on residual hearing as well as the effect on speech perception over the course of time will be subject for upcoming studies. Furthermore a current evaluation of the electrode arrays tonotopy and differences between slim straight and contour advanced electrode arrays is in process.

References

1. Runge CL, Henion K, Tarima S, Beiter A, Zwolan TA (2016) Clinical Outcomes of the cochlearâ„¢ nucleus(â®) 5 cochlear implant system and smartsoundâ„¢ 2 signal processing. J Am Acad Audiol 27: 425-440.

2. Zeh R, Baumann U (2015) [Inpatient rehabilitation of adult CI users: Results in dependency of duration of deafness, CI experience and age]. HNO 63: 557-576.

3. AlSanosi A, Hassan SM (2014) The effect of age at cochlear implantation outcomes in Saudi children. Int J Pediatr Otorhinolaryngol 78: 272-276.

4. Beyea JA, McMullen KP, Harris MS, Houston DM, Martin JM, et al. (2016) Cochlear implants in adults: Effects of age and duration of deafness on speech recognition. Otol Neurotol .

5. Gordon KA, Ebinger KA, Gilden JE, Shapiro WH (2002) Neural response telemetry in 12 to 24 month old children. Ann Otol Rhinol Laryngol Suppl 189: 42-48.

6. Abbas PJ, Brown CJ, Shallop JK, Firszt JB, Hughes ML, et al. (1999) Summary of results using the nucleus CI24M implant to record the electrically evoked compound action potential. Ear Hear 20: 45-59.

7. Wesarg T, Arndt S, Aschendorff A, Laszig R, Zirn S (2014) Intraoperative audiological-technical diagnostics during cochlear implant surgery. HNO 62: 725-734.

8. Potts LG, Skinner MW, Gotter BD, Strube MJ, Brenner CA (2007) Relation between neural response telemetry thresholds, T- and C-levels, and loudness judgments in 12 adult nucleus 24 cochlear implant recipients. Ear Hear 28: 495-511.

9. McKay CM, Chandan K, Akhoun I, Siciliano C, Kluk K (2013) Can ECAP measures be used for totally objective programming of cochlear implants? J Assoc Res Otolaryngol 14: 879-890.

10. Christov F, Munder P, Berg L, Bagus H, Lang S (2016) ECAP analysis in cochlear implant patients as a function of patient's age and electrode- design. Eur Ann Otorhinolaryngol Head Neck Dis 1: S1-S3.

11. Moura AC, Goffi-Gomez MV, Couto MI, Brito R, Tsuji RK, et al. (2014) Longitudinal analysis of the absence of intraoperative neural response telemetry in children using cochlear implants. Int Arch Otorhinolaryngol 18: 362-368.

12. Carvalho B, Hamerschmidt R, Wiemes G (2015) Intraoperative neural response telemetry and neural recovery function: a comparative study between adults and children. Int Arch Otorhinolaryngol 19: 10-15.

13. Kutscher K, Goffi-Gomez MV, Befi-Lopes DM, Tsuji RK, Bento RF (2010) Cochlear implant: Correlation of nerve function recovery, auditory deprivation and etiology. Pro Fono 22: 473-478.

14. King JE, Polak M, Hodges AV, Payne S, Telischi FF (2006) Use of neural response telemetry measures to objectively set the comfort levels in the Nucleus 24 cochlear implant. J Am Acad Audiol 17: 413-431.

15. Mittmann P, Todt I, Ernst A, Rademacher G, Mutze S, et al. (2016) Electrophysiological detection of scalar changing perimodiolar cochlear electrode arrays: A long term follow-up study. Eur Arch Otorhinolaryngol.

16. Chen JK, Chuang AY, Sprinzl GM, Tung TH, Li LP (2013) Impedance and electrically evoked compound action potential (ECAP) drop within 24 h after cochlear implantation. PLoS One 8: e71929.

17. Tanamati LF, Bevilacqua MC, Costa OA (2009) Longitudinal study of the ecap measured in children with cochlear implants. Braz J Otorhinolaryngol 75: 90-96.

18. Brown CJ, Abbas PJ, Etlert CP, O'Brient S, Oleson JJ (2010) Effects of long-term use of a cochlear implant on the electrically evoked compound action potential. J Am Acad Audiol 21: 5-15.

19. McRackan TR, Gifford RH, Kahue CN, Dwyer R, Labadie RF, et al. (2014) Cochlear implantation in Ménière's disease patients. Otol Neurotol 35: 421-425.

20. Samy RN, Houston L, Scott M, Choo DI, Meinzen-Derr J (2015) Cochlear implantation in patients with Meniere's disease. Cochlear Implants Int 16: 208-212.

21. Miyagawa M, Nishio SY, Usami S (2016) A comprehensive study on the etiology of patients receiving cochlear implantation with special emphasis on genetic epidemiology. Otol Neurotol 37: e126-e134.

22. Kraaijenga VJ, Smit AL, Stegeman I, Smilde JJ, van Zanten GA, et al. (2015) Factors that influence outcomes in cochlear implantation in adults, based on patient related characteristics - a retrospective study. Clin Otolaryngol.

23. Nehmé A, El Zir E, Moukarzel N, Haidar H, Vanpoucke F, et al. (2014) Measures of the electrically evoked compound action potential threshold and slope in HiRes 90K(TM) users. Cochlear Implants Int 15: 53-60.

24. Lazard DS, Vincent C, Venail F, Van de Heyning P, Truy E, et al. (2012) Pre-, per- and postoperative factors affecting performance of postlinguistically deaf adults using cochlear implants: A new conceptual model over time. PLoS One 7: e48739.

A Pilot Study of Induction Triplet Chemotherapy Followed by Minimally Invasive Surgery for Stage 3-4 Resectable Oropharyngeal Cancer

Krishna Rao[1,2,3,4*], **Kathy Robinson**[4], **James Malone**[4,5], **Cathy Clausen**[6], **Bruce Shevlin**[6] and **K Thomas Robbins**[4,5]

[1]*Department of Internal Medicine, Southern Illinois University School of Medicine, USA*

[2]*Division of Hematology/Oncology, Department of Internal Medicine, Southern Illinois University School of Medicine, USA*

[3]*Department of Medical Microbiology, Southern Illinois University School of Medicine, USA*

[4]*Simmons Cancer Institute at SIU, Southern Illinois University School of Medicine, USA*

[5]*Division of Otolaryngology Head and Neck Surgery, Department of Surgery, Southern Illinois University School of Medicine, USA*

[6]*St. John's Hospital Department of Radiation Oncology, Springfield, IL, Southern Illinois University School of Medicine, USA*

*****Corresponding author:** Krishna Rao, Simmons Cancer Institute at Southern Illinois University School of Medicine, 315 W. Carpenter St., PO Box 19678, Springfield, IL 62794-9678, USA; E-mail: krao@siumed.edu

Abstract

The current study reports the results of an open label pilot study evaluating a novel treatment protocol for patients with locally advanced head and neck cancer. Patients received induction chemotherapy and those who had a clinical complete response to induction chemotherapy were offered trans-oral nidusectomy for the primary lesion and neck node dissection. If a pathologic complete response was achieved, patients were then observed. Patients not achieving a clinical or pathologic complete response to induction therapy were subsequently treated with chemoradiation.

Keywords: Induction; Head and neck cancer; Chemotherapy

Introduction

Three modalities of therapy have established roles in the treatment of carcinoma of the head and neck: surgery, radiation therapy, and chemotherapy. The choice of which modality to use depends upon many factors such as the site and extent of the primary lesion, the likelihood of complete surgical resection, the presence of lymph node metastases, and the associated acute and long term toxicities. Traditionally, smaller lesions (stage T1-T2) are effectively treated with surgical excision or irradiation whereas more advanced disease (stage III-IV) is treated with combined surgery and radiation therapy. The use of such combined modality therapy represents an important advancement in the treatment of this disease [1-3]. However, even when surgery and radiation therapy are used concomitantly, only a minority of patients with advanced regional disease are cured; and the subsequent morbidity related to radiation, including xerostomia, dysphonia, and dysphagia, is a major problem among survivors [4].

The use of a third modality, chemotherapy, has provided an additional option for improved survival when combined with radiation therapy. Of particular note is the ECOG trial in which IV cisplatin administered concomitantly with radiation therapy was more effective than radiation alone and equally effective as polychemotherapy combined with split course radiation therapy [5]. Cisplatin has received the greatest attention over the past 2 decades particularly in its combination with 5-fluorouracil.

Whereas the tumoricidal effects of combination regimens may be greater, this potential advantage is partly negated by the higher rates of normal tissue toxicity, particularly if it is combined with radiation therapy.

Chemotherapy's greatest impact has been for locally advanced disease when used in combination with radiation therapy. However, more recent trials using an induction triplet chemotherapy regimen prior to concomitant chemoradiation have demonstrated even better results for local-regional disease control and overall survival. In the TAX 324 study with a minimum of 2 years of follow-up (3 years for 69% of patients), significantly more patients survived in the triplet chemotherapy group versus the doublet chemotherapy group (hazard ratio for death, 0.70; P=0.006). Estimates of overall survival at 3 years were 62% in the triplet group and 48% in the doublet group; the median overall survival was 71 months and 30 months, respectively (P=0.006) [6]. An important observation of the induction triplet chemotherapy regimen is that there was an unprecedented high proportion of patients treated who had a complete response of their disease upon the completion of the induction phase, even before chemoradiation [7]. Despite the improvements in disease control and survival that have been shown with chemoradiation protocols for advanced head and neck cancer, there continues to exist the problem of treatment toxicity and its impact on quality of life. Whereas the major toxic effects of chemotherapy are acute and mostly reversible, the adverse sequelae of radiation therapy are both acute and chronic. Long term effects such as xerostomia, fibrosis, strictures, and soft tissue or bone necrosis can be highly devastating or even morbid [8,9]. The development of an effective treatment protocol that does not rely on radiation therapy would be a major advancement in terms of improving quality of life parameters.

One treatment strategy for patients with advanced head and neck cancer who prove to be highly sensitive to chemotherapy is to combine the modalities of polychemotherapy and conservation surgery 4 with the goal of avoiding radiation therapy. For those patients whose primary disease is classified as T2-3 (resectable), and who have a complete response following induction therapy, it is feasible to perform an organ preservation tumor nidusectomy at the primary site to verify that the clinical complete response is truly a pathological complete response. Similarly, the clinical complete response observed for the associated nodal disease, can be verified pathologically by performing a selective neck dissection without causing significant morbidity. Both tumor nidusectomy and selective neck dissection has been shown to be an effective adjuvant in this setting. Building on these observations, we conducted a novel protocol in patients with locally advanced head and neck cancer. Patients received induction chemotherapy and those that had a clinical complete response to induction chemotherapy were offered nidusectomy and neck node dissection. If a pathologic complete response was achieved, patients were then observed. Patients not achieving a clinical or pathologic complete response to induction therapy were treated with chemoradiation.

Materials and Methods

This was an open label, non-randomized, pilot study. After obtaining approval from the Springfield Committee for Research Involving Human Subjects (SCHRIS), we proceeded forward with this study. The study was also registered at clinicaltrials.gov and assigned a study number of NCT 01111942. Between May 2006 and May 2010, a total of 4 adult patients were enrolled in the study after obtaining written informed consent. Patients eligible for the study included those with biopsy proven, previously untreated, stage III-IV (T1, T2, T3) (N0-N2) squamous cell carcinoma of the oropharynx staged according to AJCC guidelines. Patients with T4 tumors or N3 neck disease were excluded as were patients with a prior history of malignancy, excluding basal and squamous cell carcinoma of the skin and carcinoma in situ of the cervix. The oropharynx subsite was selected for this trial as tumors in the region are very amenable to surgical access and potential nidusectomy.

Prior to chemotherapy, at the time of examination under anesthesia and panendoscopy, the interface between the soft tissue involvement of the tumor and the surrounding normal mucosa was tattooed with India ink. This served to mark the site of future nidusetomy. All subjects enrolled received induction chemotherapy with docetaxel, cisplatin, and 5-fluorouracil. Induction chemotherapy was given over 3 cycles, each cycle consisting of 21 days.

Following induction triplet chemotherapy, subjects were restaged by physical examination and radiological imaging. If there was an unequivocal absence of evidence for residual disease (i.e. an apparent complete response), the subject underwent conservation surgery and neck node dissection under general anesthesia.

Using a transoral approach, the region that was previously involved by the primary tumor was excised. The amount of tissue removed was intended to be minimal and accessed directly without major exposure techniques. The intent of conservation surgery was to remove the residual abnormal (scar) tissue in the region originally occupied by the cancer rather than to perform an oncologic resection in which 1-2 cm margins around the tumor are included. The lymph node groups at risk were removed en bloc based on neck level or sublevel. For subjects with positive nodal disease prior to induction therapy, this included the neck level that was involved and at least one neck level distal to the pattern of flow for the lymphatic drainage. For subjects at risk for bilateral nodal involvement (base of tongue, posterior pharyngeal wall, and soft palate) the levels at risk were also removed. Post-surgery,

patients were then carefully monitored for maintenance of disease remission.

All subjects with clinical or radiological evidence of persistent disease and who failed to achieve a clinical complete response to induction triplet chemotherapy as evidenced by physical examination and CT/PET scan subsequently underwent concomitant chemoradiation. Radiation therapy consisted of 6 conventional standard beam or IMRT to the involved areas according to NCCN guidelines at the discretion of the treating physician. Suggested total dosage was 5600 to 7000 Gy. Carboplatin was administered weekly during radiotherapy at an AUC dosage of 1.5.

Quality of life measurements were performed on all patients FACT H and N, UW-QOL,[10] and MDADI questionnaires. Subjects were followed for 24 months after cessation of study treatment, progression of disease with subsequent treatment with a non-study treatment, or until death.

The study protocol permitted enrollment to 10 patients of which at least 1 of the first five needed to achieve a complete clinical and pathologic response to induction TPF therapy in order to continue the study and enter 5 additional patients.

Results

A total of four male patients were enrolled in the study. Enrollment of the fifth patient was elusive due to the rurality of the patient population and long travel distance for protocol based therapy, which potentially included daily radiation treatments.

The age of the patients ranged from 55 to 67, with an average of 60.75 years. Subsites of involvement included the tonsil (50%) and base of tongue (50%). Three patients had T2 lesions while one patient had a T3 lesion. Nodal status ranged from N1 (50%) to N2b (50%). All four patients had HPV positive disease. Characteristics are noted in Tables 1 and 2.

Characteristics	Number or Percent
Enrolled in Study	4
Average Age	60.75
Gender	----
Male	100%
Female	0%
Ethnicity	----
European	100%

Table 1: Patient characteristics.

N1	N2b
T2	1
T3	1

Table 2: Tumor characteristics of patients.

	Mild	Moderate	Severe	Life Threatening	Fatal
Alopecia	100%	3			
Anemia		1			
Anorexia	3	3	2		
Ascites		1			
Atrial Fibrillation		1			
Low Hematocrit		1			
Low RBC		1			
Bands				1	
Bruising	1				
Constipation	2				
Cough	1				
Creatinine Elevated	2	1	1		
Dehydration		2	1		
Diarrhea	3	4	1		
Distention/Bloating of Abdomen		1	1		
Dizziness	1	1			

Table 3: List of toxicities and grading with number of patients exhibiting the toxicity listed in each cell.

One of the four patients received only one cycle of TPF and had to stop due to nephrotoxicity. Of the remaining three who completed protocol therapy, one patient did achieve a complete clinical response and went to surgery. Pathology from the surgery showed evidence of residual carcinoma, and received chemoradiation. The other two patients, not having achieved a clinical complete response, received chemoradiation with weekly carboplatin. All four patients are alive and disease free with over 24 months of follow-up.

Grade 3 or higher toxicities included anorexia (50%), renal failure (25%), dehydration (25%), diarrhea (25%), abdominal distension and bloating (25%), fatigue (25%), hypocalcemia (25%), hypokalemia (50%), hypomagnesemia (25%), hyponatremia (25%), hypophosphatemia (25%), hypotension (25%), infusa-port site infections (75%), insomnia (25%), lymphopenia (25%), anxiety (25%), depression (50%), nausea (50%), neutropenia (75%), neutropenic fever (25%), small bowel obstruction (25%), salivary gland changes (25%), sepsis (25%), thrombosis (25%), and vomiting (50%). Adverse events that were serious i.e. required hospitalization included atrial fibrillation, dehydration, diarrhea, depression, neutropenic fever, nausea, salivary gland changes, sepsis, thrombosis, and vomiting. All toxicities are outlined in Table 3.

Discussion

The role of taxanes and the use of triplet induction chemotherapy in head and neck cancer still remain controversial due to the conflicting results of several randomized studies. Positive studies, which motivated us to perform this present study, include TAX 323 and TAX 324. Initially, Investigators at the Dana Farber Cancer Institute conducted a series of Phase II studies evaluating the addition of docetaxel to PF-based chemotherapy. Consistently, high complete response rates (42%-61%) and overall response rates (91%-100%) were noted [11]. Based on these studies, TAX 324 was conducted [6]. Five hundred and one patients (all of whom had stage III or IV disease with no distant metastases and tumors considered to be non-resectable or were candidates for organ preservation) were randomly assigned to receive either TPF or PF induction chemotherapy, followed by chemoradiotherapy with weekly carboplatin therapy and radiotherapy for 5 days per week. The primary end point was overall survival.

With a minimum of 2 years of follow-up, significantly more patients survived in the TPF group than in the PF group. Estimates of overall survival at 3 years were 62% in the TPF group and 48% in the PF group; the median overall survival was 71 months and 30 months, respectively. There was better locoregional control in the TPF group than in the PF group, but the incidence of distant metastases in the two groups did not differ significantly. The EORTC 24971/ TAX 323 study used a slightly different dosing scheme for the TPF regimen and conducted a similar study. Importantly, the study omitted concurrent chemotherapy with the radiation, and the radiation was delivered either as fractionated or hyperfractionated therapy. A total of 358 patients underwent randomization, with 177 assigned to the TPF group and 181 to the PF group. At a median follow-up of 32.5 months, the median progression-free survival was 11.0 months in the TPF group and 8.2 months in the PF group. Treatment with TPF resulted in a reduction in the risk of death of 27%, with a median overall survival of 18.8 months, as compared with 14.5 months in the PF group. The authors concluded that induction chemotherapy with the addition of docetaxel significantly improved progression-free and overall survival in patients with non-resectable squamous cell carcinoma of the head and neck [12].

Licitra L et al. [13] reported their experience of primary chemotherapy in resectable oral cavity squamous cell carcinoma. Patients were randomized to receive either initial surgery or neoadjuvant (induction) chemotherapy with three cycles of cisplatin and 5-FU followed by surgery. The study noted a pathologic complete response rate of 27% at the primary site after the neoadjuvant chemotherapy. Thirty-three percent of patients had a pathologic complete response or near complete response at both the primary site and regional lymph nodes. Although the addition of neoadjuvant treatment did not impact overall survival, it did have some intriguing effects. "Less demolitive surgery (31% vs 52%)" was required in the surgery arm without an increased rate of positive margins and less postoperative radiotherapy (33% vs 46%) was used. Additionally, Haddad et al. [7] reported the results of pathologic complete responses in head and neck cancer patients treated with triple induction chemotherapy followed by chemoradiation. The study noted that, post TPF induction, primary site biopsy was negative in 89% (64/72) of patients. Neck dissection was performed in patients with N3 disease and those who did not achieve a clinical complete response. Twenty-two of twenty-nine patients (76%) achieved a pathologic complete response post all treatment. Holsinger et al. [14] conducted a study using triple induction chemotherapy with paclitaxel, ifosfamide, and cisplatin (TIP) in patients with stage III and stage IV laryngeal squamous cell carcinoma. Patients received three cycles of TIP. Patients with a partial response received conservation laryngeal surgery while those achieving a complete pathologic response received an additional three cycles of TIP. Thirty-seven percent of patients achieved a pathologic complete response. Nearly all of those patients (90%) maintained a durable remission. Of the remaining patients, laryngeal preservation was possible in 83% and only 16% of patients required post-operative radiation.

Our own study failed to substantiate the expected pathologic complete response rates of other studies, despite a 100% HPV positivity rate. However, minimally required surgery was performed on one patient who remains in complete remission. Thus, the benefit of neoadjuvant chemotherapy may be the reduction in the performance of functionally impairing surgery. Additionally, as suggested by the Holsinger study, it may be that neoadjuvant chemotherapy and conservative surgery may be as effective as surgery and radiation or chemoradiation in selected head and neck cancer patients. The statistical design of the study was also rigorous. Although the failure to recruit a fifth patient had impaired the original design of the study, we think that these negative results still do remain valid and provide important information for future trial design.

The amount of acute toxicity encountered in our study was high, which made it difficult for patients to complete the three cycles of triplet chemotherapy. Other studies using the triple induction regimen have reported high rates of acute toxicity as well. Schrijvers et al. [15] reported their outcomes and noted diarrhea (70%), stomatitis (65%), nausea (83%), and vomiting (70%) at dose level II of cisplatin (100 mg/m2). Nearly 15% of patients experienced nephrotoxicity. Patients on the DECIDE trial were noted to have grade 3/4 mucositis (50%), dysphagia 12%), and infection (11.2%) [16]. The PARADIGM study, which used a slightly different induction regimen of docetaxel, hydroxyurea, and 5- fluorouracil, noted no difference in rates of mucositis, pain scores, xerostomia, and PEG tube use with patients randomized to receive induction chemotherapy [17]. The intriguing benefit of induction chemotherapy may, in fact, be the reduction in subsequent radiation intensity in the HPV positive setting. The Phase II ECOG 1308 study enrolled HPV positive patients and treated them with a three cycle induction regimen of carboplatin, paclitaxel, and cetuximab followed by chemoradiation with weekly cetuximab and reduced dose intensity modulated radiation therapy (IMRT) of 54 Gy, if the patient had achieved a clinical complete response after induction chemotherapy. Late toxicities were minimal, and the results in this group of patients were excellent with an 84% progression free survival at 23 months and a 95% two year survival. We believe that the toxic effects of induction chemotherapy, both short term and long term, should not be underestimated and thorough patient counseling is necessary prior to activating such a treatment approach.

References

1. Adelstein DJ (2007) Concurrent chemoradiotherapy in the management of squamous cell cancer of the oropharynx: current standards and future directions. Int J Radiat Oncol Biol Phys 69: S37-39.

2. Adelstein DJ (1998) Recent randomized trials of chemoradiation in the management of locally advanced head and neck cancer. Curr Opin Oncol 10: 213-218.

3. Adelstein DJ (2000) Mature results of a phase III randomized trial comparing concurrent chemoradiotherapy with radiation therapy alone in patients with stage III and IV squamous cell carcinoma of the head and neck. Cancer 88: 876-883.

4. Goldstein NE, Genden E, Morrison RS (2008) Palliative care for patients with head and neck cancer: "I would like a quick return to a normal lifestyle". JAMA 299: 1818-1825.

5. Al-Sarraf M, LeBlanc M, Giri PG, Fu KK, Cooper J, et al. (1998) Chemoradiotherapy versus radiotherapy in patients with advanced nasopharyngeal cancer: phase III randomized Intergroup study 0099. J Clin Oncol 16: 1310-1317.

6. Posner MR, Hershock DM, Blajman CR, Mickiewicz E, Winquist E, et al. (2007) Cisplatin and fluorouracil alone or with docetaxel in head and neck cancer. N Engl J Med 357: 1705-1715.

7. Haddad R (2003) Docetaxel, cisplatin, and 5-fluorouracil-based induction chemotherapy in patients with locally advanced squamous cell carcinoma of the head and neck: the Dana Farber Cancer Institute experience. Cancer 97: 412-428.

8. Hassan SJ, Weymuller EA Jr (1993) Assessment of quality of life in head and neck cancer patients. Head Neck 15: 485-496.

9. Langerman A, Maccracken E, Kasza K, Haraf DJ, Vokes EE, et al. (2007) Aspiration in chemoradiated patients with head and neck cancer. Arch Otolaryngol Head Neck Surg 133: 1289-1295.

10. Rogers SN, Gwanne S, Lowe D, Humphris G, Yueh B, et al. (2002) The addition of mood and anxiety domains to the University of Washington quality of life scale. Head Neck 24: 521-529.

11. Haddad R, Tishler R, Wirth L, Norris CM, Goguen L, et al. (2006) Rate of pathologic complete responses to docetaxel, cisplatin, and fluorouracil induction chemotherapy in patients with squamous cell carcinoma of the head and neck. Arch Otolaryngol Head Neck Surg 132: 678-681.

12. Vermorken JB, Remenar E, van Herpen C, Gorlia T, Mesia R, et al. (2007) Cisplatin, fluorouracil, and docetaxel in unresectable head and neck cancer. N Engl J Med 357: 1695-1704.

13. Licitra L, Grandi C, Guzzo M, Mariani L, Lo Vullo S, et al. (2003) Primary chemotherapy in resectable oral cavity squamous cell cancer: a randomized controlled trial. J Clin Oncol 21: 327-333.

14. Holsinger FC, Kies MS, Diaz EM Jr, Gillenwater AM, Lewin JS, et al.(2009) Durable long-term remission with chemotherapy alone for stage II to IV laryngeal cancer. J Clin Oncol 27: 1976-1982.

15. Schrijvers D, Van Herpen C, Kerger J, Joosens E, Van Laer C, et al. (2004) Docetaxel, cisplatin and 5-fluorouracil in patients with locally advanced unresectable head and neck cancer: a phase I-II feasibility study. Ann Oncol 15: 638-645.

16. Cohen EE, Karrison TG, Kocherginsky M, Mueller J, Egan R, et al. (2014) Phase III randomized trial of induction chemotherapy in patients with N2 or N3 locally advanced head and neck cancer. J Clin Oncol 32: 2735-2743.

17. Haddad R (2013) Induction chemotherapy followed by concurrent chemoradiotherapy (sequential chemoradiotherapy) versus concurrent chemoradiotherapy alone in locally advanced head and neck cancer (PARADIGM): a randomised phase 3 trial. The Lancet Oncology 14: 257-264.

Permissions

All chapters in this book were first published in OTOLARYNGOLOGY, by OMICS International; hereby published with permission under the Creative Commons Attribution License or equivalent. Every chapter published in this book has been scrutinized by our experts. Their significance has been extensively debated. The topics covered herein carry significant findings which will fuel the growth of the discipline. They may even be implemented as practical applications or may be referred to as a beginning point for another development.

The contributors of this book come from diverse backgrounds, making this book a truly international effort. This book will bring forth new frontiers with its revolutionizing research information and detailed analysis of the nascent developments around the world.

We would like to thank all the contributing authors for lending their expertise to make the book truly unique. They have played a crucial role in the development of this book. Without their invaluable contributions this book wouldn't have been possible. They have made vital efforts to compile up to date information on the varied aspects of this subject to make this book a valuable addition to the collection of many professionals and students.

This book was conceptualized with the vision of imparting up-to-date information and advanced data in this field. To ensure the same, a matchless editorial board was set up. Every individual on the board went through rigorous rounds of assessment to prove their worth. After which they invested a large part of their time researching and compiling the most relevant data for our readers.

The editorial board has been involved in producing this book since its inception. They have spent rigorous hours researching and exploring the diverse topics which have resulted in the successful publishing of this book. They have passed on their knowledge of decades through this book. To expedite this challenging task, the publisher supported the team at every step. A small team of assistant editors was also appointed to further simplify the editing procedure and attain best results for the readers.

Apart from the editorial board, the designing team has also invested a significant amount of their time in understanding the subject and creating the most relevant covers. They scrutinized every image to scout for the most suitable representation of the subject and create an appropriate cover for the book.

The publishing team has been an ardent support to the editorial, designing and production team. Their endless efforts to recruit the best for this project, has resulted in the accomplishment of this book. They are a veteran in the field of academics and their pool of knowledge is as vast as their experience in printing. Their expertise and guidance has proved useful at every step. Their uncompromising quality standards have made this book an exceptional effort. Their encouragement from time to time has been an inspiration for everyone.

The publisher and the editorial board hope that this book will prove to be a valuable piece of knowledge for researchers, students, practitioners and scholars across the globe.

List of Contributors

Simple Patadia and Saurin Shah
MS ENT, SR Neuro-otology, Department of Neurosurgery, SGPGIMS, India

Amitkumar Keshri
MS ENT, Assistant Professor, Department of Neurosurgery, Neuro-otology, SGPGIMS, India

Arun Shrivastava
MCh Neurosurgery, Associate Professor, Department of Neurosurgery, SGPGIMS, India

Neelam Sood and Nisha Sehrawat
Department of Pathology, Deen Dayal Upadhyay Hospital, New Delhi, India

Irmi Wiest, Klaus Friese, Annika Stiasny, Tobias Weißenbacher, Darius Dian, Udo Jeschke and Bernd Kost
Department of Obstetrics and Gynecology – Klinikum Innenstadt, Germany

Christoph Freier
Department of Obstetrics and Gynecology – Klinikum Innenstadt, Germany
Division of Clinical Pharmacology, LMU, Germany

Christoph Alexiou and Marina Pöttler
Department of Otorhinolaryngology, Head and Neck Surgery, Section for Experimental Oncology and Nanomedicine (SEON), Germany

Doris Mayr
Department of Pathology, LMU, Germany

Peter Betz
Department of Legal Medicine, FAU, Germany

Jutta Tübel
Department of Orthopedics, TUM, Germany

Steffen Goletz
Glycotope, Germany

Beqir Abazi, Bajram Shaqiri and Halil Ajvazi
Department of ENT – Ophthalmology, Regional Hospital Centre of Gjilan, Kosovo

Pajtim Lutaj and Pjerin Radovani
Department of ENT – Ophthalmology, University Hospital Clinical Centre "Mother Teresa", Tirana, Albania

Mohammed A. Gomaa, Osama G. Abdel Nabi, Abdel Rahim A. Abdel Kerim and Ahmed Aly
Faculty of Medicine, Minia University, Minia, Egypt

Singh G, Banda NR and Kandya A
Department of Pedodontics and preventive dentistry, Modern dental college and research centre, Indore, India

Patel A
Department of Oral and maxillofacial surgery, Modern dental college and research centre, Indore, India

Takafumi Yamano
Section of Otorhinolaryngology, Department of Medicine, Fukuoka Dental College, Japan
Department of Otorhinolaryngology, Fukuoka University School of Medicine, Japan

Hitomi Higuchi, Tetsuko Ueno and Takashi Nakagawa
Department of Otorhinolaryngology, Fukuoka University School of Medicine, Japan

Tetsuo Morizono
Department of Otorhinolaryngology, Fukuoka University School of Medicine Nishi Fukuoka Hospital, Japan

Amtul Salam Sami
ENT and Allergy Department, Royal National Throat, Nose and Ear Hospital, University College London Hospitals, London, UK

Nida Ahmed
King's College London School of Medicine at Guy's, King's College and St Thomas' Hospitals, London, UK

Kimihiro Okubo
Department of Otorhinolaryngology, Nippon Medical School, Japan

Terumichi Fujikura
Department of Otorhinolaryngology, Nippon Medical School, Japan
Department of Otolaryngology, Tokyo Woman's Medical University Medical Center East, Japan

Aparna Upadhye Chavan and Gajanan Namdeorao Chavan
Department of Anesthesia, Jawaharlal Nehru Medical College, Maharashtra, India

Bibek Gyanwali, Hongquan Wu, Meichan Zhu and Anzhou Tang
Department of Otolaryngology-Head and Neck Surgery, First affiliated Hospital of Guangxi Medical University, Nanning Guangxi, People's Republic of China

Neela Doddi, Bassem Mettias and Alexi Usanov
Department of ENT, Princess of Wales Hospital, UK

Minakshi Gulia and Neelam Sood
Department of Pathology, Deen Dayal Upadhyaya Hospital, New Delhi, India

Hamed Sajjadi
Stanford University School of Medicine, San Jose, CA, USA

Haruna Yabe, Koichiro Saito, Kosuke Uno, Takeyuki Kono and Kaoru Ogawa
Department of Otolaryngology-Head and Neck Surgery, Keio University School of Medicine, Tokyo, Japan

Hiroshi Morisaki
Department of Anesthesiology, Keio University School of Medicine, Tokyo, Japan

Martin M, García J, Lopez M, Hinojar A, Manzanares R, Fernandez L, Prada J and Cerezo L
Hospital Universitario de La Princesa, Madrid, Spain

Atsunobu Tsunoda, Koichi Tsunoda, Takuro Sumi, Seiji Kishimoto and Ken Kitamura
Department of Otolaryngology and Head and Neck Surgery, Tokyo Medical and Dental University, Japan

Schweta Singh and Anupam Mishra
Department of Otolaryngology and Head and Neck Surgery, King George Medical University, Lucknow (UP), India

Wei Zhong Ernest Fu, Ming Yann Lim and Li-Chung Mark Khoo
Department of Otolaryngology, Tan Tock Seng Hospital, Singapore

Khoon Leong Chuah and Khoon Leong Chuah
Department of Pathology, Tan Tock Seng Hospital, Singapore

Raja Meganadh Koralla
MAA Research Foundation, Somajiguda, Hyderabad, Telangana, India

Madhavi Jangala and Santoshi Kumari Manche
MAA Research Foundation, Somajiguda, Hyderabad, Telangana, India
Institute of Genetics and Hospital for Genetic Diseases, Osmania University, Hyderabad, Telangana, India

Jyothy Akka
Institute of Genetics and Hospital for Genetic Diseases, Osmania University, Hyderabad, Telangana, India

Muhammad Sami Jabbr, Jamal Kassouma, Hussain Talib Salman and Gamal Youssef
Dubai Health Authority, Dubai Hospital, Albaraha, Alkhalij Street, Dubai, UAE

Pritha Pal and Ajanta Halder
Department of Genetics, Vivekananda Institute of Medical Sciences, Ramakrishna Mission Seva Pratishthan, 99 Sarat Bose Road, Kolkata, West Bengal, India

Ranjan Raychowdhury
Department of Otolaryngology, Vivekananda Institute of Medical Sciences, Ramakrishna Mission Seva Pratishthan, 99 Sarat Bose Road, Kolkata

Hassan Haidar, Rashid Sheikh, Aisha Larem, Ali Elsaadi, Hassanin Abdulkarim, Sara Ashkanani and Abdulsalm Alqahtani
Otolaryngology Department, Hamad Medical Corporation, Doha, Qatar

Ilmari Pyykkö
Hearing and Balance Research Unit, Field of Otolaryngology, School of Medicine, University of Tampere, Tampere, Finland

Jing Zou
Hearing and Balance Research Unit, Field of Otolaryngology, School of Medicine, University of Tampere, Tampere, Finland
Department of Otolaryngology-Head and Neck Surgery, Center for Otolaryngology-Head & Neck Surgery of Chinese PLA, Changhai Hospital, Second Military Medical University, Shanghai, China

Santhosh Gaddikeri and Yoshimi Anzai
Department of Radiology, University of Washington Medical Center, USA

Amit Bhrany
Department of Head and Neck surgery, University of Washington Medical Center, USA

Lingamdenne Paul Emerson
Department of ENT, Arogyavaram Medical Centre, Madnapalle, Andhra Pradesh, India

Dabo Liu
Department of Otorhinolaryngology, Guangzhou Women and Children's Medical Center, Guangzhou, China

Chao Cheng
Pediatric Center, Southern Medical University Zhujiang Hospital, Guangzhou, China

Jiahui Pan and Susu Bao
School of Computer Science, South China Normal University, Guangzhou, China

Suela Sallavaci and Ylli Sallavaci
Service of Otorhinolaryngology, University Hospital Center "Mother Teresa", Tirana, Albania

Ervin Toci
Department of Epidemiology and Health Systems, Institute of Public Health, Tirana, Albania

Gentian Stroni
Service of Infectious Diseases, University Hospital Centre "Mother Teresa", Tirana, Albania

Tufan T, Erkoc MA, Yilmaz MB, Comertpay G and Alptekin D
Department of Medical Biology, University of Cukurova, Adana, Turkey

Mehmet Akdag, Ismail Onder Uysal, Salih Bakir, Fazıl Emre Ozkurt, Suphi Muderris, Ediz Yorgancılar and Ismail Topcu
Department of Otolaryngology, Faculty of Medicine, Dicle University, Turkey

Myriam Jrad, Farouk Graiess, Selma Behi, Rym Bachraoui, Ghazi Besbes and Habiba Mizouni
Department of Radiology, La Rabta Hospital, Jabberi 1017, Tunis, Tunisia

Cristina Caroça
Department of Otolaryngology, NOVA Medical School, Universidade Nova de Lisboa, Campo Mártires da Pátria 130, 1169-056 Lisboa, Portugal
Hospital CUF Infante Santo, 34, 6°, 1350-079 Lisboa, Portugal
Centre for Toxicogenomics and Human Health (ToxOmics), Faculty of Medical Sciences, NOVA Medical School, Universidade Nova de Lisboa, Campo Mártires da Pátria 130, 1169-056 Lisboa, Portugal

João Paço
Department of Otolaryngology, NOVA Medical School, Universidade Nova de Lisboa, Campo Mártires da Pátria 130, 1169-056 Lisboa, Portugal
Hospital CUF Infante Santo, 34, 6°, 1350-079 Lisboa, Portugal

Paula Campelo
Hospital CUF Infante Santo, 34, 6°, 1350-079 Lisboa, Portugal

João Pereira de Lima and Susana Nunes Silva
Centre for Toxicogenomics and Human Health (ToxOmics), Faculty of Medical Sciences, NOVA Medical School, Universidade Nova de Lisboa, Campo Mártires da Pátria 130, 1169-056 Lisboa, Portugal

Elisabete Carolino
Escola Superior de Tecnologia da Saúde de Lisboa, Av. Dom João II Lote 4.69.01, 1990-096 Lisboa

Helena Caria
BioISI - Biosystems & Integrative Sciences Institute, Faculty of Science of the University of Lisbon, R. Ernesto de Vasconcelos, 1749-016 Lisboa, Portugal
ESS/IPS, School of Health, Polytechnic Institute of Setúbal, Campus do IPS Estefanilha, 2910-761 Setúbal, Portugal

Gus J Slotman
Director of Clinical Research, Inspira Health Network, Vineland

Shanmugam VU, Vidyachal Ravindra, Ruta Shanmugam, Mariappan RG, Balaji Swaminathan and Prem Nivas
Department of ENT, RMMCH, Annamalai University, Chidambaram, India

Dhanashekaran C and Srinivasan SK
Department of Aneasthesia, RMMCH, Annamalai University, Chidambaram, India

Takatsugu Mizumachi, Tomohiro Sakashita, Yusuke Hishimura, Tomohiko Kakizaki, Akihiro Homma and Satoshi Fukuda
Department of Otolaryngology - Head and Neck Surgery, Hokkaido University Graduate School of Medicine, Sapporo, Japan

Tomoko Mitsuhashi
Department of Surgical Pathology, Hokkaido University Hospital, Sapporo, Japan

Pedersen M, Akram BH and Agersted AA
The Medical Center Ear, Nose, Throat and Voice Unit, Østergade 18, 3 DK 1100 Copenhagen, Denmark

Aseel Almeqbel
Department of Hearing and Speech Sciences, Faculty of Allied Health Sciences, Health Sciences Center, Kuwait University, Kuwait

Federico Maria Gioacchini, Daniele Monzani, Livio Presutti and Matteo Alicandri-Ciufelli
Otolaryngology Department, University Hospital of Modena, Modena, Italy

Elisabetta Genovese
Audiology Unit, Otolaryngology Department, University Hospital of Modena, Modena, Italy

Kamal N Rattan
Department of Paediadtric Surgery, PGIMS, Rohtak, India

Bikramjeet Singh
Department of Plastic Surgery, PGIMS, Rohtak, India

Priya Malik
Department of Otolaryngology, PGIMS, Rohtak, India

Hirotaka Hara, Kazuma Sugahara, Takefumi Mikuriya, Makoto Hashimoto, Shinsaku Tahara and Hiroshi Yamashita
Department of Otolaryngology, Yamaguchi University Graduate School of Medicine, Ube, Japan

Mohamad A. Bitar
Department of ENT Surgery, The Children's Hospital at Westmead, Sydney Medical School, University of Sydney, Sydney, Australia

Wu Gang, Li Zong-Ming, Han Xin-Wei, Wang Zhong-Gao, Jiao De-Chao, Ren Ke-Wei and Zhu Ming
Department of Interventional Radiology, the First Affiliated Hospital of Zhengzhou University, Zhengzhou 450052, China

Jyoti Ranjan Das, Debabrata Biswas and Ajay Manickam
Rg Kar Medical College, Kolkata, India

Omar Shafic Ayub
Department of Orthodontics and Dentofacial Orthopedics, Dentistry, Federal University of Mato Grosso do Sul - UFMS, Campo Grande, Brazil

Bruno Ayub
University of Franca - UNIFRAN, Franca, Brazil

Priscila Vaz Ayub
Orthodontics at the São Paulo State University - UNESP, Araraquara, Brazil

Dirceu Barnabé Ravelli
Orthodontics, São Paulo State University - UNESP, Araraquara, Brazil

Paulo Domingos Ribeiro
Department Surgery and Traumatology, Disciplines Sacred Heart University - USC, Bauru, Brazil

Margareth da Silva Coutinho
Department of Dentistry at the Federal University of Mato Grosso do Sul - UFMS, Campo Grande, Brazil

Aseel Almeqbel
Department of Hearing and Speech Sciences, Faculty of Allied Health Sciences, Health Sciences Center, Kuwait University, Kuwait

Catherine McMahon
Linguistics Department, Faculty of Human Sciences, Macquarie University, the Hearing Cooperative Research Centre (CRC), Sydney, Australia

Zeyad Mandour, Remon Kalza and Samy Elwany
Department of Otolaryngology, Alexandria Medical School, Alexandria, Egypt

Florian Christov, Patrick Munder, Laura Berg, Judith Arnolds, Heike Bagus, Stephan Lang and Diana Arweiler-Harbeck
Uniklinik Essen, HNO, Essen, Germany

Krishna Rao
Department of Internal Medicine, Southern Illinois University School of Medicine, USA
Division of Hematology/Oncology, Department of Internal Medicine, Southern Illinois University School of Medicine, USA
Department of Medical Microbiology, Southern Illinois University School of Medicine, USA
Simmons Cancer Institute at SIU, Southern Illinois University School of Medicine, USA
Division of Otolaryngology Head and Neck Surgery, Department of Surgery, Southern Illinois University School of Medicine, USA

Kathy Robinson
Simmons Cancer Institute at SIU, Southern Illinois University School of Medicine, USA
James Malone and K Thomas Robbins
Simmons Cancer Institute at SIU, Southern Illinois University School of Medicine, USA
Division of Otolaryngology Head and Neck Surgery, Department of Surgery, Southern Illinois University School of Medicine, USA

Cathy Clausen and Bruce Shevlin
St. John's Hospital Department of Radiation Oncology, Springfield, IL, Southern Illinois University School of Medicine, USA

Index